Chapple's Principles of Wound Care and Healing

Peter Charlesworth • Michael F. Klaassen

Chapple's Principles of Wound Care and Healing

The Physiological Challenge

Springer

Peter Charlesworth
Retired Vascular and General Surgeon
Auckland, New Zealand

Michael F. Klaassen
Plastic and Reconstructive Surgeon
Private Practice
Sydney, NSW, Australia

ISBN 978-3-031-53103-3 ISBN 978-3-031-53104-0 (eBook)
https://doi.org/10.1007/978-3-031-53104-0

This Springer imprint is published by the registered company Springer Nature Switzerland AG
The registered company address is: Gewerbestrasse 11, 6330 Cham, Switzerland

Dedicated to my daughter Raven,
whose devotion to living things has always
been inspirational to me.

[Dr Joan Chapple's original 2003 dedication]

Foreword

In 1951, after leaving the operating theatre having completed a pneumonectomy for cancer on King George VI, surgeon Sir Clement Price-Thomas was asked whether he had closed the chest. He is said to have replied 'I haven't stitched up a chest for 25 years and I am not about to start practising now'. This cavalier attitude to wounds was standard in that era. Juniors were left to close surgical wounds. Casualty departments were staffed by house surgeons, and minor surgical procedures were delegated to junior doctors with little or no training in wound care. Surgical textbooks provided only cursory coverage of this topic, and frequent wound breakdown and delayed healing were accepted as inevitable. This book, first self-published in preliminary form in 1994 and based on Dr Joan Chapple's many years' experience in a soft tissue clinic at Auckland Hospital in New Zealand, addresses these deficiencies.

Joan Chapple and I were contemporaries at Otago University Medical School, and she was a loyal friend of our family for the rest of her turbulent life. She was one of 9 women in our class of 86 who graduated in 1957, being awarded distinction in surgery. She subsequently trained in Auckland, gaining Fellowship of the Australasian College of Surgeons in General Surgery in 1963. At that time most young surgeons trained in Britain. She was the second woman to achieve specialist status in surgery in New Zealand. Her first interest was in hand surgery, and she spent a year visiting departments around the world, notably at the Christian Medical College in Vellore, India. She worked there with the celebrated British surgeon Paul Brandt who was pioneering tendon transplantation in the hands of lepers.

Joan returned to a position in the Plastic Surgical Unit at Middlemore Hospital under William Manchester, later Sir William. Her later dismissal under controversial circumstances and her subsequent appointment to a soft tissue clinic at Auckland Hospital are discussed in detail in the first chapter of this revision of her book.

Suffice it to say here that her unconventional views, social, political, and surgical, were never fully accepted by many in the highly conservative surgical hierarchy of the time, and that this detracted from full acceptance of her ideas. Despite this, she inspired a generation of young doctors and nurses to treat wounds in much more logical and scientific ways.

Joan was an indomitable idealist, and a loyal and outstandingly generous friend. Her work may well have had greater significance than she could have achieved as a hand surgeon. I believe that the principles encompassed in this revision of her book will still resonate with the current generation of doctors and nurses.

Auckland, New Zealand Alan Kerr

Preface

The Editors' project to introduce Dr Joan Chapple's previously self-published book *Wound Care and Healing: The Physiological Challenge* (2003) to a wider, modern readership has gained momentum in a faltering fashion over a period of several years. One of them (MFK) first became aware of the book in 2013, when he was given a copy by Dr Chapple's daughter Raven, whom he had interviewed during preparation for a presentation on the topic of women in plastic surgery. Subsequently, the Editors first discussed the potential for the book in 2016, but an approach to the representative of Dr Chapple's estate for permission to sensitively re-write and formally publish it was rebuffed.

The idea remained in abeyance for some time, until a chance meeting with Dr Alan Kerr by one of the Editors (PC), while walking his dog in a local park. Knowing that Dr Kerr was a longstanding close friend of Dr Chapple and her daughter and had delivered the eulogy at the memorial service following Dr Chapple's death, the Editor discussed with him the concept of the project, and the difficulties that had thus far been encountered in obtaining permission to proceed with it. Thanks to the generous assistance of Dr Kerr, the Editors then re-entered into discussion with the Trustees of Dr Chapple's estate and after several months of negotiations, formal permission was granted for them to proceed with the suggested re-publication of the book.

Because of the previous experience of one of the Editors (MFK) in publishing several books through Springer Nature, the concept of rewriting Dr Chapple's book was submitted to that company and after their evaluation, a contract to publish the book was signed in June 2022. This was a moment of significant satisfaction for the Editors, since it was known that historically, Dr Chapple had previously approached a number of medical publishers about the book, without success.

Both of the Editors encountered Dr Joan Chapple professionally from the early 1970s; one (PC) as a medical student and later as a consultant surgeon, and the other (MFK) as a plastic surgical trainee. While they were superficially aware of her complex background and her marginalisation by the plastic surgical fraternity of the day, they did not really know her, or the subtleties of her story. Those people who did know Joan Chapple well say that the style of writing in her book eerily evokes her voice and conversational delivery in real life. The Editors have tried hard to conserve this 'voice' in their revision of her book, making grammatical or stylistic changes only where essential, and omitting only a few passages containing potentially distracting 'political' comment.

Dr Chapple's original book, self-published in 2003 and based on a preceding version in 1994, was produced in a relatively unsophisticated fashion. The text and extensive range of accompanying clinical photographs were completely separated, making coherent reading continuity very difficult. Accordingly, in re-transcribing the book, the Editors have integrated the original clinical images into the relevant chapters, positioned adjacent to their references in the text. In some cases, original short chapters containing related material have been combined into a single, new chapter. For clarity of the principles described, some images appear in more than one chapter.

International experts have been invited to contribute short commentaries at the end of chapters relevant to their respective fields of expertise. Their observations demonstrate not only how Dr Chapple's once innovative and poorly accepted philosophies of wound care and healing have generally stood the test of time, but also where knowledge or treatment methods have advanced, and where significant ongoing challenges in the subjects remain.

Finally, while Dr Chapple was well known in Auckland where she had many devotees, particularly among nurses and general medical practitioners, her work and accomplishments were probably not widely appreciated elsewhere. Accordingly, the Editors have introduced a new chapter in her book, entitled 'Who Was Joan Chapple?'. In this, we have endeavoured to provide a broad description of Dr Chapple's background for a modern, international readership. Information for this chapter was provided from interviews with her surviving family, close friends, and medical professionals who worked with her in a range of roles, as well as from details already in the public domain.

Auckland, New Zealand — Peter Charlesworth
Sydney, NSW, Australia — Michael F. Klaassen

Acknowledgements

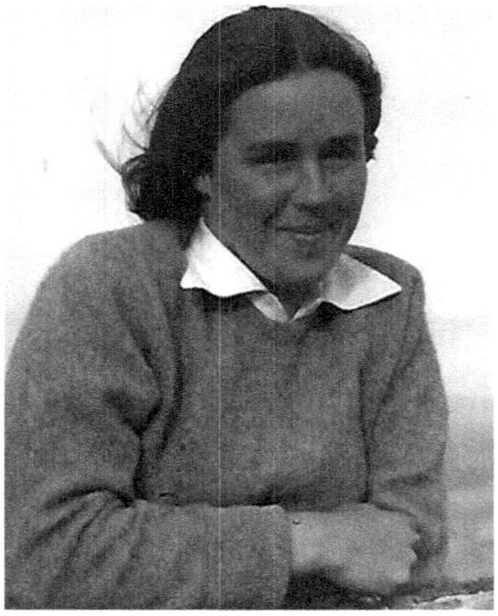

Joan Shirley Chapple [1934-2013]

The editors wish to thank:

Raven Chapple, Joan's daughter, for generously gifting an original copy of *Wound Care and Healing: The Physiological Challenge* to MFK in 2014, receipt of which was the initial stimulus for the process that eventually led to this new edition. Joan's original self-published manuscript was dedicated to Raven and that dedication has been retained. We also acknowledge the support and permission to re-issue the late Dr Joan Chapple's work from the Trustees of her estate, including Dr Ian Scott, Judge Janey Forrest, Diana Smallfield, and Raven Chapple.

Ken Choe of Auckland's Presentation Design and Print, who provided the digital image files used in Joan's original book.

Daniela Heller, Rosemarie Unger, Nandini Priya M, and all the team at Springer Nature for their expertise and advice in achieving international publication for the re-issue.

All the friends, family, and colleagues of Dr Joan Chapple who agreed to be interviewed by the editors for the book, including Dr Alan Kerr, FRACS, Dr David Morris, FRACS, Dr Earle Brown, FRACS, Dr Onkar Mehrotra, FRACS, Dr Patrick Beehan, FRACS, the late Dr JJ de Geus, FRACS, the late Dr John H. Williams, FRACS, Dr Pat Clarkson, FRACP, Dr Kaye Ottaway, FANZCA, Pauline O'Brien, RN, Jefferson Chapple and Cody Chapple, John Chapple, Pat Chapple, Di Smallfield, and George Farrant. Sarah Lang [former NZ Herald journalist] for her 2008 Lifestyle article.

All the chapter commentary contributors who are listed on a separate page including Murray Beagley, Peter Bovey, Rosanne Bovey, Ian Burton, Demetrius Evriviades, James Frame, Lisa Hansen, James Klaassen, Sophie J. Klaassen, Swee Tan, Natalie Tanner, Mark Thomas, Adam White, Richard Wong She, and Fiona Wood.

Contents

Editors and Contributors

About the Editors

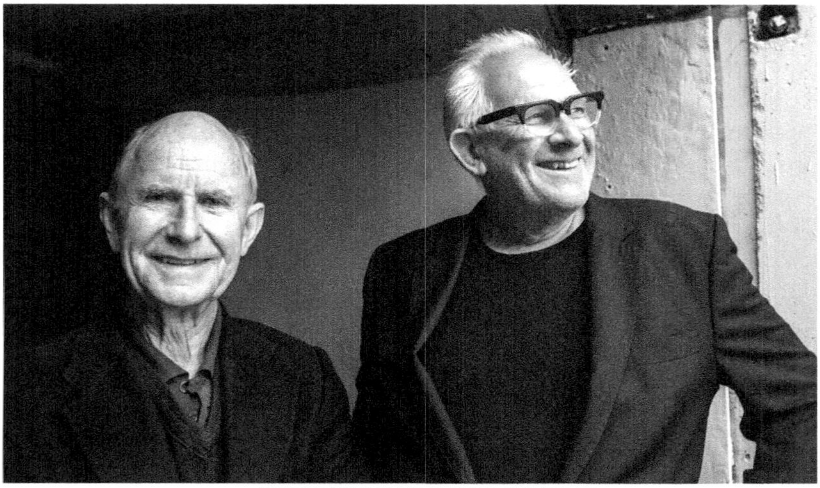

Drs Peter Charlesworth and Michael F. Klaassen

Peter Charlesworth, BSc, MBChB, FRACS Vascular and General Surgeon (Retired)

Peter graduated in the inaugural class of the University of Auckland School of Medicine in 1973 and subsequently undertook surgical training at Middlemore, Auckland, and Waikato hospitals. During this period, he had twelve months' plastic surgical experience, which strongly influenced his later practise, but he naively declined an offer from Professor William Manchester to pursue a career in the field. In his final year of training, he was appointed Chief Surgical Resident, working under Professors E M Nansen and G L Hill. Following the completion of his surgical Fellowship, he had a one-year clinical and research appointment as a Lecturer in Surgery, University of Auckland. He then had three year's overseas postgraduate training, completing a Fellowship in Surgical Metabolism at Columbia Presbyterian Medical Centre, New York, NY, a Vascular Fellowship at Massachusetts General Hospital, Boston, MA, and twelve months of General and Vascular surgery as Senior Registrar at St James's University Hospital,

Leeds, UK. On his return to New Zealand, he had a four-year appointment as a full-time General and Vascular surgeon at Middlemore Hospital, Auckland, followed by a number of part-time consultant appointments at other Auckland hospitals, eventually entering full-time private practice. After 30 years of medical practice, for various reasons his passion for surgery died and he retired, retraining, in Kent, UK in the craft of antique furniture restoration, a pursuit which he likens to plastic surgery with wood.

Michael F. Klaassen, ONZM, MBChB, FRACS Plastic and Reconstructive Surgeon

Michael graduated from the University of Otago Medical School in 1980 and after stints in general surgery, orthopaedic surgery, and surgical research completed his training in plastic and reconstructive surgery in 1990. Then followed overseas fellowships at the Queen Victoria Hospital, East Grinstead, England, and Canniesburn Hospital, Glasgow, Scotland, before a decade as a consultant plastic surgeon at Waikato Hospital, Hamilton, New Zealand. Always restless, he then took his family to Australia for nearly 5 years in Sydney at St George Hospital, Kogarah, and for the last 15 years he has been based in Auckland, mainly in private practice with services provided to many provincial centres as well as his urban practice. Latterly his focus has been on extreme facial cancer with regular tours of surgical duty to the Queensland Plastic Surgery Clinic in Townsville, North Queensland, Australia.

Contributors

Murray Beagley, FRACS, Dip Hand Surg *Plastic and Reconstructive Surgeon Middlemore and Starship Hospitals, Auckland, New Zealand.*

Murray works within the Hand Surgery Unit treating mainly adult and paediatric hand disorders. His private practice also has a focus on hand surgery. He graduated from Otago Medical School in 1987 and qualified as a plastic surgeon in 2000. His studies after gaining Fellowship to the Australasian College of Surgeons took him to the UK where he worked with David Elliot and Paul Smith, two of the world's leading hand surgeons. During his time overseas he sat the European Hand Surgery Diploma, where he was the best candidate in the exam and was awarded the Churchill Livingstone medal. As well as complex hand surgery he subspecialises in skin cancer and cosmetic surgery, including genito-plastic surgery. He is a previous Director of Training and Selector for advanced training in plastic surgery and has partaken in Interplast missions to Fiji as a volunteer surgeon.

Peter Bovey, FRACS *General Surgeon, Townsville, North Queensland, Australia.*

Peter is a general surgeon in Townsville, North Queensland, where he has worked since 1990. He was born and raised in Brisbane where he completed his surgical training before settling in Townsville. A true general surgeon with extensive practice in skin cancer surgery, he formerly retired from all surgery in September 2023.

Rosanne Bovey, RN Dip App Sci (Nursing Management - Hons) *Nurse, Townsville, North Queensland, Australia.*

Rosanne is a Registered Nurse and Clinical Nurse Consultant for Dr Michael Klaassen, plastic surgeon, and Dr Peter Bovey, general surgeon, Queensland Plastic Surgery, Townsville, Australia.

Ian D. Burton, FRACS *General Surgeon, Gisborne, New Zealand.*

Ian qualified as a general surgeon in 1985 with FRACS, before working in the UK and Sultanate of Oman for four years. He has worked in Gisborne New Zealand for 30 years, the last 10 being in private practice. He was on the Executive Committee of the New Zealand Association of General Surgeons for 14 years.

Demetrius Evriviades, FRCS *Plastic and Reconstructive Surgeon, Royal Centre for Defence Medicine and the New Queen Elizabeth Hospital, Birmingham, UK.*

Demetrius qualified in medicine from Liverpool Medical School and before his surgical training he completed his initial training in General Practice. He has completed research into the treatment of chemical burns and qualified in plastic & reconstructive surgery in 2007. He served 22 years in the RAF medical branch and was the former Head of the Department of Plastic Surgery at University Hospitals Birmingham NHS Trust. He is currently working as a cosmetic plastic surgeon in Dubai during his sabbatical.

James Frame, FRCS *Plastic Surgeon, School of Medicine, Anglia Ruskin University, Essex, UK.*

James qualified in Medicine from St Bartholomew's Hospital in 1977 and was appointed as a consultant plastic surgeon to the NHS in 1990. He was a visiting professor to a number of international plastic surgery and burns units around the world, including Singapore, Australia, the Middle East and the USA, and retired from the NHS in 2001 to focus on research and teaching in Aesthetic Surgery.

Lisa Hansen, Dip Phyt, Adv Dip MT *Senior Hand Therapist, Waikato, New Zealand.*

Lisa is senior hand therapist who qualified in Auckland in 1986 and gained further qualifications in Manipulative Therapy, Acupuncture, and Hand therapy. She established Lisa Hansen Physiotherapy clinic in 1997 and has enjoyed managing and working in the four locations of the clinic in the Waikato.

Alan Kerr, CNZM, FRACS *Retired Cardiothoracic Surgeon, Auckland, New Zealand.*

Alan was born in Takaka, Nelson, in 1935 and educated at Nelson College and Otago University Medical School, graduating in 1957. Following 3 years as house surgeon and registrar in Wellington, he joined the Green Lane Hospital staff as a Research Fellow in cardiac surgery in 1961 and gained FRACS in general surgery in 1965. After 2 years at the University of Alabama

Medical School as a research fellow and later chief resident in cardiac surgery, he became a cardiothoracic and vascular surgeon at Green Lane Hospital from 1969 until retirement in 2002. He initially had a leading role in the development of coronary artery surgery in NZ and later a major interest in heart surgery for children. He was made a Companion of the NZ Order of Merit in 1996, and became Honorary Clinical Professor of Surgery of the Auckland School of Medicine in 1997. In 2002 he was awarded the inaugural Colin McRae medal by the Australasian College of Surgeons for service to surgery in New Zealand. Since retirement he has worked as a volunteer helping develop paediatric cardiac services in Palestine.

James Klaassen, MBChB *Advanced Trainee, Emergency Medicine, Melbourne, Victoria, Australia.*

James is a final year trainee in Emergency Medicine. He graduated from the University of Auckland with MBChB in 2015 and is currently working in the Emergency Department of Sunshine Hospital, Melbourne, Australia, as a late phase trainee with the Australasian College of Emergency Medicine.

Sophie J. Klaassen, FANZCA *Anaesthetist, Royal Women's Hospital and Prince of Wales Hospital, Sydney, Australia.*

Sophie is a consultant anaesthetist in Sydney, Australia. She graduated from Australian National University, Canberra, in 2010 and completed her anaesthetic training at Canberra Hospital, Westmead Hospital, and Prince of Wales Hospital. In 2022 she completed a fellowship in Obstetric Anaesthesia at the Royal Women's Hospital, Randwick, and was appointed as a VMO there and at the neighbouring Prince of Wales Hospital early in 2023. Her main interests are in obstetric perioperative care and pain management.

Swee Tan, ONZM, MBBS, PhD, FRACS *Consultant Plastic Surgeon, Hutt Hospital and Executive Director, Gillies McIndoe Research Institute, Wellington, New Zealand.*

Swee graduated from the University of Melbourne Medical School in 1986 and qualified as a plastic and reconstructive surgeon in New Zealand in 1992. Following Craniofacial Fellowships at Oxford and Boston, he was appointed consultant plastic and cranio-maxillofacial surgeon at Hutt Hospital in 1995, where he was the Director of Plastic Surgery (2000-2006) and Director of Surgery (2007-2013). He founded the Centre for the Study & Treatment of Vascular Birthmarks in 1996 and was awarded a PhD by the University of Otago in 2001 for his work in infantile haemangioma. He is the Founder and Executive Director of the Gillies McIndoe Research Institute. He is a past President of the Australian and New Zealand Head and Neck Cancer Society, and the Founder and Chair of the Head and Neck Cancer Foundation Aotearoa. His research focuses on vascular anomalies, cancer, and fibrotic conditions. Swee is an author of 225 book chapters and peer-reviewed journal articles and a recipient of 20 science prizes and 25 honours and awards, including Wellingtonian of the Year—Science and Technology, KEA World Class New Zealand Award, and ONZM.

Natalie Tanner, FCPodS *Podiatrist and Podiatric Surgeon, Dunedin, New Zealand.*

Natalie is a Dunedin-based senior podiatrist who trained in the UK as a podiatric surgeon. Natalie joined the team of 2 podiatrists at Knox Podiatry in Dunedin in 2021 from the UK where she worked as both a private and NHS senior podiatrist. Natalie has also spent 12 years training and working as a podiatric surgeon and is a Fellow of the Royal College of Podiatry in Podiatric Surgery, UK. Her last role in the UK was as a specialist registrar in Podiatric Surgery under a joint Orthopaedics and Podiatric Surgical unit which specialised in limb salvage. She lives with her partner Iain on a lifestyle property near Lawrence, Otago, and was recently appointed to the Podiatrists Board of New Zealand by the Minister of Health.

Mark Thomas, FRACP MD *Associate Professor of Medicine and Senior Infectious Diseases Specialist University of Auckland, Auckland, New Zealand.*

Mark is an infectious disease specialist who trained in Auckland and London. He worked as a specialist infectious diseases physician at Auckland City Hospital between 1988 and 2021. He continues to work in the School of Medical Sciences in the University of Auckland.

Adam White, BSc Physiotherapy *Senior Hand Therapist, Waikato Hospital, Hamilton, New Zealand.*

Adam is a senior hand therapist who qualified at the London Hospital, UK, in 1985 and has worked in numerous hospitals in the UK and private practice. He has worked in the Hand Therapy Department at Waikato Hospital, Hamilton, New Zealand, for the last 27 years.

Richard Wong She, CNZM, FRACS *Plastic and Reconstructive Surgeon, Middlemore Hospital, Auckland, New Zealand.*

Richard is a plastic and reconstructive surgeon working at Middlemore Hospital, Auckland, New Zealand. He qualified as a plastic surgeon in 2005. He has specialised in burn care and was the first Clinical Leader for Burns at the National Burn Centre of New Zealand it opened in 2006. He continues to be involved as a member of the Burn Team, which treats the most severely injured burn patients from throughout New Zealand and across parts of the Pacific.

Fiona Wood, AM, FRCS, FRACS *Plastic and Burns Surgeon, Fiona Stanley Hospital and Perth Children's Hospital, Perth, Australia; Director of the Burns Service of Western Australia.*

Fiona graduated from St Thomas's Hospital Medical School in London [1981]. She has been a burns surgeon and researcher for over 30 years. She is the co-founder of the first skin cell laboratory in Western Australia, Winthrop Professor in the School of Surgery at the University of Western Australia, and co-founder of the Fiona Wood Foundation [formerly the McComb Foundation].

1 Who Was Joan Chapple?

The nuances of Dr. Joan Chapple's life story will be unknown to the vast majority of readers of this book. Although she had a significant influence on both co-editors, at various stages in their respective surgical careers, at the time, neither was more than superficially cognisant of the complexities of her background. Therefore, in the course of re-writing this book, the co-editors also decided to conduct a series of detailed interviews with surviving family members, longstanding close friends, and medical professionals who had worked with Joan Chapple, in an attempt to present a more relatable picture of her life and career, as well as the person that she was. There is no doubt that she was a unique and enigmatic human being.

Joan Chapple was born in 1934 to Kingsley and Winifred Chapple in Te Puke, New Zealand, where her parents were sole teachers at Te Matai Native School in rural Bay of Plenty. She had two older siblings, James and Jocelyn, and subsequently, two younger ones, John and Jefferson (Fig. 1.1). When Joan eventually attended this same small school, she and her siblings were almost the only Pākehā (New Zealanders of European descent) in the school roll of otherwise Māori children. This intimate contact with other cultural values, life in the rural community, and the related attitudes of her parents likely had a profound influence on her ultimate personality. In particular, these factors almost certainly contributed to her empathy for the underprivileged and the deep kindness she constantly displayed in dealings with her friends and patients.

Joan also attended Te Puke District School, Rotorua Girls High School and finally Epsom Girls Grammar School (EGGS) in Auckland. She was a Prefect at EGGS in 1951, became an accomplished cellist and competed for the school in tennis, hockey, and swimming. Joan completed her Medical Intermediate year at Auckland University in 1952 and was accepted into Otago Medical School in 1953, where, in a student demographic vastly different from today's, she was among only a handful of women in a class of nearly 100. A female classmate recalled her as a rather quiet person, who did not interact a great deal with other women students. In the 1954 Third Year Medical Class photo, Joan Chapple is seen standing with the men in the third row, on the right (Fig. 1.2). Notable classmates were Alan Kerr (later cardiac surgeon), Patricia Clarkson (later paediatric cardiologist), James Carter (later general surgeon), Malcolm Dunshea (later ENT surgeon), Peter Milsom (later general surgeon), and John Carman (later Professor of Anatomy). Joan was a capable student and under the tutelage of orthopaedic surgeon Professor Allan Aldred, she achieved distinction in surgery in her final medical school examinations and was awarded the Stanley Wilson Prize. She graduated as one of only nine women in the class.

Joan spent her first postgraduate house-surgeon year at Wanganui Hospital. Relocating to

P. Charlesworth, M. F. Klaassen, *Chapple's Principles of Wound Care and Healing*,
https://doi.org/10.1007/978-3-031-53104-0_1

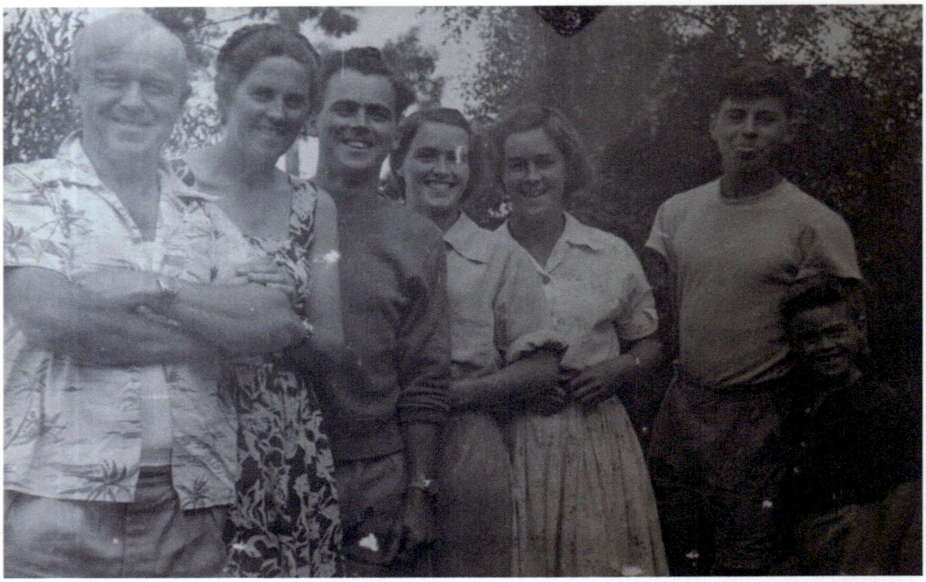

Fig. 1.1 Early photograph of the Chapple family [L to R: Kingsley, Winifred, James, Jocelyn, **Joan**, John and Jefferson Chapple]

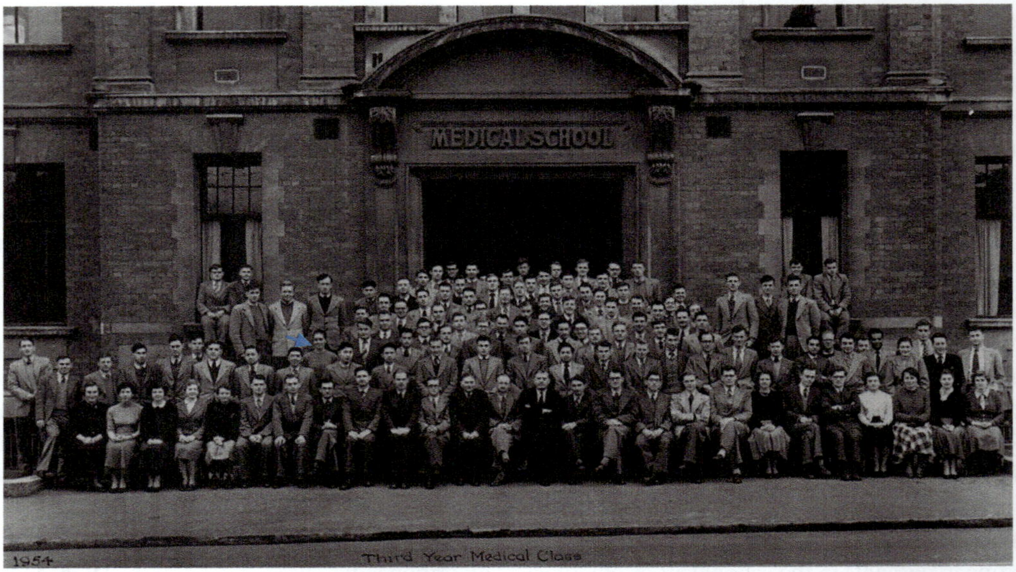

Fig. 1.2 1954 Third-year medical class, Otago University

Auckland in 1959, she continued house-surgeon training and was selected by William Manchester as a registrar in plastic surgery in 1961. She completed Fellowship of the Royal Australasian College of Surgeons (FRACS) in 1963, becoming only the second woman to gain a specialist surgical qualification in New Zealand. Following this, she pursued several months' postgraduate training with noted surgical mentors, particularly in the area of hand surgery, in Australia, India, Russia, and the United States. She was initially prevented from entering the United States when passing through Los Angeles airport, somehow targeted by the FBI due to a tenuous connection to a 'communist' meeting when she was a medical student, but after a supportive phone call with William Manchester in New Zealand, the authorities allowed her to continue her travel to New York.

On her return to Auckland, Joan was appointed as a full-time plastic surgeon at Middlemore Hospital. Here, she began to develop her profound and abiding interest in the treatment of hand and associated soft tissue injuries, perhaps to the detriment of duties in the wider general field of plastic surgery, according to others working in the Middlemore unit at the time. She acted as an itinerant consultant to other hospitals where junior doctors, particularly those working in Accident and Emergency departments, spoke highly of her dedicated support and tutelage, with respect to management of the many hand injuries they saw on a daily basis. Perhaps, these absences from Middlemore engendered resentment from her surgical colleagues there, but in any event, she encountered significant work difficulties in the male-dominated (and possibly misogynistic) surgical environment of the day. Another issue that caused friction was Joan's desire to confront, and discuss in detail, the reasons for 'unsatisfactory outcomes' of surgery, rather than focusing only on 'good results'. Speaking many years later to journalists, for articles published about her in local periodicals, Joan said that 'as the only woman, I never felt welcome in the surgical profession' [1]. One confounding anachronism was that she was prevented from attending regular meetings of the Auckland surgical fraternity, because they were held in a private club that did not allow women members. Close friends at the time reported that Joan used to return from work at Middlemore stressed and exhausted from the lack of collegial support and intolerance for her views. Perhaps her senior colleagues felt in some way threatened by her intellect, her development of unorthodox clinical concepts, and her disposition of kind connectedness to her patients.

Joan became a single mother to her daughter Raven in 1972 and applied for maternity leave. The concept of unmarried parenthood was very controversial at that time, and it remains unclear whether local attitudes to her situation and associated medical politics subsequently resulted in her position at Middlemore Hospital being formally terminated by the authorities, or whether she resigned due to the atmosphere of unpleasantness. However, she left and travelled to Wales to join her partner, Dr. Ian Scott, who was undertaking a fellowship with the Medical Research Council of Great Britain, while working as a GP in the small Welsh mining village of Glyncorrwg. Joan spent a year in Wales and later joined by her mother Winifred, the family group travelled in Europe for 3 months.

On her return to Auckland in 1975, Joan accepted a new appointment as a plastic surgeon in the Accident and Emergency department at Auckland Hospital in the city and lecturer at the nearby Auckland School of Medicine. Her hospital work narrowed to what had become her predominant interest, the management of hand and soft tissue injuries, including some burns. Nurses who worked with Joan at that time have commented not only on her technical skills and knowledge but also on her kindness, empathy, and forbearance in her dealings with staff and patients. She was actively involved in the teaching of medical students, nurses, and general practitioners, within which groups she achieved a legendary and almost cult status. Her views on healing and soft tissue injury management were widely promulgated, but not well-accepted by the entrenched traditional surgical fraternity at large. During this period, Joan honed her philosophies and concepts of physiological wound healing and began to compile an extensive written and photographic record of her clinical cases. These developed into her first book about healing and wound care, but in 1980, the first draft of the book was rejected by an Australian publisher. In 1994, after a serious illness, she retired from Auckland Hospital having published an updated version of the book, *The Management of Soft Tissue Conditions and Injuries: philosophy, principles and practice: a handbook for the care of wounds* (Allen and Hanburys 1991), based on her nearly two decades of running busy soft tissue injury clinics. The book on which the current re-edition is based,

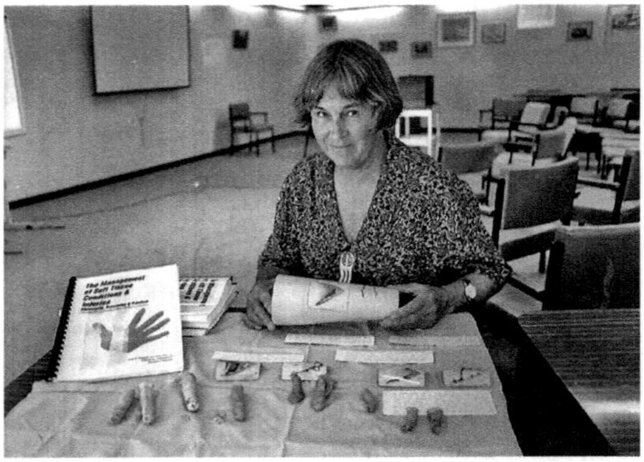

Fig. 1.3 Dr. Joan Chapple the passionate medical teacher

Wound Care and Healing: The Physiological Challenge, was self-published by Joan in 2003, and became a sentinel reference for many courses that she continued to conduct, primarily for general practitioners, nurses, and surgical trainees (Fig. 1.3). That book was dedicated to Joan's daughter Raven, and the original dedication has been retained in this edition (see frontispiece).

For many years, Joan's home was in secluded Karaka Bay in Glendowie, eastern Auckland, which is accessed by a steep path that winds down the hill from the end of Peacock Street. Boat access is also possible. The Bay looks out to the local Hauraki Gulf islands of Rangitoto, Motutapu, Browns, Motuihe, and Waiheke. The beach is on the western side of the Tāmaki River, where it flows north into the Waitemata Harbour. Historically, it was a site for one of the signings of the Treaty of Waitangi in 1840, the significance of which would not have been lost on Joan Chapple, because she was sensitive to the inequitable colonial history of the Māori in New Zealand and the plight of the underprivileged. Early in her medical career, she rented a cottage at Karaka Bay and later bought her own property there in the 1960s, including a 'boathouse', which became a place for friends to stay, after socialising or in time of need. The community at Karaka Bay was perhaps slightly non-conformist, and beach parties organised by the residents there were evidently legendary. Joan was an active participant in local community issues and shared social occasions. Junior medical staff who rented a cottage adjacent to her at Karaka Bay remember her fondly for her generous hospitality at home, but also for her passion for teaching and her enthusiastic mentoring of them when they were junior surgical residents. Joan was a humanist and saw the best in everyone. She was very astute, but humble enough to admit that she didn't have all the answers, and she was selfless beyond reproach. However, she did not hesitate to criticise strongly what she saw as the deficiencies of the health system and medical establishment of her time.

Between 1995 and 2001, Joan looked after her elderly mother Winifred in Takapuna, Auckland, organising care rosters with her siblings. Winifred died in 2001. The same year, Dr. Joan Chapple was made a Companion of the New Zealand Order of Merit (CNZM) for services to medicine and the community, the award being presented by the Governor General of New Zealand, Dame Sylvia Cartwright. When interviewed about the honour, Joan was quietly proud, but said that what she would really like was for her soft tissue philosophies and techniques to be accepted 'for the difference it would make to patients, not for personal glory' [2].

Dr. Joan Chapple died in 2013 at the age of 79 from recurrent pelvic cancer, at the Mercy Hospice in Auckland, surrounded by her family. Prior to this, she had been nursed by her long-standing close friend and medical classmate Dr. Alan Kerr and his wife Hazel. A memorial service was held for Joan at the Girl Guides Hall, Glendowie, on the edge of Churchill Park Farm, near Karaka Bay. In 2019, the New Zealand Medical Journal and the Royal Australasian College of Surgeons magazine *Cutting Edge* published an obituary for Joan, written by Dr. Alan Kerr and Raven Chapple. The final lines state:

'Joan was a compassionate and caring doctor and a generous and loyal friend. Her gender and

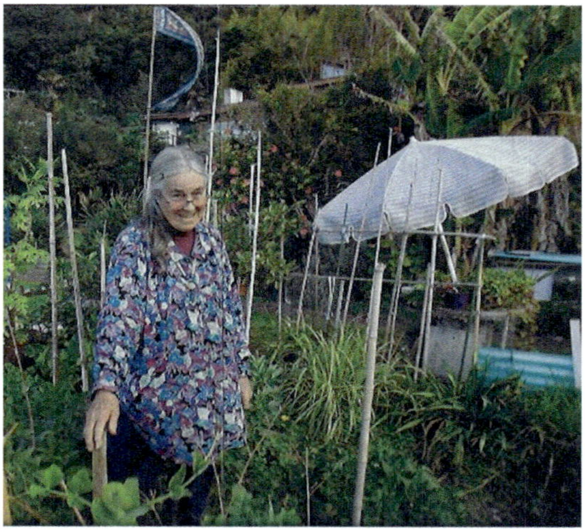

Fig. 1.4 Dr. Joan Chapple [1934–2013], retired plastic surgeon and gardener

her unconventional attitudes may have restricted her from reaching her full potential as a surgeon, but she was in many ways ahead of her time. Her achievements were significant, and she will be remembered with affection and respect' [3] (Fig. 1.4).

References

1. NZ Herald Lifestyle "Thinking Outside the Square". Accessed 23 June 2008.
2. Ibid.
3. http://www.nzma.org.nz/journal/read-the-journal/all-issues/2010-2019/2019/vol-132-no-1489-1-february-2019/7807.

2 Summary of Chapple's Principles for Wound Care and Healing

Summary

1. After injury or surgery there is always a 24–48 h interval of temporary reactive swelling in the tissues.
2. The transient reactive swelling reflects the disordered physiology, which may be profound.
3. Co-ordinated repair processes follow to bring about healing and remodelling of the affected tissues, which may continue for months and years.
4. All wounds will eventually heal, but not without circulation.
5. An adequate circulation is the key to recovery and healing.
6. Venous insufficiency is more common than arterial ischaemia and just as detrimental to the healing.
7. Haematomata can be avoided by precise haemostasis during surgery.
8. Pain is a protective sensation and has multifactorial causes, which must be worked out so that the correct management is selected for pain control.
9. Flaps and grafts are distinguished by their circulatory dynamics and physiology.
10. First Aid for wounds involves elevating the bleeding part, applying focal pressure to stop the bleeding, tourniquet use for blood loss leading to shock, and resting the patient as flat as possible.
11. When evaluating wounds, the history and mechanism of injury provide the necessary information required for management decisions.
12. Acute treatment depends on the anatomical and physiological damage but includes anaesthesia, meticulous cleansing and haemostasis, and the consideration of the question 'Is tissue missing or displaced?'
13. Local anaesthetic use requires knowledge of pharmacology, potential drug toxicity, and regional anaesthetic applications.
14. Cleansing of wounds is a mechanical process using hydrostatic pressure and may also involve serial surgical debridement.
15. The craft of suturing requires experience, judgment, and knowledge of alternative approaches.
16. Wound dressings have different roles, including absorption of seepage, support of the inflamed tissues, prevention of desiccation of exposed living cells, and occlusive protection from the environment.
17. Rehabilitation after injury should be a seamless process with the goals being a rapid recovery and restoration of full function.
18. Hand injuries are common and involve specialised structures in a confined space; management is aimed at restoring full hand function.

P. Charlesworth, M. F. Klaassen, *Chapple's Principles of Wound Care and Healing*,
https://doi.org/10.1007/978-3-031-53104-0_2

19. Infection is often caused by pathogenic bacteria colonising compromised, dirty wounds, haematomas, or dead tissue. Antibiotic resistance is a growing problem that we must all be aware of.
20. Particular sites on the body and certain causative agents give rise to difficult and unusual wounds.
21. Ingrown toenails can be managed increasingly with conservative approaches, using surgery mostly as a backup for failed conservative measures.
22. Burns are the most preventable of injuries, and prevention is the best approach to them.

Commentary by Michael F. Klaassen ONZM, FRACS—Co-editor with Peter Charlesworth FRACS

Joan Chapple's principles of Wound Care & Healing are fundamental and simple. Under the classification of general principles, they would be considered EXECUTIONAL Principles [1].

Her principles are the bedrock of Wound Care & Healing, both then and now. They remain a starting point for constructing solutions to the everyday wound challenges faced by doctors, nurses, and associated health professionals—be they vascular surgeons or podiatric surgeons!

Professor Robert A. Chase [b. 1923] of Stamford University, a leading teacher of plastic surgery and a contemporary of Joan Chapple, once stated 'A principle develops through a period of gestation, it is not born fully developed. Once born, a principle continues to evolve and to become more refined'. Professor Chase was famous for his hand surgery and Joan Chapple would have probably visited him at some stage in her career. Her 22 principles stated above certainly have evolved in the way Robert Chase predicted.

An even earlier pioneer of surgery, Professor William Halstead [1852–1922] of Johns Hopkins Hospital, Baltimore described his Seven Tenets of Halstead [in the 1890s]:

1. Handle tissue gently.
2. Achieve meticulous haemostasis.
3. Preserve vascularity.
4. Ensure strict asepsis.
5. Ensure good approximation of tissues.
6. Close the wound without tension.
7. Avoid dead space.

When you read these, you may recognise the recurring theme and fundamental principles so eloquently described by Joan Chapple almost a century later. The future will reveal many changes to technique, wound dressings and stem cell science but the bedrock principles will remain.

Reference

1. Klaassen MF, Brown E. General principles. In: An examiner's guide to professional plastic surgery exams. Springer Nature; 2018.

3 The Healing Process

Summary

Dr Joan Chapple started her self-published book in 2003 with a number of hypotheses:

1. Injury initiates a series of coordinated living responses. The human body endeavours to return to a pre-existing image in terms of both structure and function. Remodelling of the tissue continues to achieve further improvement for months and years after the initial healing.
2. Living cells need to be nurtured in a moist and non-toxic environment.
3. The speed and quality of recovery/repair after injury depends on the circulation. The human body recovers and heals with or without treatment but never without circulation.
4. After injury there is always a 24–48 h interval of temporary reactive swelling reflecting the physiological damage. Very few clinicians actually get to see wounds at this stage to appreciate the extent of the process or allow for it safely in their primary treatment. The low-pressure venous sector of the circulation is the most vulnerable to an increase in tension.
5. Most necrosis after injury arises from venous stasis rather than arterial deprivation. Venous insufficiency, reflected by increasing throbbing pain as tension increases, is likely to be associated with a sluggish recovery and infective complications, even if tissue survives.
6. Standard treatment with immediate restoration of the appearance as the priority rather than the physiological needs of tissue often reduces the circulatory throughput. Standard techniques which do this have nevertheless continued to be legitimised because healing eventually occurs.
7. Whenever dressing pressure is used for final haemostasis it immediately also reduces the circulation in the vicinity of the wound/flap. Dressings that are initially firm become tighter as swelling increases, reducing circulation even further. Already disadvantaged tissues are of course always the first and most seriously affected by an increase in tension.
8. Infection is usually associated with inadequate cleansing and/or haematoma. This is particularly a problem with poorly nourished or dead tissue.
9. Meticulous cleansing and haemostasis, followed by accurate alignment of tissue, elevated posturing to reduce wound tension, measures to assist venous drainage, and dressings designed to accommodate swelling provide safer and more optimal conditions for tissue recovery and uncomplicated healing.

P. Charlesworth, M. F. Klaassen, *Chapple's Principles of Wound Care and Healing*,
https://doi.org/10.1007/978-3-031-53104-0_3

10. It is essential to clearly distinguish initially between flap and graft circulatory requirements. All flaps need special circulatory consideration. If skin is recognised initially as being without sufficient perfusion to survive, it can usually be assisted to pick up enough new capillary attachments to survive as a graft. The techniques involved in this form of grafting are readily accessible to all those who are treating wounds.
11. Each wound deserves to be considered and treated individually, with all treatment regarded as doing things for tissues rather than to them.

All injuries trigger innate responses. Transient reactive swelling, reflecting the disordered physiology, reaches its peak during the first 48 h. Coordinated repair processes follow to bring about healing and remodelling of the affected tissues can continue for months or years.

Every injury initiates a series of responses from living tissues. There is bleeding and bruising from damaged blood vessels, followed by non-specific swelling in the vicinity. This increases to a maximum within about 48 h and diminishes again over the next few days. Although nothing seems to be happening in these early days, a great deal is going on. Cells are recovering and both local and general responses are being organised. By about 5 or 6 days, skin cells at the edge of a full-thickness wound are starting to divide and migrate across living tissue in continuity to restore surface integrity. The key factor in all this is always the quality of perfusion available. New capillaries also begin to proliferate from damaged blood vessels within a few days, producing pink and highly vascular *granulation tissue* on any unhealed surface. This is an ideal layer on which skin cells can migrate to bring about healing. Once epithelial cells meet, they first of all reconstitute the intact basal layer of epidermis, but thereafter they proliferate vertically. The original, single layer of cells thickens up to several and these mature, then flatten and lose their nuclei as they move towards the surface. This process is merely re-establishing normal skin behaviour where layers of dead cells are flaking off in order to protect the body surface from wear and tear. Ordinarily, epithelial cells take about a month to reach the surface. Connective tissue cells in the injured subcutaneous tissues have also been multiplying and laying down fibres which strengthen the deeper aspects of the wound.

Left entirely to nature, healthy acute wounds usually produce a protective covering of adherent clot or fibrin over any exposed living tissue, with a surface that dries in the air. Skin cells from the edges, nourished on the moist living tissue beneath this scab, divide and migrate beneath it to re-establish a healed skin layer at which stage the scab falls off [1]. Unhealed raw surfaces remain vulnerable to desiccation, which can produce a surface slough needing to be separated off before a living surface can be produced again (Fig. 3.1).

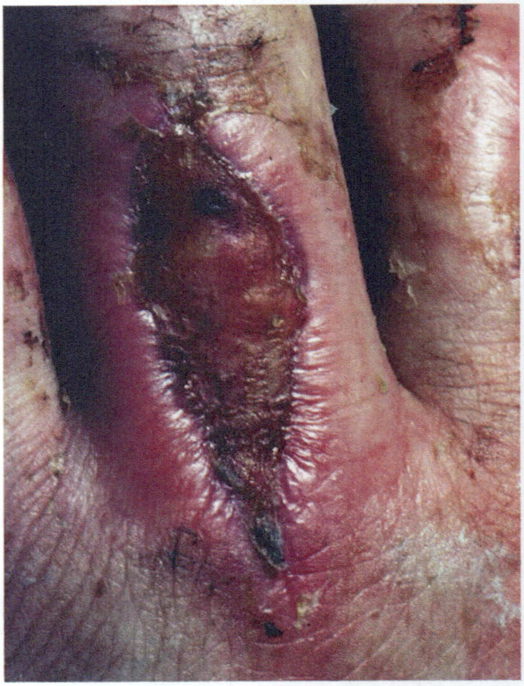

Fig. 3.1 This unhealthy wound now has a dry surface, which cannot support healing until it granulates again

Healing is achieved three times as fast if surfaces are kept moist at all times. Repeated drying of raw surfaces may discourage healing altogether, especially in the case of chronic ulcers, where tissues are always struggling to produce enough viable tissue to support epithelial migration. Occlusive dressings not only protect surfaces from desiccation but also keep bacteria out and stop wounds sticking to bedding and clothing.

The **optimum therapeutic approach to injured tissue must be the physiological one**, helping living tissues to do what only they can do. Exposed and injured tissues need a moist, non-toxic environment and an active circulation in order to recover and heal. Both sutures and dressings have the potential to restrict the circulation, especially during the period of reactive swelling. The accurate redisposition of tissues disrupted by injury is a much more appropriate concept of helping, rather than dragging or pulling everything accurately together in a standard closure, however, tidy the repair looks. If tissues are accurately controlled within broad and gentle constraints, a good deal of further closure will often occur as tissue swells and there is likely to be further improvement as swelling subsides. A more complete closure with tapes can generally be achieved after 3 or 4 days. Closure in this way is best regarded as a persuasive process much more akin to gardening than to precision engineering.

If the skin edges can be safely closed initially, or brought together by tapes or secondary suturing within the next few days, surface healing is completed within days. Small gaps or small losses heal quickly as long as there is healthy tissue on which epithelial cells can migrate. Larger defects will take longer to heal and may be helped by skin grafting. Significant delay in healing will allow the development of additional granulation tissue which turns into scar tissue, but it must also be remembered that the death of tissue following inappropriate suturing also delays healing and is often associated with infection, which produces additional diffuse, as well as local scarring (Figs. 3.2 and 3.3).

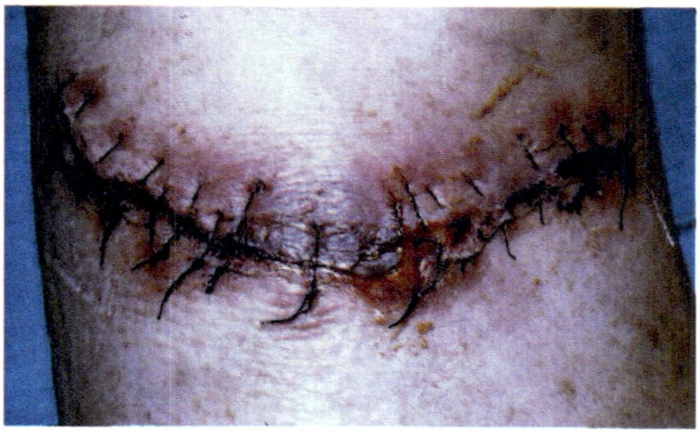

Fig. 3.2 Broad proximally based knee flap showing circulatory problems caused by sutures. Infection is already present. Taping this flap wound have been a much safer option but the knee would have needed splinting

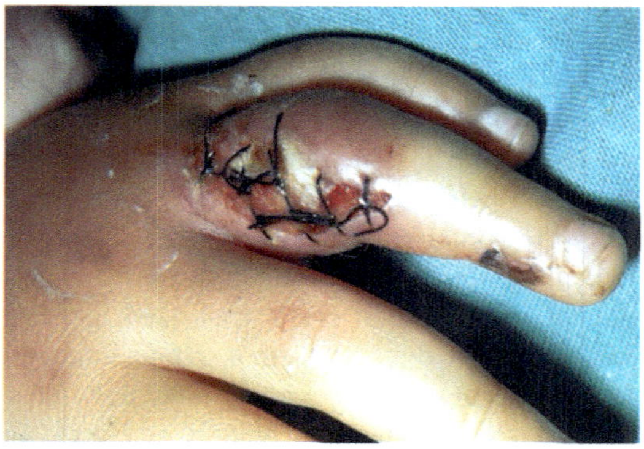

Fig. 3.3 This unhealthy infected wound has followed the inappropriate suturing of a crushed finger. The underlying fracture became infected. The eventual result was poor

Once surface healing is complete, the deeper layers continue to remodel the subcutaneous architecture, attempting also to re-create the interdigitating relationship of dermis with epithelium which helps to stop skin shearing off. Connective tissue cells lay down additional fibres beneath the epithelium in a new scar that becomes bulky and vascular for several months and also shrinks. Very new scar is rather brittle and the epithelium over it may also be particularly unstable at first. Eventually, however, scar tissue softens and lengthens, as well as becoming less vascular and less irritable. Maturation and remodelling of scars continue to improve them further for several years, eventually completing the reaction of the body to the stimulus of the original injury.

Human beings seem to need to attribute healing to treatment, a misconception that has become the basis for all sorts of therapies and much conventional medicine. The body has its own efficient homeostatic mechanisms and highly coordinated repair processes, so ascribing these to external ministrations is outrageous. Proprietary applications and dressings, despite the extravagant claims of drug companies, never do any of the healing either, but merely provide an environment in which it can occur and not necessarily even the best one. Healing will never be done by anything other than living tissue, ideally in physiological conditions.

It is just as fallible to base treatments on the questionable assumption that doing something is always better than doing nothing. Patients are always in the vulnerable position of wondering whether there is something more that could or should be being done and will readily embrace everything on offer, just in case they miss out on something important. Wounds have their own agenda for healing at every stage, and the very best that can be done for them is to tune into their needs as accurately as possible, doing only those things that are genuinely helpful and none of those which could possibly be meddlesome or inappropriate.

An even more difficult concept for people to grasp is that all setbacks are quite contrary to the innately constructive behaviour of normal living tissue. All complications have definite and mostly discernible causes and must never be explained away by statistics or bad luck. There can be important relationships between primary wound care techniques and the subsequent health of wounds.

Continuing the process of looking after these factors is what the acquisition of expertise is all about. Additional surgical procedures always add to the original tissue injury, so the technicalities and timing of these are also highly relevant. The most appropriate attitude to all complications is to assume that they do have causes and to keep looking for the explanations. Striving to prevent them happening on another occasion must always include a review of everything untoward. The reorganisation of health services in the name of efficiency unfortunately has now promoted one-off interventions and the avoidance of personal responsibility through the use of protocols, standardisation, and risk-management policies. All of these of course mitigate very efficiently against the development of personal expertise and true professionalism.

Healing is truly part of a master plan, with the human body running comprehensive and coordinated short- and long-term agendas and doing the best it can to eventually return itself to a preexisting body image in both function and appearance. While this aspect of healing is undoubtedly one of the most fascinating, it is also presently one of the least understood. Faced with this highly organised miracle, we should all acknowledge that we are to a great extent merely bystanders in the arena of wound healing. The answers presently remain in the genes.

Editors' Note *As an illustrative clinical case of venous insufficiency, MFK recently had a classic example of throbbing, swelling, and red hand in a patient 6 days post excision of a squamous cell carcinoma from the dorsum of his non-dominant hand and attempted repair with a keystone perforator island local flap (Fig. 3.4a–c).*

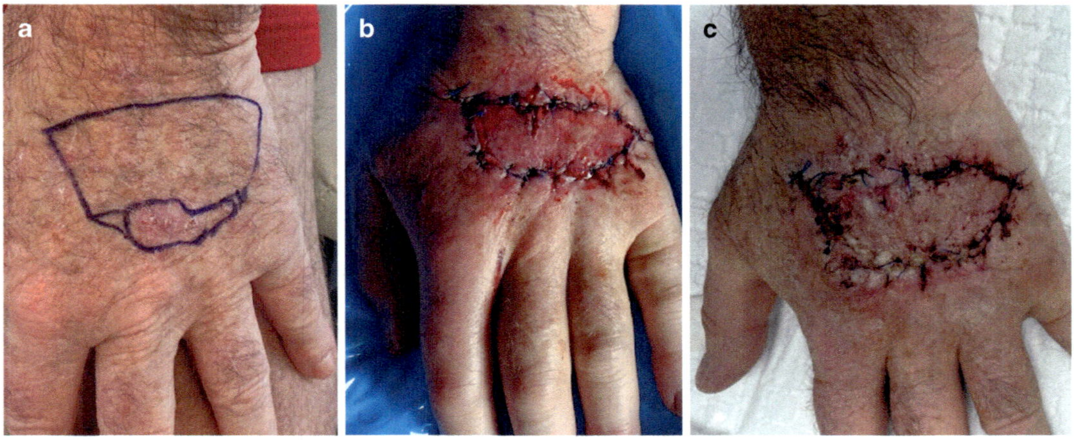

Fig. 3.4 (**a–c**) 71-year-old man 6 days post wide excision of an SCC from the dorsum of his left non-dominant hand who re-presented with throbbing hand pain, redness in the local keystone flap, cellulitis, and finger swelling. He required release of some sutures and intravenous antibiotics to settle his cellulitis and infection. He did not elevate his hand enough post-surgery and the dressings were too tight. (**c**) 17 days post-surgery when the venous insufficiency & sepsis have resolved

Commentary by Professor Fiona Wood AM, FRCS, FRACS

Understanding the healing process underpins the practise of plastic and reconstructive surgery. In this chapter, Dr Joan Chapple clearly outlines the key practical elements for consideration. Meticulous attention to detail with knowledge of the likely natural history of the wounded area will drive optimal outcome. Inflammation is an essential healing response and will result in temporary oedema. The oedema will limit circulation if unchecked, which in turn will increase the risk of necrosis and further tissue loss and infection.

Attempting healing by primary means in an environment of tension and oedema will increase the risk of complications. The use of the knowledge of healing by secondary intention as a temporising strategy allows for oedema control and natural wound modulation by contraction, such that delayed primary closure can give the desired outcome. The concept of oedema control, and appropriate strategies to facilitate healing, are clearly demonstrated by clinical cases within this chapter.

The consideration of long-term healing and scar maturity articulated by Dr Joan Chapple is vitally important as it helps us guide our patients in expectations of their recovery of function. This chapter provides a very solid foundation, with principles that will enable predictable clinical outcomes.

Restoration of skin integrity requires a source of cells capable of differentiation in a framework for cell migration, such that the cells express the appropriate phenotype. The skin is maintained by self-organisation over a lifetime, but apart from trivial injuries, the capacity to regenerate is overwhelmed. Repair by regeneration, not scar repair, is the ultimate goal. Research into understanding how to guide cells to express the appropriate phenotype may provide the answer, and as stated in the chapter, the answer may be in the genes.

Reference

1. Winter GD. Formation of a scab and the rate of epithelialisation of superficial wounds in the skin of the young domestic pig. Nature. 1962;193:293–4.

Commentary by Professor F… Wood AM, FRCS, FRACS

4 Circulation

Summary
The precise details of the circulation relevant to a wound are critical to recovery and healing. Many long-lasting or permanent sequelae arise out of circulatory insufficiency during the period of reactive swelling following injury. Venous insufficiency is potentially just as lethal to tissues as ischaemia, but much more common and frequently overlooked. Fortunately, there are several ways to assist venous drainage. When sufficient circulation cannot be demonstrated in an isolated tissue flap, the next technical consideration must be the reattachment of the flap as a graft, to provide access to a new capillary perfusion.

When the heart is inefficient or the blood pressure or volume is reduced significantly, the fall-off in general circulatory efficiency usually constitutes a medical emergency. When circulatory insufficiency is localised to a wound, the response by professionals tends to be much less dramatic, although for affected tissues, the deprivation may be extreme. The restoration and maintenance of maximum circulation to all injured tissues should always be addressed as a priority.

Tissue can die from either venous or arterial insufficiency, or survive if sufficient throughput is maintained. This is further illustrated in Chap. 10 on Flaps and Grafts. The low-pressure venous system of the circulation is the most vulnerable to restriction with venous death of tissue being around 20 times more common than arterial necrosis. It is surprising therefore that venous congestion and insufficiency does not command anything like the clinical attention it deserves or commentary in the literature. White, bloodless ischaemic tissue invariably excites much more comment and action than blue, congested tissue which for no reason at all is assumed to be better off because it has blood in it, even if this is going nowhere (Figs. 4.1, 4.2, 4.3, and 4.4).

The term ‘blood supply’ remains widely used in place of circulation or perfusion, indicative of thinking that has not yet encompassed the concepts of flow, throughput, or drainage.

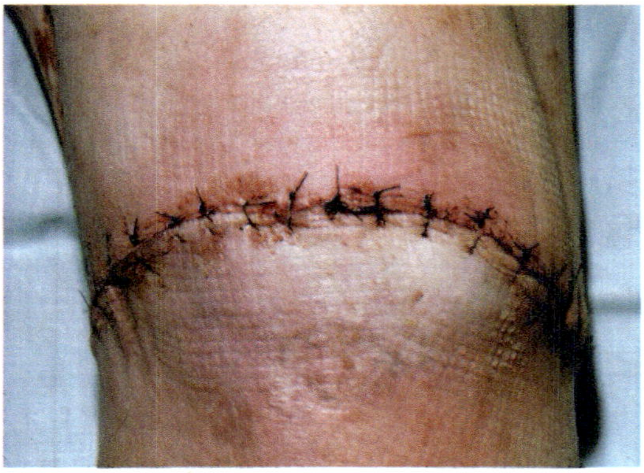

Fig. 4.1 Sutured distally based knee flap showing true ischaemia [arterial insufficiency]

P. Charlesworth, M. F. Klaassen, *Chapple's Principles of Wound Care and Healing*,
https://doi.org/10.1007/978-3-031-53104-0_4

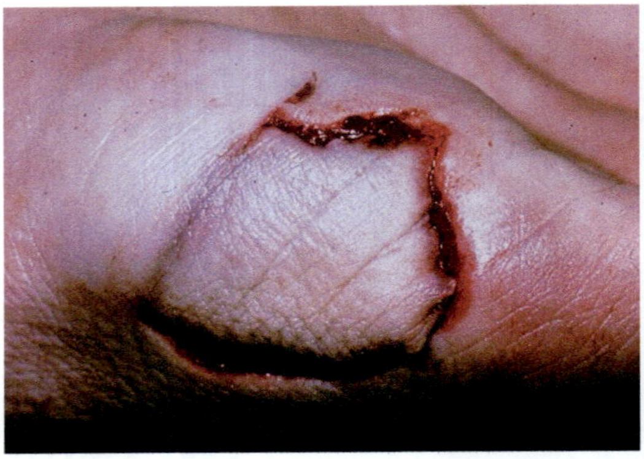

Fig. 4.2 This thickish flap has insufficient arterial input. It will therefore die as a flap, but will survive if it can be given a second chance, reapplied as a graft

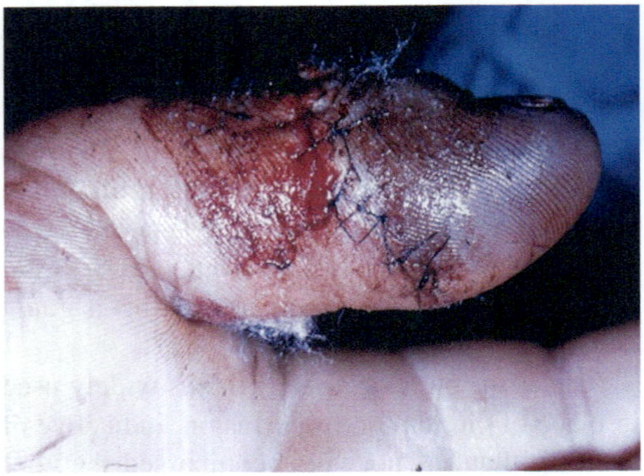

Fig. 4.3 Venous congestion of a thumb-tip. All suturing has jeopardised *the continuity* of circulation. This thumb-tip did not survive

Tissue without enough intrinsic circulation can usually pick up new capillary attachments from adjacent living tissue quickly enough to survive as a graft if it is treated appropriately. This alternative can be readily provided for dislodged and separated skin, and any flap that is bound to die otherwise.

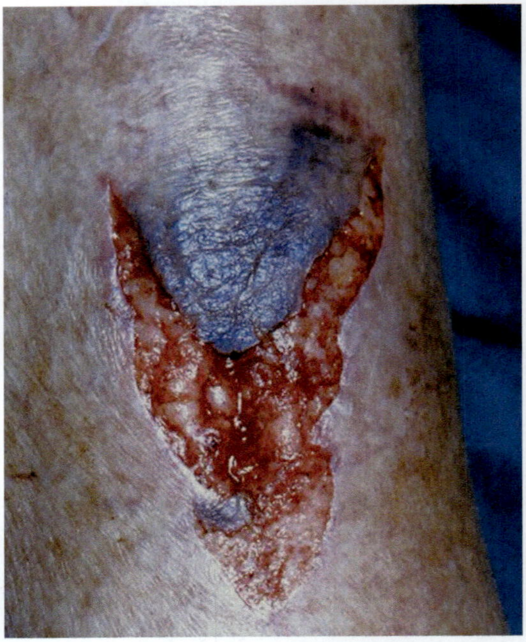

Fig. 4.4 Venous stasis in a leg flap. Such skin is likely to die unless defatted, stretched, and re-applied as a graft

Understanding Tissue Circulation

Tissue dies when it has insufficient circulation to keep it alive. There are two distinct ways this predicament can come about:

1. **Arterial insufficiency,** i.e. diminished or absent blood supply, ischaemia (Figs. 4.1 and 4.2).
2. **Inadequate venous drainage.** Congestion can progress to stasis and thrombosis. Venous insufficiency is a much more common clinical problem than ischaemia (Figs. 4.3 and 4.4).

Tissue also has two distinct modes of survival:

1. **Flap survival**—retaining sufficient flow through existing vessels in continuity.
2. **Graft survival**—secured by new capillary attachments to adjacent living tissue.

The close scrutiny of tissue appearance and behaviour in these four categories is the only way to accumulate meaningful information. If confusion exists about how, why, where, when, or whether tissue has survived or died, there is no possibility of determining what to do on another occasion to improve the chances of tissue survival and success. The concepts of flap and graft survival are not just the esoteric distinctions for plastic surgeons, but are at the heart of designing appropriate treatment for all wounds.

Measures to Assist Venous Drainage

The recognition of venous distress is particularly important because there are several technical responses that can assist venous drainage and markedly improve the circulation, and therefore the chances of tissue survival.

1. **Encouraging free drainage** of serosanguinous fluid from the wound by gravity, instead of having it build up tension in the locality. Posturing the wound to do this is usually very simple. Drains are unnecessary unless wound closure is watertight or there is no skin wound, in which case continuous suction drainage needs to be inserted.
2. **General elevation.** This assists venous drainage by gravity but specific postures may be necessary to assist blood from congested tissues to drain by gravity towards any remaining attachment. It may help to draw the flap on the other side or the other limb, as patients themselves need to understand the detailed posture and its importance.
3. **Reduction of tension and pressure** in the vicinity of the wound by:
   (a) Posturing adjacent joints to relax congested tissues, which assists attenuated veins to regain their maximum calibre and flow.
   (b) Aiming for accurate re-disposition rather than coercive closure, in order to minimise focal and general tension.
   (c) Meticulous haemostasis so that external haemostatic pressure can be avoided in the final dressings [see Chap. 16 on Bleeding, Haemostasis, and Tourniquets]. Congestion can be relieved sometimes by stroking or squeezing blood out of the congested edges. Pricking congested tissues with a needle repeatedly or attaching leeches are additional measures which have been used to remove stagnant blood. Such manoeuvres allow new arterial blood to flow through the area immediately and may be repeated as necessary to help tide the tissue along until sufficient circulatory throughput is re-established. Such measures can realistically only be carried out under very close supervision. It is quite surprising how little flow is actually needed to keep tissues alive. Ironically, it is probably this very resilience of tissue which has allowed mediocre techniques and treatments to persist.

Tissue Without Circulation

Vascular surgery is only applicable where sizeable vessels have been affected and the circulation to a limb or whole digit is cut off and can be repaired. This is specialist in-patient treatment territory with both arteries and veins requiring repair by microsurgical techniques.

Tissue without circulation is usually skin. This tissue may be physically separated from the body or still attached to it. It may suffer from arterial or venous insufficiency or both, but it will die unless provided with an opportunity to survive as a graft. This is done by removing fat and placing the skin accurately against or onto living tissue and immobilising it there to facilitate rapid capillary re-attachment. Survival depends on the vitality and area of the bed, the volume of tissue requiring sustenance and on technical expertise rather than luck. The detailed techniques are described in Chap. 10 on Flaps and Grafts.

Tissue with Both Flap and Graft Requirements

Diverse circulatory needs sometimes occur within the same wound. It is important to recognise these and endeavour to provide for them. Unless detailed observations are recorded in these situations, it is difficult, if not impossible, to retrospectively evaluate the results or evolve improved techniques. Unless both venous and arterial insufficiency are clearly distinguished and the equally fundamental differences between flap and graft survival fully appreciated, it is extremely difficult to acquire expertise as distinct from numerical encounters. **Follow-up and continuity of care must therefore always become an integral part of real learning.** Unfortunately, hospital managers do not usually appreciate this.

Circulatory Deprivation

When the Circulation Is Restricted Gradually

In vascular diseases and aging, there is a gradual decline in the vitality of all tissues, with atrophic changes and slow, difficult recovery after injury, which can be the precursor or background to many leg ulcers.

Long-Term or Permanent Interruption of Circulation

Injury can lead to tissue death, but necrosis can also come about as a result of swelling within fixed constraints during the period of reactive swelling. If this is deep within wounds, the body will either deal with it by phagocytosis or by extruding dead material in abscess or sinus formation (Fig. 4.5).

Dead tissue is a nuisance until it separates, frequently becoming a source of infection and causing delay in healing (Figs. 4.6 and 4.7).

Unfortunately, the tissue adjacent which is expected to assist in its rejection is often itself nearly dead. Separation of slough is accordingly

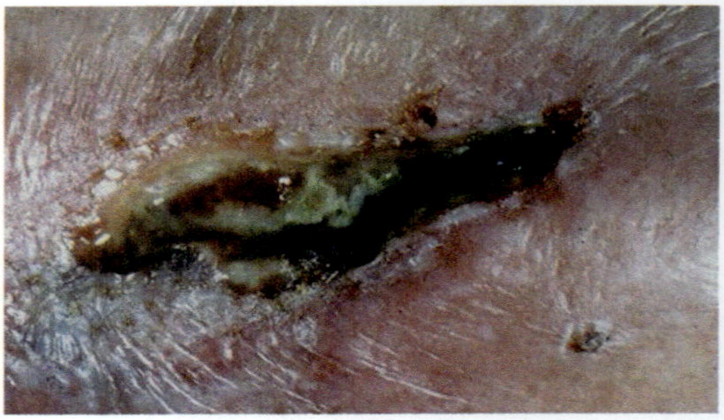

Fig. 4.5 Deep slough following operation through a previous scar. Subcutaneous sutures were used, and there has also been a haematoma within the wound

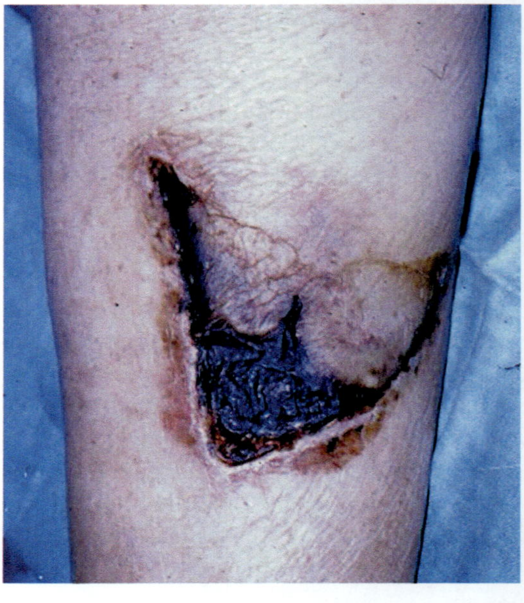

Fig. 4.6 Typical venous necrosis following suture of triangular leg flap. Note further zone of partial-thickness loss

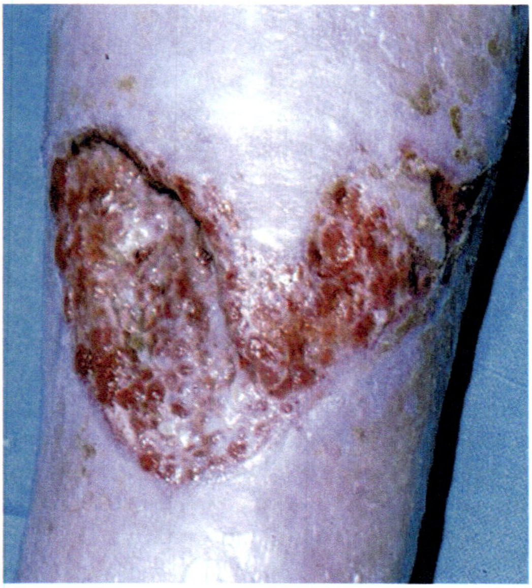

Fig. 4.7 Ragged raw surface on the lower leg a month after proximally-based flap had been sutured back and died

often slow and can be helped by serial excision/debridement. Just how living tissue immediately recognises dead tissue as no longer acceptable and responds by rejecting it as a foreign body remains a very interesting and unanswered question.

Temporary Short-Term Interruption of Circulation

The use of a tourniquet, or short-term distortional injuries or pressure, do not necessarily have permanent sequelae. Restoration of the circulation is followed by hyperaemia and sometimes by a period of transient oedema, but the effects are usually reversible.

When Circulation Is Compromised During the Period of Reactive Swelling

All adverse tissue responses and outcomes are customarily attributed solely to the injury. Within this approach, there is little or no incentive to examine the possibility that some or all of them may be related to the treatment itself. If we are determined, however, to be actually helpful and avoid circulatory risks, it is necessary to **disentangle the inevitable effects of injury from those produced by treatment interventions.** This after all should be the arena of professional input and expertise.

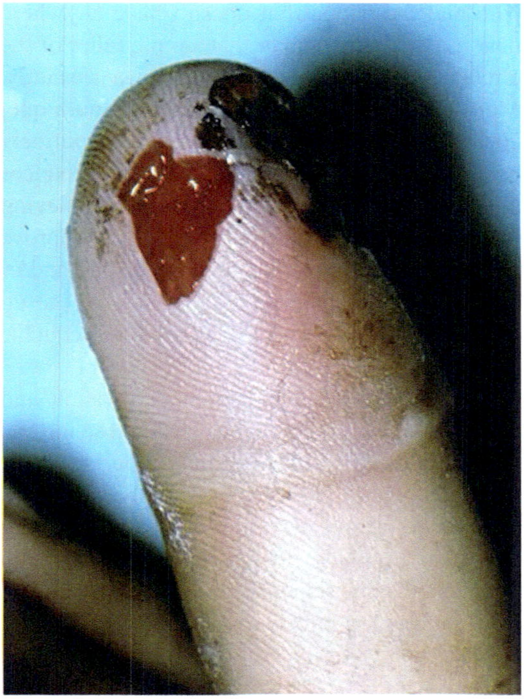

Fig. 4.8 This shallow fingertip wound was bandaged very firmly for 3 days to stop the bleeding. The finger was very painful throughout

The earliest indication that all is not ideal for tissue perfusion is the level and quality of the pain that the patient experiences. Increasing, throbbing, intolerable pain is characteristic of obstructions reflecting back to the pulsatile part of the circulation. The poor perfusion of nerves may itself further lower the pain threshold (Fig. 4.8).

Circulatory pain after acute injuries is unfortunately, commonly managed not by reviewing treatment or splitting tight bandages and plasters or snipping tight suture but by administering large doses of powerful analgesics, often intravenously and with pain pumps. This dulls both the pain and the patient but doesn't have anywhere near the dramatic benefit that simple relief of the circulatory problem can often have instantly. Many operations are performed under tourniquet control with bleeding and haematoma routinely prevented by pressure bandaging. This produces a huge dilemma, in that subsequently relieving pain or tension by loosening bandages to improve the circulation also risks causing bleeding and/or haematoma. Mostly patients just have to put up with both the pain and the circulatory sequelae (Fig. 4.9).

Both bleeding and haematoma are visible and instantly recognised complications and so long as neither of these occur, the assumption is usually made that everything is fine. Both these complications are clearly prevented by firm bandaging which is probably why this has become so entrenched in the standard professional approach. Consideration is rarely, if ever, given to the fact that the much less visible reduction in perfusion, which is readily produced by firm bandaging, can make its own separate contribution to poor outcomes and permanent sequelae.

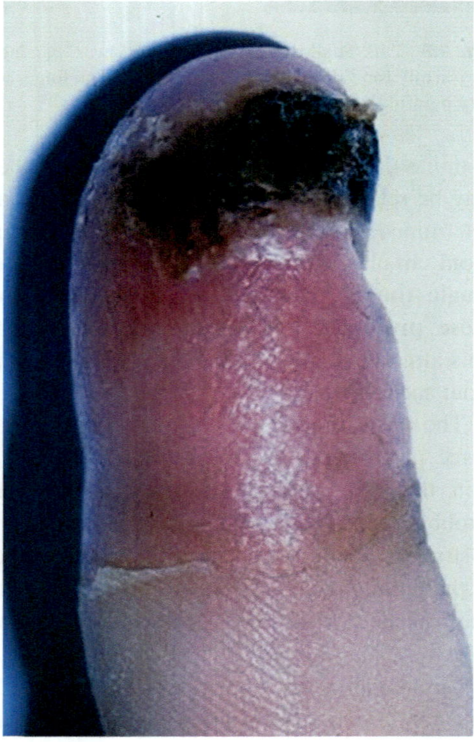

Fig. 4.9 Three weeks later, the full extent of the bandage injury is evident. The loss of both bulk and sensation persisted

It is preferable to avoid the use of a tourniquet altogether. Elevation during treatment reduces bleeding and allows progressive and straightforward haemostasis to be achieved without a tourniquet. If a tourniquet has to be used, it is best to release it and stop bleeding before the final bandaging is applied. The use of a suction drain for 24 h is always preferable to tight bandaging in the prevention of subsequent accumulations of blood. **For lower limb injuries, a double bandage technique must always be an essential part of the post-operative management.** Once haemostasis has been achieved, maximum circulation is maintained within non-tight dressings regardless of swelling, as long as the limb is elevated. The temporary additional and firm bandaging is used to prevent bleeding and haematoma during the restricted periods of ambulation permitted during the first 2–3 days. This is detailed in the instructions for double bandage technique in the Appendix.

When post-operative pain is excessive and increasing, there comes a point where the possibility of serious permanent circulatory sequelae outweighs the risks of reducing dressing tension (Figs. 4.10, 4.11, and 4.12).

If bleeding or haematoma are encountered, the wound may have to be re-opened so that they can be dealt with.

Serious and unrelieved early circulatory deprivation debilitates tissue, with oedema persisting for weeks rather than resolving after the first few days (Fig. 4.13). This woody oedema tends to evolve into diffuse fibrosis with eventual atrophy of the subcutaneous tissues, often as significant as the injury itself in the production of long-term symptoms and disability. Using pressure dressings in an attempt to either forestall or treat swelling of the injured tissue is a deeply flawed concept, as it profoundly reduces perfusion to cells. If maximum circulation can be provided within non-tight dressings, with joint function protected by splintage, even marked early swell-

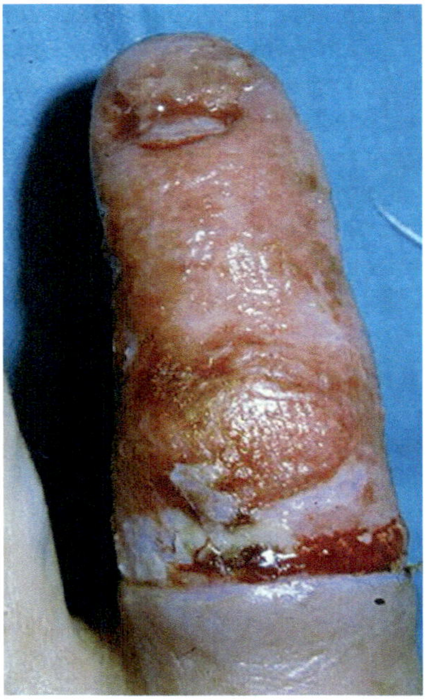

Fig. 4.10 Nutritional injury to a finger from a tight Elastoplast around the base of a dressing after a crushed nail injury 10 days earlier

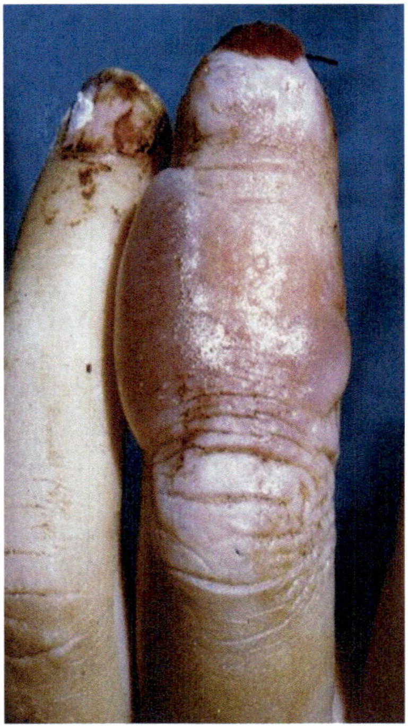

Fig. 4.11 Blistering caused by a tight Elastoplast around the base of a bandage

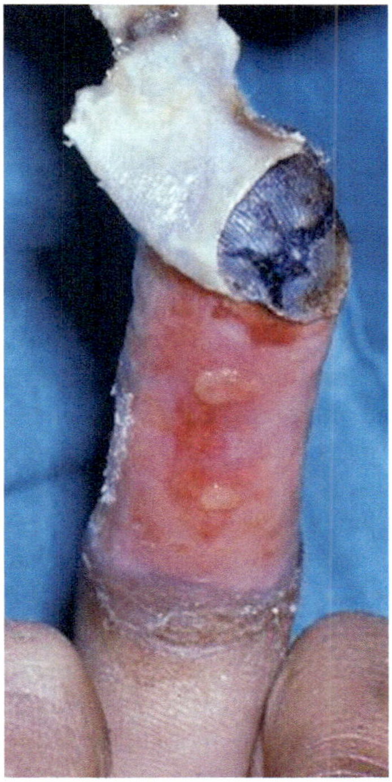

Fig. 4.12 Gangrene of a crushed pulp after a tight basal Elastoplast has caused a more extensive injury

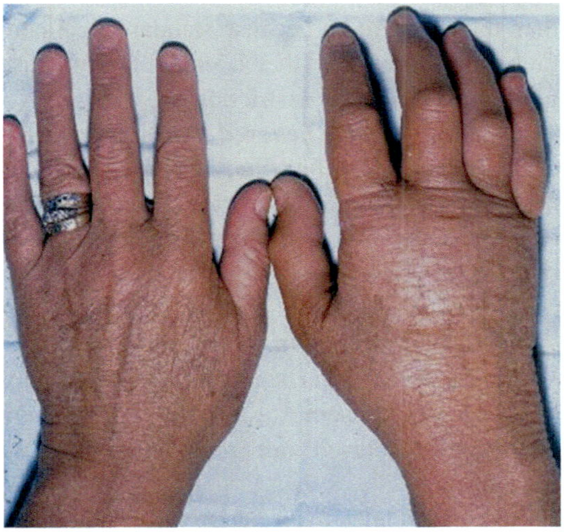

Fig. 4.13 Persistent swelling of the right hand 3 weeks after a carpal tunnel decompression caused by tight initial bandaging. This patient never regained full flexion or full use of her hand

ing usually resolves quickly, reducing the risk of long-term sequelae.

Skin debilitated by circulatory insufficiency often blisters or peels initially in a partial-thickness manner. Such skin may eventually become shiny and scaly with the originally oedematous subcutaneous compartment often dwindling away. Joints become prominent and sometimes also stiffen in this process. Excessive wound pain and painful movement discourages early mobilisation, and this situation may go on to become a disabling pain syndrome. It is often salutary, in the retrospective elucidation of pain syndromes, to ask patients about their pain history and analgesic requirements in the first few days after injury or operation. They usually have a nightmarish and important story to tell.

Long-term neuralgias and cold sensitivity are other common neurovascular sequelae. The sensitivity of the circulation to cold and dependency may persist for many months, with tissues tending to go blue and swelling readily. This is a common aftermath of many lower limb injuries. While all of these things can and do occur when injuries themselves have reduced the perfusion, they occur much more often and are more severe than they need to be because standard treatment fails to acknowledge that it can actually cause important circulatory restriction.

Dr Joan Chapple believed that the incidence of long-term woody oedema, atrophy, and painful sequelae after limb injuries could be markedly reduced by avoiding any circulatory restriction from sutures, tight bandages, or restrictive plaster casts during the first 48 h after injury or operation.

After severe trauma, surgical procedures other than cleansing, haemostasis, and repositioning may be best delayed until reactionary swelling has subsided.

Sequelae related to circulatory deprivation are not anticipated after minor trauma or elective surgery and the fact that they sometimes do occur allows the circulatory effects of treatment to be disentangled from the aftermath of the injury itself. For instance, persistent oedema and disabling neurovascular pain in the hand and fingers, not unknown after carpal tunnel decompression surgery or other minor procedures around the hand, must be ascribed to the use of tourniquets, tight dressings, and/or possibly haematoma in the wound, as they are unlikely to be due to the trauma of surgery per se.

A safer alternative technique for carpal tunnel decompression is to use local anaesthetic, operate with the hand elevated and without a tourniquet, achieving absolute haemostasis, so that tight bandaging is never required. The median nerve circulation and symptoms are relieved immediately by the operation. After 5 days in a sling, with the wrist splinted comfortably in a functional position, the patient can start using their hand again. Patients treated like this need very little pain relief, never develop swollen or disabled hands and rarely if ever need formal rehabilitation.

This analysis of circulatory sequelae can be confirmed in any physiotherapy or pain clinic by the sorry stories of most of the long-term or ‘problem’ patients. When we eventually manage to prioritise and maximise circulation after all trauma and surgical procedures, there will be a revolutionary improvement in the quality of results achieved, in all wounds and in all branches of surgery. Treatment will not only be much less painful but Dr. Chapple believed there would be a spectacular reduction in the incidence of complications, most of which she also thought had a circulatory basis.

Commentary by Dr Swee T. Tan ONZM, MBBS, PhD, FRACS

Wound healing either following direct closure of a defect or by transfer of tissue as a flap that brings along its own blood supply or a graft that relies on a vascularised bed is fundamental to the practice of plastic surgery. It depends on a normal circulation with adequate arterial inflow and venous outflow that sustains perfusion of the capillary bed to provide nutrients and oxygenation to the tissue. This is particularly relevant in an injury in which the traumatised tissue is already compromised.

The prescient observations and espousal of important principles of wound care by the late Dr Joan Chapple are artfully conveyed and retold by the editors with superb case studies in this chapter.

A vital element of wound management is the care of the injured tissue or body part, and to abrogate or minimise further injury, with an eye on rehabilitation with eventual restoration of form and function. This includes avoidance of further circulatory compromise by iatrogenic injury (such as inappropriate application of a tourniquet, excessively tight wound closure and dressings) and mitigation of the secondary effects of trauma (such as tissue oedema) by elevation and/or splinting of the affected part. In their retelling of Dr Chapple's approach, the editors highlight some of the pitfalls of wound management with numerous case studies that are helpful to both students and the experienced.

The text underscores the detrimental effect of inappropriate use of tourniquet. Whilst it plays an important role in controlling life-threatening bleeding in certain situations, local pressure of the bleeding point is far more effective. The cases in which ischaemia and/or the loss of tissues or body parts caused by excessively tight dressings are devastating and unforgettable.

The often-unappreciated presence and consequences of venous insufficiency are highlighted, and mitigation strategies are presented. Advice is also offered on the management of flap lacerations with ischaemia by converting the devitalised flap into a skin graft, placed on a vascularised bed.

This chapter, along with the wisdom contained in the rest of the book, conveys the vital principles and sound guidance, to all who are involved, on optimal wound management for their patients.

5 Avoidance of Complications (Haematoma, Pain, and Infection)

Summary
The spectre of wound disruption caused by haematoma, complicated frequently by pain and infection, has probably contributed to the unfortunate tendency to bandage wounds firmly. The effects of this on the local circulation, as swelling increases, are rarely if ever acknowledged. A much safer alternative is afforded by achieving haemostasis as an integral part of treatment, so that haemostatic bandaging is never needed. Non-watertight closure of wounds assisted by gravity drainage reduces the risk of haematoma. In closed wounds or spaces such as degloved areas, vacuum drainage can be used for 24 h to prevent accumulations of fluid. The control of bleeding is best achieved by elevation and focal pressure, not by the application of a tourniquet. Complete haemostasis, achieved progressively during treatment, is a specific goal because it means that final dressing tension no longer has to be haemostatic and maximum perfusion of tissue is achieved during the period of reactive swelling. Pain is a protective sensation. Responding to its underlying causes is much more appropriate than simply giving pain relief.

This chapter is a condensation of three separate chapters in Joan Chapple's original manuscript where her sense of humour really comes to the fore! Her antagonism towards the age-old custom of packing was before the new era of negative wound pressure devices [VAC and SNAP] which are effectively functional packing with physiological wound-healing enhancement properties.

Haematoma

Blood accumulating within the tissues can produce a space-occupying collection pressing on both deep tissues and the overlying skin (Figs. 5.1 and 5.2). Blood can sometimes track off along planes and into loose tissues to cause bruising at a distance. A sizeable haematoma is usually well worth draining. The skin over a tense collection is very often anaesthetic already, but may require the injection of local anaesthetic to enable a 1–2 cm incision to be made through skin only, in the direction of the skin creases or the lines of relaxed skin tension [1]. If this does not open into

P. Charlesworth, M. F. Klaassen, *Chapple's Principles of Wound Care and Healing*,
https://doi.org/10.1007/978-3-031-53104-0_5

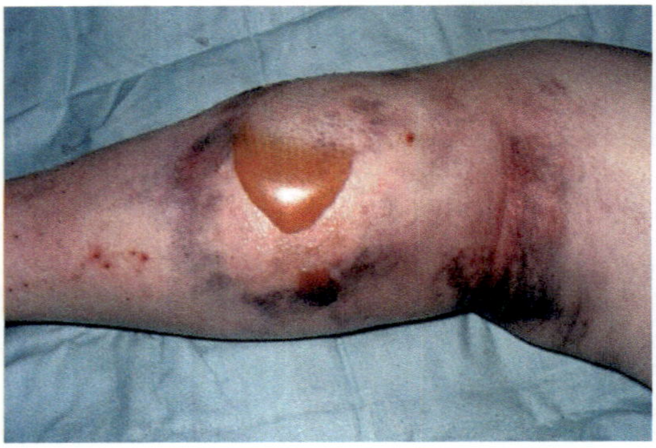

Fig. 5.1 Skin blistering from poor nourishment due to tension from a deep-seated haematoma, 10 days after injury

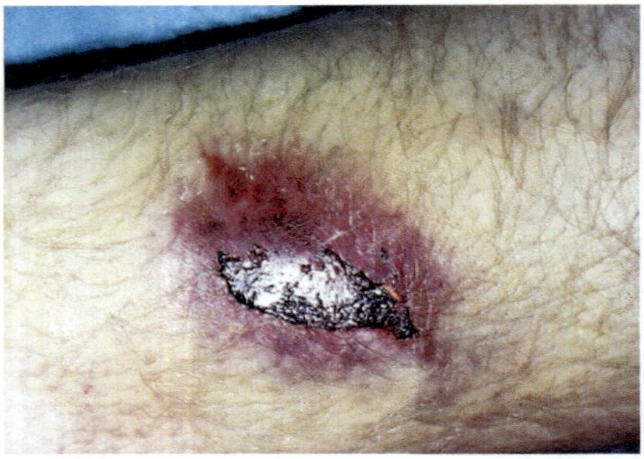

Fig. 5.2 Necrosis of skin over an unrelieved haematoma in the lower leg, 2 weeks after injury

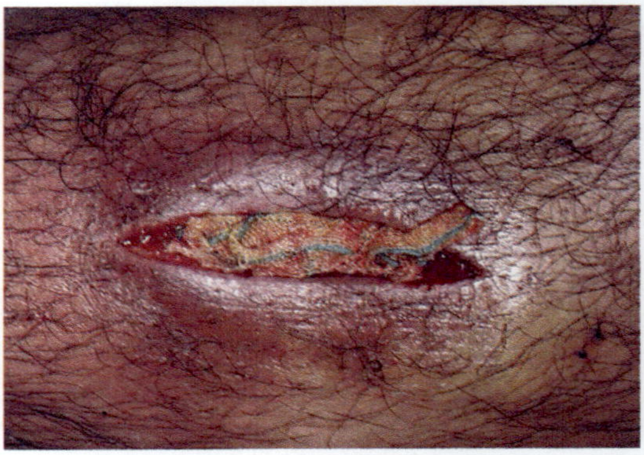

Fig. 5.3 Packing in wound after evacuation of a haematoma 3 days previously. Such packing merely maintains the open cavity

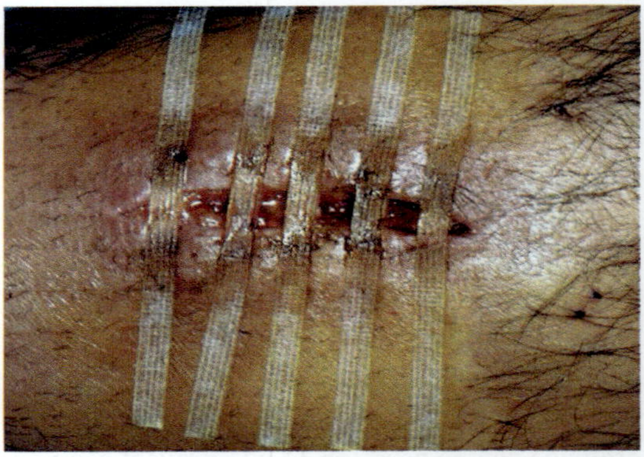

Fig. 5.4 After removal of packing, wound closure is being encouraged with tapes. This image is 3 days after image Fig. 5.3

the haematoma, deeper drainage should **not** be carried out with scalpel or scissors, but made using closed instruments and with a spreading or stretching of the tissues until the collection is encountered. This technique will never damage either vessels or nerves. The haematoma can then be evacuated with jiggling pressure or with a curette. It sometimes helps to eventually clean out the cavity using gauze swabs over a finger, although this needs to be done gently. Where it seems possible that the skin could snap closed immediately, a strip of Penrose rubber drain or ribbon gauze may be left through the wound for a day or so. Drainage of deep haematoma may need additional or general anaesthesia. The main thing is to relieve pressure and encourage displaced tissues to return to their original situation as soon as possible. Continuing drainage should be assisted by gravity and posturing. Both haematomas and abscesses go on draining until they have got rid of whatever they need to, and then they heal.

Packing haematoma cavities after drainage is unhelpful because it maintains tissue displacement and often obstructs continuing drainage (Figs. 5.3 and 5.4).

Packing can be distressing to remove and the disturbance often starts bleeding off again. Most professionals seem to find repacking irresistible. Packing ceremonies can sometimes continue diligently for months, causing irritation, pressure, and continually frustrating the healing (Fig. 5.5).

Packing is one of those regimes which tend to become perpetuated. Someone has to actually decide that it is counterproductive and stop doing it.

Haematomas which get neither infected nor drained may resolve by becoming organised slowly into scar tissue. Not to drain a closed haematoma that is threatening to devitalise skin can however be very regrettable (Figs. 5.6 and 5.7).

Dead skin separates slowly and the associated haematoma often gets infected. The walls and base of the cavity are usually also debilitated, and it can take weeks or months for the cavity to fill in to support surface healing (Fig. 5.8). It is clearly better to intervene surgically early rather than too late.

The effect of post-operative haematomas within closed wounds is comparable with their behaviour beneath intact skin. They are a potent source of undue tension and pain, which should be diagnosed and evacuated. Haematomas related to open wounds generate less tension. They are also best removed, especially where they are disrupting or displacing tissue (Figs. 5.9 and 5.10).

They also provide a wonderful culture medium for infection. Haematomas beneath flaps do not necessarily interfere with flap circulation until they are large. On the other hand, every tiny collection of blood accumulating between a graft and its bed will cause graft failure at that site, unless evacuated within a few days (Figs. 5.11 and 5.12).

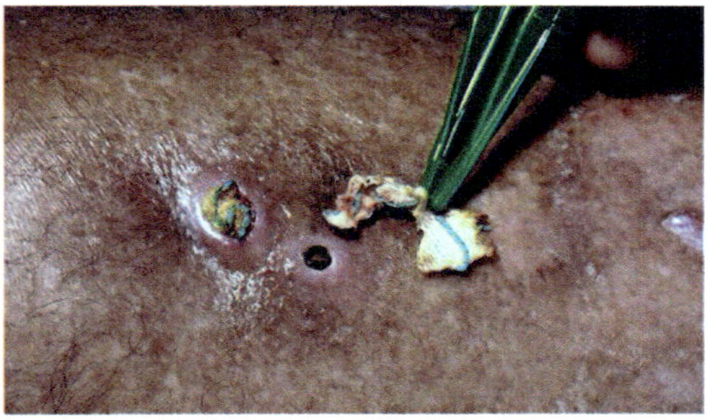

Fig. 5.5 Removal of ribbon gauze from several cavities produced initially by streptococcal abscess. This packing had continued for months. These sinuses healed within days of stopping the packing

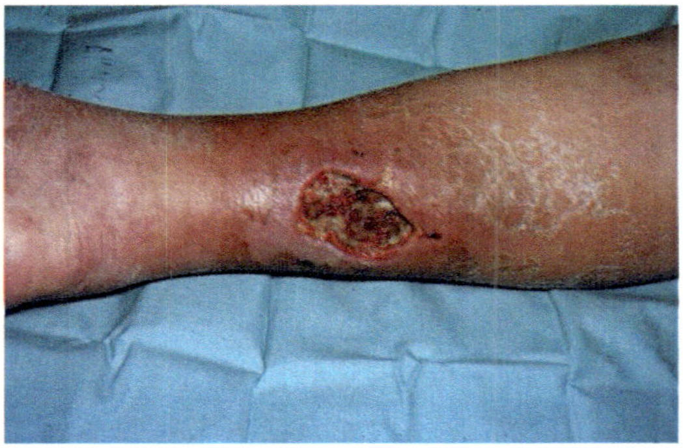

Fig. 5.7 Unhealthy deep leg ulcer 6 weeks after the treating doctor made a decision not to decompress a tense haematoma because the patient was 94 years old

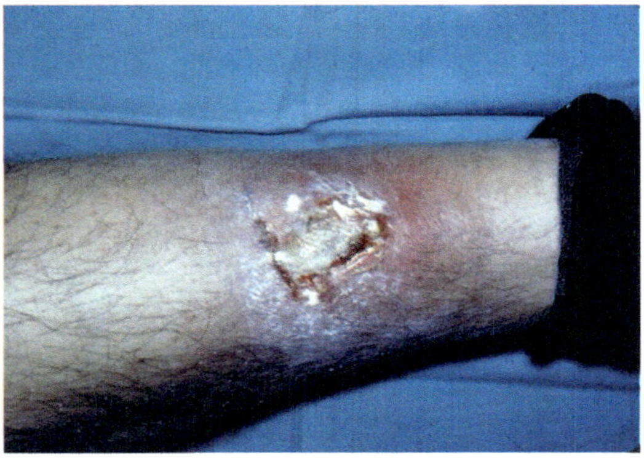

Fig. 5.6 Loss of tissue down to bone, following an unrelieved haematoma. Infection is well established 3 weeks later

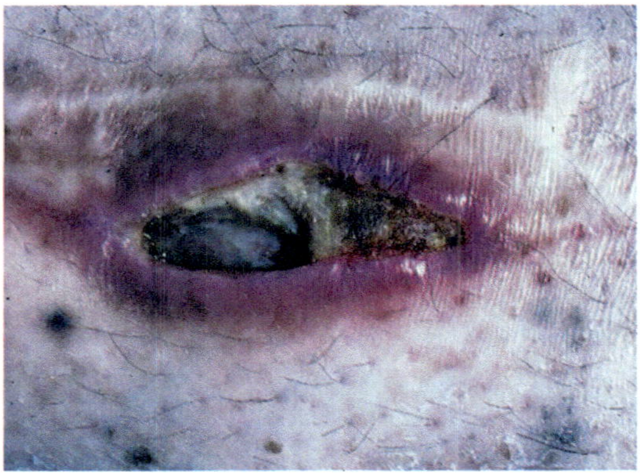

Fig. 5.8 The end result of a deep haematoma after surgery though scarred tissue. The cavity wall was particularly unhealthy and healing took many months

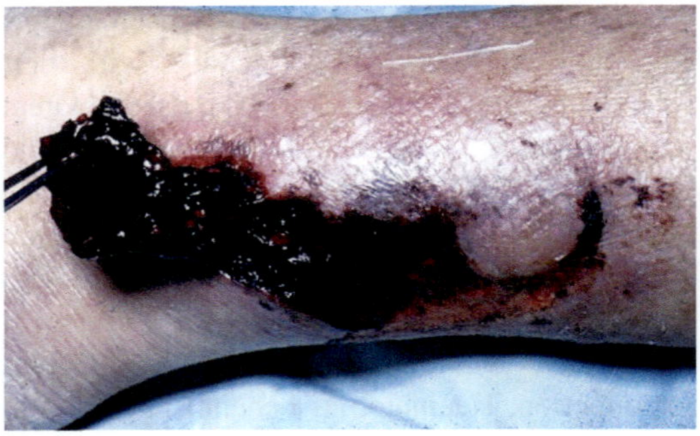

Fig. 5.9 Extensive clot beneath a laterally based leg flap at 5 days. Most of the flap is fortunately surviving

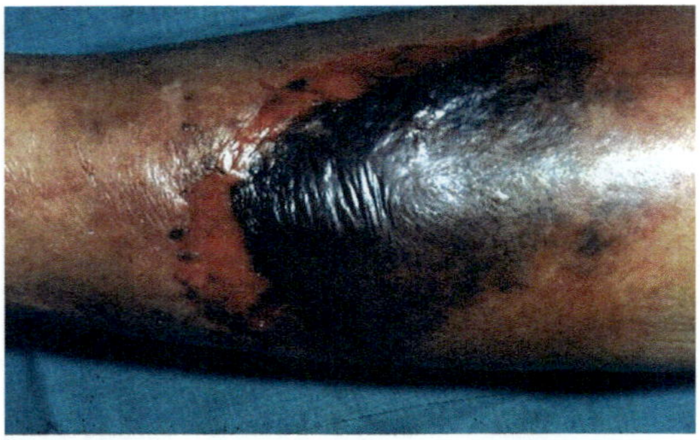

Fig. 5.10 Haematoma adding to a serious venous insufficiency in a leg flap. The result at 5 days is disastrous, This patient was 'mobilised' without a firm bandage applied to prevent bleeding and haematoma

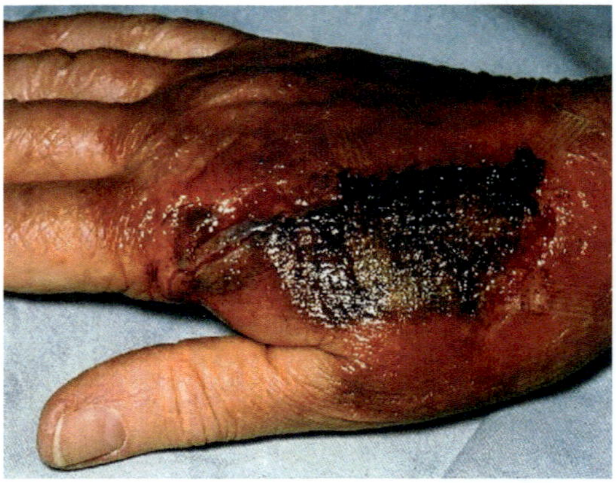

Fig. 5.11 Five-day appearance of replaced skin that has a confluent haematoma beneath it

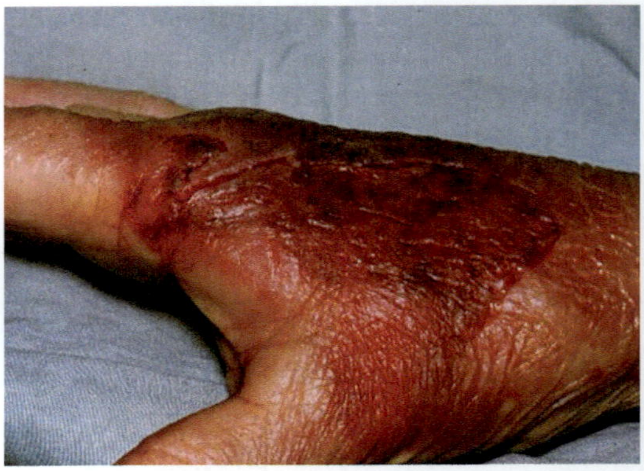

Fig. 5.12 The changed appearance on the same day as Fig. 5.11 after blood was removed. All fat was trimmed off, and the reapplied skin was then held with tapes. It all survived

Diffuse extravasated blood, although it usually absorbs eventually, is always associated with increased local oedema which adds its toll to tension. It is therefore worthwhile spending a little time retrieving this by sponging bruised tissues with damp saline swabs before closing open wounds.

Prevention of Haematoma

Painstaking attention to achieving absolute haemostasis before dressing the wound is by far the best insurance against haematoma. The use of a tourniquet is a technique that makes it extremely difficult if not impossible to achieve haemostasis without using either firm pressure after its removal or a suction drain. Suction drains for 24–48 h can be of assistance in preventing haematoma after tourniquet use, beneath degloved skin or in oozy situations and are much safer than pressure dressings. Haemostatic dressings, while they can usually prevent bleeding and haematoma, inevitably get tighter during the phase of reactive swelling and progressively reduce the circulation. This adversely affects outcomes for both flaps and grafts. In the leg, these effects are much more noticeable, as circulation is often marginal to begin with. Immaculate haemostasis, the making of fenestrations [cuts] and accurate modest pressure [with tie-over dressings], should prevent haematoma beneath grafts.

One of the editors [MFK] has recently adopted the Auersvald haemostatic net sutures for flaps, skin grafts, and undermined wounds with a reduction in the incidence of post-surgery haematomas. This technique was taught to him in 2019 for cervicofacial lift techniques by Dr Daniel Labbé of Caen, France [2].

If collections do occur beneath grafts, they should be evacuated at the earliest opportunity by a tiny incision or snip and blotting with a damp saline swab. The Double Bandage recovery regime delivers the best of both worlds thereafter in lower limb situations, i.e. unimpeded circulation except for the short intervals of dependency when firm bandaging is used to prevent bleeding and haematoma [See Appendix].

Pain

The perception of pain is subjective. People have individual thresholds that can vary with anxiety levels and fatigue. There are distinct types of pain associated with injury.

Pain Caused by Trauma to Nerves and Nerve Endings

This starts immediately after injury as an intense searing, sharp, cutting, stinging, aching, and sometimes fluctuating pain, aggravated by moving or disturbing the injured part. It is at its peak during the first few hours after injury and is greatly relieved by analgesics, which should initially be given intravenously as early as possible and according to need. This pain becomes steadily less intrusive and more intermittent over the next few days, when it can usually be adequately managed with oral analgesia.

Tension/Pressure Pain

While this may not be particularly prominent at the beginning unless there is a tense haematoma or tight bandages, it increases as reactive swelling increases tension within the tissues. It is continuous and pulsatile because circulation is somewhat obstructed. When severe, it is often complained as 'this-is-killing-me' kind of pain. It is comparatively difficult to relieve adequately with drugs but can be markedly reduced if tight dressings, relentless splints and/or any tight sutures are removed. If severe throbbing pain is not relieved by these simple measures, surgical exploration, drainage of haematoma, decompression, or even fasciotomy may at times be needed. This type of pain always indicates impaired perfusion and any pressure or tension above venous pressure can produce or worsen it (Fig. 5.13).

The arterial circulation is endeavouring to push blood through tissues against venous obstruction, and the nerve endings are quite correctly interpreting this as a life-threatening impasse. Once tissue actually dies, pain subsides unless invasive sepsis supervenes. With primary arterial insufficiency, anaesthesia follows rapidly, and throbbing tension pain in thin dislodged skin or white flaps is not a feature. See Pain Disability Chart/Appendix.

Infective or Inflammatory Pain

Invasive sepsis can also cause throbbing pain. Typically, infective pain takes over and increases as injury pain would ordinarily be subsiding or complicates the wound at some later stage. Infection usually arises on the basis of inadequate cleaning, haematoma, or dead tissue, and bacterial invasion is associated with prolonged inflam-

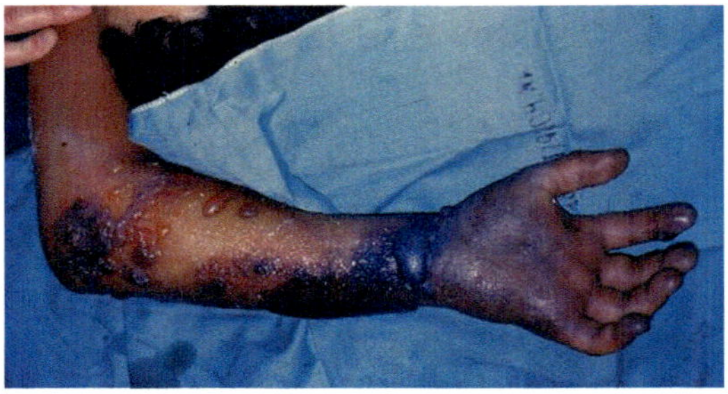

Fig. 5.13 Gangrene of hand and forearm 10 days after a tight turn of crepe bandage at the elbow was used to apply an initial plaster slab to a fractured forearm. The venous return was obstructed at the elbow and the loss of vitality necessitated a below-elbow amputation. This is venous gangrene

mation. Inflammatory pain is partly a tension pain associated with swelling, but also has neurovascular and toxic aspects to it. It is also impossible to numb inflamed tissue with local anaesthetic or topical spray. Analgesics seem to make more of an impression in inflammatory pain than they do on the relentless pain of reactive swelling, perhaps because it is usually somewhat less excruciating.

Editors' Note *There are recognised benefits from the use of a 'pre-emptive' technique for commencing analgesia administration. Also, it should be strongly emphasised to patients that their pain will be significantly better controlled if they follow a regimen of taking the nominated analgesic(s) 'by the clock', whether or not they are in pain at the time, at least for the first few days.*

Infection and Antibiotics

Normal skin and its appendages harbour a multiplicity of benign microscopic organisms described by laboratories as 'skin flora'. A normal person needs repeated contact with a range of environmental organisms in order to maintain a high level of personal immunity against infection. To use antibacterial soaps on the skin or disinfectants regularly around the household is therefore probably ill-advised. It is not possible to sterilise skin without also damaging it, which means that ordinary washing procedures are adequate. Thorough soap and water hand-washing, especially preparing and eating food and after toileting plus a sensible approach to dealing with contaminated material, is usually all that is required. The recent climate of obsessive cleanliness with the exaggerated fear of infection is a commercial invention. In the home, ventilation, drying, ordinary washing, and sunshine remain the best forms of sterilisation. Diluted household oxidising bleaches are useful and effective bactericidal agents for disinfecting soiled clothing, bedding, and surfaces. In a clinical context, routine and regular hand-washing before and after procedures, the use of sterile disposable gloves, and strict sequential sterile techniques should remove the risk of introducing infection or cross-infection to wounds.

Intact skin provides a barrier to bacteria. When skin is broken, there is an opportunity for bacteria to thrive in a warm, moist environment nourished by body fluids. 'Skin flora' are always present but do not normally interfere with healing or become invasive. Other organisms that prevent healing or proliferate to produce clinical signs and symptoms of infection are called **pathogenic.** These may be present consistently or intermittently on skin but are not necessarily a problem, until the skin is breached. Gram positive streptococci and/or staphylococci cause most skin and wound infections. Both can prevent healing and can also become invasive and dangerous. In diabetes and other conditions where circulation is reduced or the immune system is ailing, there is a greatly increased risk of infection. Such patients need to be taught how to look after their feet and nails and how to avoid broken skin so that they do not allow the initial entry of pathogenic bacteria.

Infection rarely becomes established in a healthy wound, so prevention needs to focus on the meticulous cleansing of wounds, maximising the circulation and preventing haematoma. The use of antibacterial preparations within wounds is inappropriate. All antibacterial solutions damage living tissue, which makes it more vulnerable to infection. If the solutions are diluted so as not to harm cells, they then fail to kill bacteria. Those that are spirit-based or bactericidal, like hydrogen peroxide, actually denature living protein making it more likely that pathogens will colonise the dead tissue.

In the pre-antibiotic era, even minor infections had the potential to kill people. Treatment was understandably preoccupied with preventing infection because there was no treatment. It is not surprising that cleansing, haemostasis, and maximising the circulation all featured prominently at that stage. Since the advent of antibiotics, we have become very much less vigilant. We have come to regard infection as more of a treatable nuisance than a disaster. This era of complacency is passing. As well as an increasing incidence of infections, which have become resistant to the common antibiotics, we are also quite rapidly running out of effective treatment alternatives. Sooner rather than later, it seems essential that all the earlier preventive measures and more appropriate clinical techniques will be revived.

Prophylactic Antibiotics

The most troublesome and aggressive pathogenic skin organisms of all are Gram positive haemolytic streptococci. These are found on the skin and in people's throats, particularly where skin hygiene and health are poor and people are living in overcrowded conditions. They can invade through any breach in the skin. Streptococci are the main cause of many troublesome infections, such as impetigo [school-sores] and cellulitis, and can colonise other skin conditions, e.g. eczema, bites, or scabies. It is a wise precaution to give prophylactic antibiotics to an injured individual when there are any indications that there are any of these skin infections already in the household. Antibiotics are always indicated whenever skin is reapplied as a graft, as haemolytic organisms prevent the early fibrinous attachment that precedes capillary revascularisation. If indicated, antibiotics should be started as early as possible, not given as an afterthought. If wounds are clean and well-nourished there is otherwise so little chance of infection that prophylactic antibiotics are not needed routinely.

The use of broad-spectrum prophylactic antibiotics is justifiable where the development of any infection would be disastrous, e.g. where joint spaces, tendon sheaths, and open bone injuries are involved. Immobilisation is also important in preventing infection in all these situations. When wound contamination has been heavy and/or tissue vitality is depressed, antibiotics also become more and more relevant. Specific antibiotic regimes may be needed to counter anaerobic organisms and/or Gram negative pathogens.

When the wound is simple, prophylactic antibiotics can be stopped after 3–5 days if everything is improving. The course can be extended for more complicated wounds or if a wound is not settling. When the initial wound has been deep and dirty, with severely damaged tissue, it is wise to have a longer period of antibiotic cover, checking with the wound swabs as necessary. Most patients with these more severe injuries will be admitted to hospitals, where prophylactic antibiotics will initially be given intravenously.

Tetanus Prophylaxis

The ideal is to have a population that is fully immunised with a 3-dose course of Tetanus Toxoid. Most patients with the majority of wounds then need only a booster injection. When the wound is minor and the immunisation status is not known, a first dose of Tetanus Toxoid can be given with a written instruction to their GP to complete the course. A dirty puncture wound should be treated by giving Tetanus Toxoid promptly, with the wound explored under local anaesthesia and dirty tissue cleansed or excised. A clean deep puncture wound, which may not need exploring, nevertheless sometimes warrants a course of antibiotics as well as Toxoid. When the immunisation status is uncertain and the wound is considered unfavourable, a thorough wound toilet and debridement is urgent, with prompt Tetanus Toxoid administered and intravenous antibiotics providing additional security. Tetanus immunoglobulin is sometimes given in addition, to patients at particular risk, after ascertaining that there is not an allergic history. Such patients need to be closely supervised in hospital for several days.
(see Commentary on modern tetanus prophylaxis at chapter end)

Treatment of Invasive Infection

If infection is becoming invasive, patients are usually aware of increasing throbbing pain 12–24 h ahead of visible inflammation. They therefore always need to be able to report back if their wound pain or general state is causing concern. The modern organisation of medical services by efficient managers can make this kind of arrangement increasingly difficult. Wound infection requires several different approaches. It is really important to remove sutures as this immediately relieves any circulatory impairment they may be causing, allows better drainage, and removes their foreign-body effect. It is also important to evacuate haematomas and excise/debride dead tissue. In pre-antibiotic times, excision of slough, drainage, and immobilisation was all that could be done to combat infection, and these are still very useful measures. Depending on the severity and spread of the infection, antibiotics may need to be given immediately or possibly deferred until a swab result is available. It is a useful concept to consider the battle between infection and the human body as on a see-saw which can be tipped at any stage favourably or unfavourably, for or against the body by several different factors. Once improvement commences, it is however nearly always maintained, and in simple wounds, once pain has gone, the antibiotics can usually be stopped.

Haemolytic streptococci are always lurking and are one of the most important causes of wound infection. Proliferation and invasion occurs rapidly, adding to early wound pain and swelling. Instead of wounds starting to settle down around day 3, they feel and look worse and worse with lymphangitis and lymphadenitis developing rapidly (Figs. 5.14 and 5.15).

At their worst, streptococci are capable of causing rapidly spreading cellulitis, destructive 'flesh-eating' complications, necrotising fasciitis, toxaemia, septicaemia, and sometimes death (Fig. 5.16).

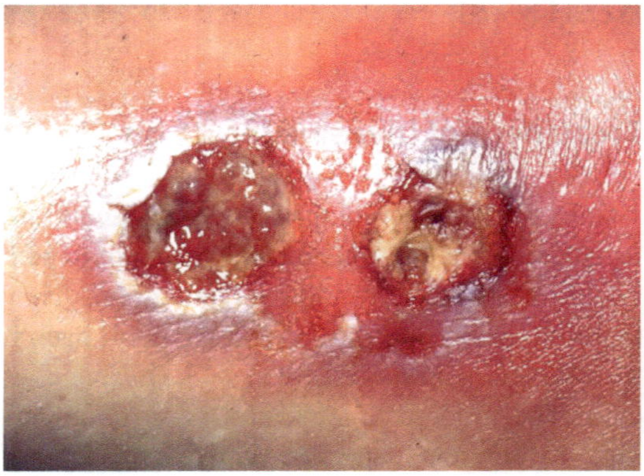

Fig. 5.14 Typical streptococcal 'school-sores' with some cellulitis. Systemic antibiotics are needed and will be immediately effective

Blood should be immediately taken for blood culture, and antibiotic treatment should be commenced forthwith. Penicillin is particularly effective against streptococci, but in the absence of a swab result and presence of spreading infection, this often needs to be backed up with broader spectrum antibiotics. The only organisms capable of producing swifter general toxicity are anaerobes of the gas-gangrene family. Tetanus may take a little longer to develop but it is also potentially lethal. Early appropriate antibiotic treatment can be life-saving and should be given

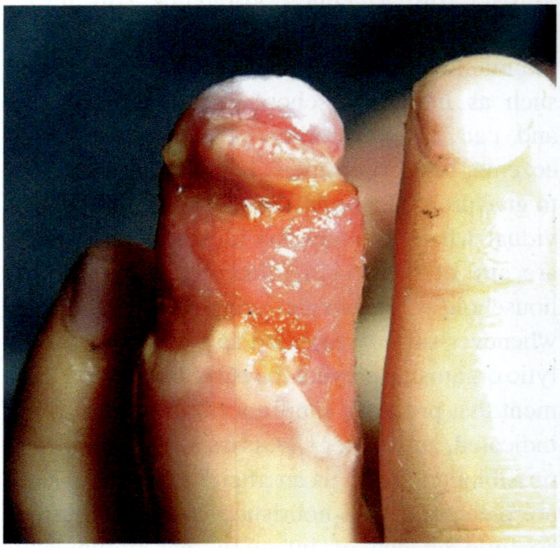

Fig. 5.15 Destructive streptococcal cellulitis, complicating a crush injury in a child's finger. The finger healed uneventfully following antibiotic use

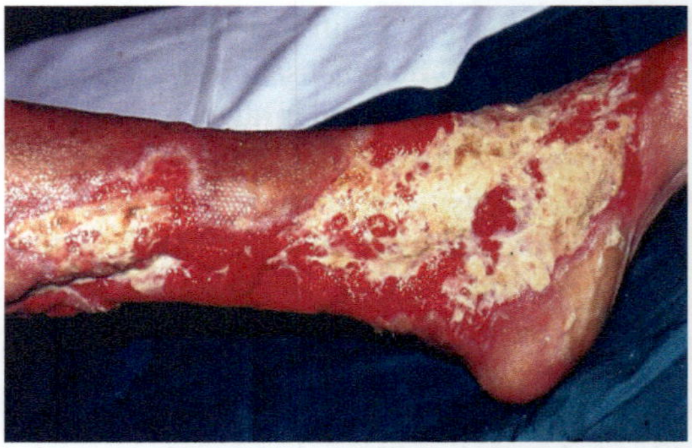

Fig. 5.16 Extensive and deeper streptococcal destruction of skin and subcutaneous tissue, 6 weeks after severe cellulitis. Adherent dead tissue is still present. Grafting will be needed

intravenously when there are any symptoms or signs of these very serious infections.

Haemolytic staphylococci can also cause invasive wound infection and septicaemia but not quite so rapidly as streptococci, and they do not usually cause lymphangitis. These days, staphylococci may be resistant to many common antibiotics and the taking of swabs at the earliest opportunity assists in management. Blood culture is indicated in any patient who is generally unwell or feverish and broad spectrum antibiotics should be started. It is estimated that around 90% of staphylococci found in hospitals are now resistant to ordinary Penicillin.

Treatment for invasive infection arising in chronic ulcers should ordinarily be able to be based accurately on swab results.

Signs and Symptoms of Resolving Infection

The important signs and symptoms that the body is gaining ascendancy over invading organisms, with or without antibiotics, is bringing an infection under control are:

1. A reduction in pain. This occurs up to 24 h ahead of any visible change. The first question for every returning patient is to ask how their wound feels compared with yesterday or 2–3 days ago. It is most unwise to be telling patients something at variance with how their wound feels and if there is a clinical uncertainty as to which direction infection is heading, close supervision is important.
2. The body temperature starts to return to normal if it has been elevated, and general toxicity starts to recede.
3. Local swelling reduces progressively. Shiny, tight skin starts to develop wrinkles.
4. The inflammatory redness starts to become duskier instead of watery pink and the circulatory return when the skin is briefly pressed on becomes more sluggish.
5. It becomes easier to define an edge to the inflammation, rather than it fading off imperceptibly. It is as if the body has drawn up its line of defence and said 'no further'. The increasing definition of this edge, followed by its retreat, confirms a resolving infection, so it is often useful to delineate it with a skin marking pen. Patients are often able and willing to record this aspect of progress themselves.
6. Although many wound infections resolve ultimately by seepage from the wound, the resolution of infection occasionally produces a collection of pus which may need more formal drainage.

Drainage of Collections and Abscesses

In many localised infections like boils and carbuncles, there is eventually some necrotic skin produced centrally. Incision through or excision of this, taking care not to pull, push, or touch inflamed tissue, can sometimes achieve drainage without anaesthesia at all. Infected blisters can usually be drained in this way by careful excision of all the surface skin (Figs. 5.17 and 5.18).

Streptococcal cellulitis may resolve by creating a number of separate collections which may need multiple incisions. At this stage, there may no longer be any obviously inflamed tissue. Local anaesthetic can be injected along the incision line, which ideally should be along the skin creases. Use local anaesthetic with Adrenaline, inject very slowly and work from proximal to distal, so that benefit is gained from the preceding injection. Then always wait at least 5 min before starting. Deeper abscesses must be clearly fluctuant before drainage is undertaken, and general anaesthesia may be required.

In rubbery skin, such as the back, or pulp of a toe, or finger, draining an abscess needs a slightly different technique to that described above, because this skin can close prematurely. A narrow ellipse of skin is excised over the abscess, in the case of the fingers, a 2 mm wide × 3–4 mm long ellipse along the fingerprint ridges, opening into any deeper collection with mosquito forceps. Such a wound will stay open for several days and

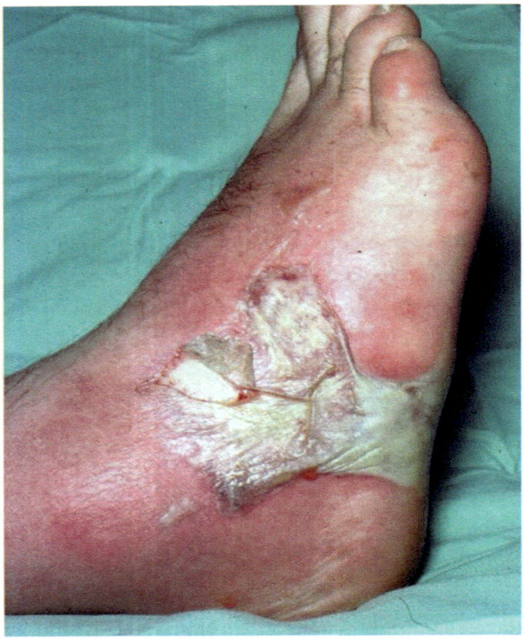

Fig. 5.17 Full-thickness burn 5 days after molten metal had run inside a boot. It is already infected

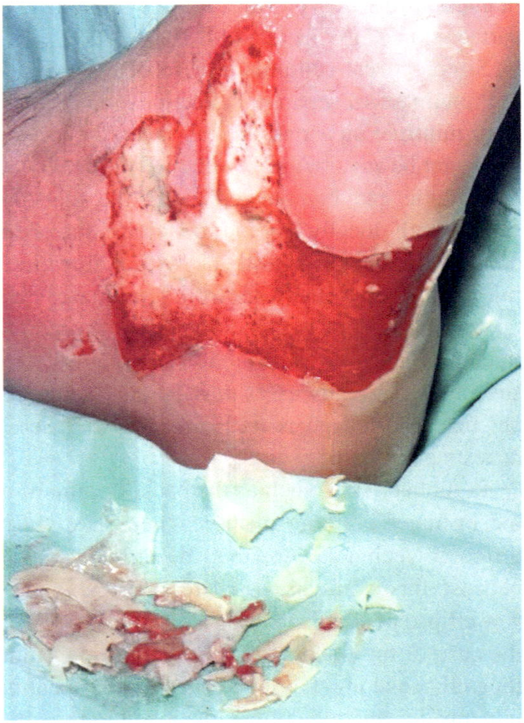

Fig. 5.18 Drainage of the blisters and excision of debris was done the same day and the infection settled promptly on antibiotics

then heal eventually. Packing is extremely painful, especially in the fingers and obstructs drainage—two good reasons not to use it.

Packing and Drainage

While packing is an age-old custom, irresistible to generations of doctors and nurses, its usefulness is very questionable. Packing consists of pushing a length of ribbon gauze into a space in the body that has been occupied by a collection of blood or pus. If one made an opening into healthy tissue and pushed ribbon gauze into it, this would very quickly create a chronically discharging if not infected wound. All packing has an active foreign-body effect, which makes it impossible for a wound to stop discharging or heal until it is discontinued (Figs. 5.19, 5.20, and 5.5).

Firm packing can be a continuing source of internal pressure in cavities where the circulation in the walls has already been marginalised by pressure. Packing supposedly works by capillarity, which isn't a particularly impressive concept of free drainage. Wounds often accumulate discharge behind ribbon gauze, with release of this as packing is removed. **[This always seemed to Dr Joan Chapple, contrary to the concept of free drainage.]** Wounds are drained by having a clear way out to the surface for fluid. They then discharge as long as they need to, assisted by

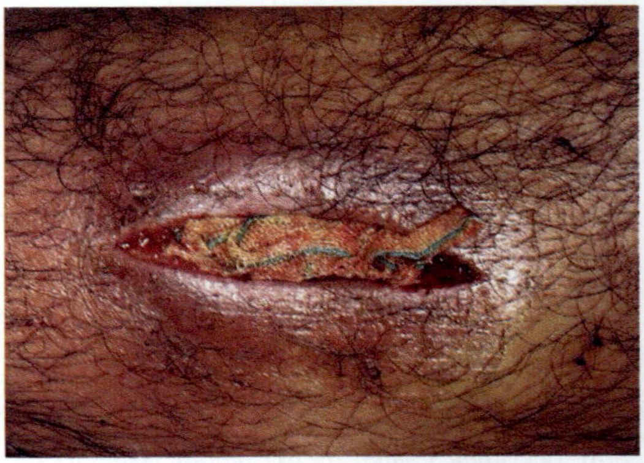

Fig. 5.19 Packing in a wound after evacuation of a haematoma 3 days previously. Such packing merely maintains the cavity

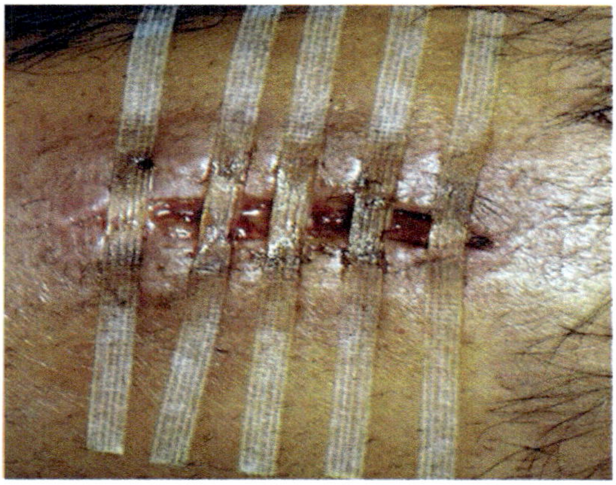

Fig. 5.20 After removal of packing, wound closure is encouraged with tapes. This image is 3 days after the image in Fig. 5.19

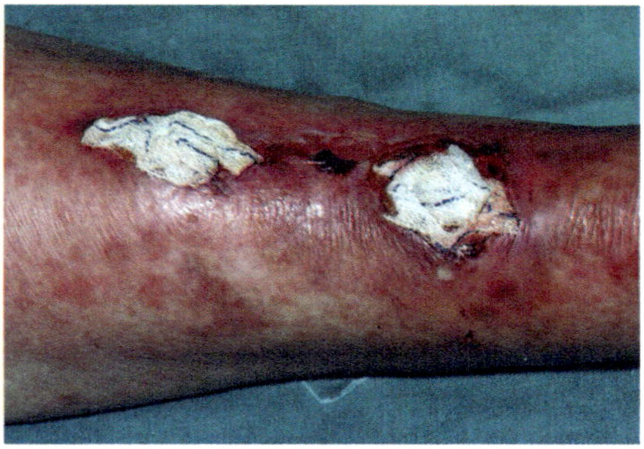

Fig. 5.21 Surface packing in place 3 days after a scraping injury to a shin. The leg was also bandaged firmly to prevent bleeding

gravity, and then they close. For deep collections, a thin rubber drain along the escape route for a few days may help in establishing an initial track to the surface. Thick rubber drains are unnecessary and uncomfortable. All drains increase the likelihood of wound infection.

There is another well-established packing ritual designed to fill hollows and ulcers with 'back and forth' layers of ribbon gauze (Figs. 5.21 and 5.22).

The circulation to such surfaces may already be diminished, especially on the lower leg and packing of this sort, followed by bandaging, has great potential to focus pressure to the raw surface and further reduce its circulation. An ulcer

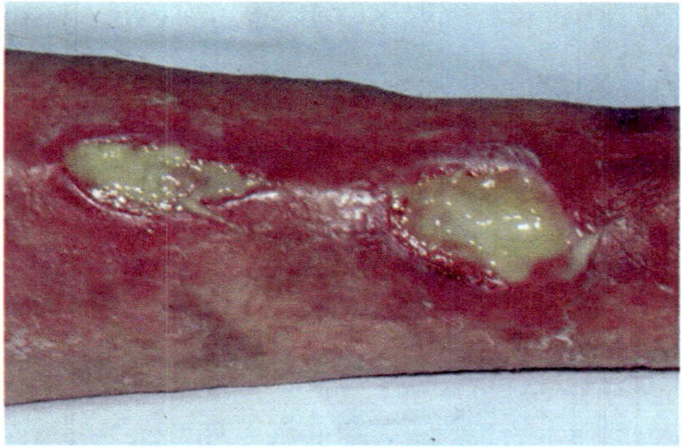

Fig. 5.22 The destructive effects of pressure on the base of these areas is evident 3 weeks later. These areas took 3 months to heal

surface is more likely to be better nourished by remaining below the general level of the surface, with any hollow filled with exudate or cream to keep it moist.

The PACKING CONCEPT seems to be part of the *'doing something is obviously better than doing nothing'* mentality that surrounds such medical treatment. There is also an irresistible tendency for most professionals to repack any wound they have just taken packing from. There even seems to be a measure of additional triumph in getting more packing back in than was put in by someone else! Packing is indeed a strangely archaic and inappropriate ritual which is hard to justify. If presented with a wound with packing already in it, the aim should always be to remove it as soon as possible, posturing the wound to drain instead by gravity.

Unhealthy Raw Surfaces and Chronic Ulcers

Surface wounds with adherent dead tissue are unhealthy and are endeavouring to get rid of this. There is no way healing can begin across dead tissue. Slough rejection is an active fibrinolytic process requiring circulation. The adjacent tissue is usually debilitated, so this process will be slow or sometimes stalled. Pathogenic bacteria are often associated with dead tissue, and if discharge is not obvious, a swab can be moistened in sterile saline before taking it. It is very important to use occlusive dressings on all chronic wounds to keep them moist.

Although antibiotics may control the signs and symptoms of infection in such a wound, healing cannot proceed until dead tissue separates and granulations are produced. Unusual opportunistic infections can become established in debilitated wounds and in patients with immune deficiency diseases. Unusual measures may be needed. Yeasts and Pseudomonas can be treated with specific antibiotics. The use of ultraviolet light from the sun may be a very effective bactericidal measure, but it is very important that this not be allowed to dry the surface. An exposure of 15 min sunlight daily, with saline being dripped on throughout is an appropriate regime. A short 3–5 day course of half or quarter strength EUSOL [Edinburgh University Solution of Lime] with the active agent being Sodium Hypochlorite on gauze swabs, covered by tulle or *Gladwrap*™ to prevent drying, can be very effective in getting rid of troublesome and often mixed pathogens.

Editors' Note *In the early 1990s, a Nursing Journal paper spelled the death knoll for EUSOL [3]. Many of us still believe it was a great wound solution product from extensive clinical experience.*

Healing can however only commence after this is discontinued. People often assume that a pink raw surface is healthy when it is inflamed by chemicals or infected with streptococci and plainly not healing. Healing of course cannot progress until the toxicity or infection is addressed. The use of Manuka Honey with its particular antibacterial properties is worth trying. Many traditional and herbal remedies have acquired their reputations by means of a useful antibacterial effect. They may be tried if patients request this as long as the wound responds favourably.

Once any wound is free of dead tissue, it should produce granulation tissue and begin to epithelialise (Fig. 5.23).

Any granulating surface that is not re-epithelialising is therefore, by definition, still an unhealthy wound and in need of further investigation. If the body is able to reject slough and produce granulations, poor circulation is not usually the basis of the non-healing.

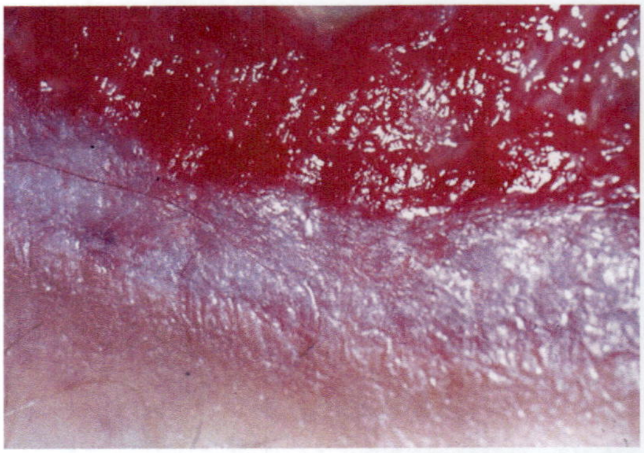

Fig. 5.23 Healthy raw surface showing a rapidly advancing epithelial edge

Non-healing of a Granulating Wound

There are six causes for non-healing of a granulating wound. Pathogenic infection is by far the most common, but once it is excluded, other possibilities must be methodically pursued.

1. Pathogenic infection (Fig. 5.24).
2. A toxic environment (Figs. 5.25 and 5.26).
3. Desiccation (Fig. 5.27).
4. Foreign-body reaction (Fig. 5.28).
5. Neoplasia (Fig. 5.29).
6. Interference with the wound/factitious wounding by the patient.

Pathogenic Infection

Streptococcal infection will produce very red and inflamed granulation tissue, which may exude clear fluid rather than pus (Fig. 5.30). The wound is usually quite painful, especially if moved, and may sting intermittently rather than throb, unless infection is also causing cellulitis.

Unless someone thinks about streptococci and takes a swab, then actively treats the infection, such wounds can remain unhealed for months or years, simply because they look clean and are assumed to be healthy (Fig. 5.31).

If healing does not resume promptly using topical antibiotics, a course of systemic antibiotics may be needed. These are essential, of course, if any invasive sepsis is also present. The development of very active local and general immunity, especially in younger patients, can prevent the invasive manifestation of infection, which would have led immediately to the diagnosis. Pseudomonas infection can be particularly troublesome in this regard, and specific antibiotics are available. **Always take a swab from a granulating wound when healing is not progressing.**

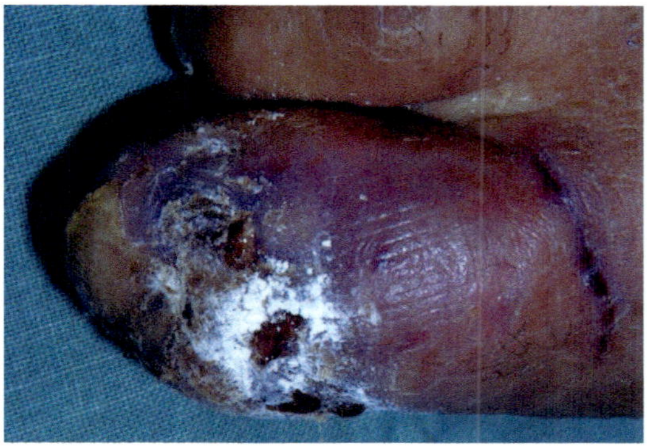

Fig. 5.27 This granulomatous wound after an ingrown toenail operation is being treated with antibiotic powder. This is a desiccating and inappropriate treatment

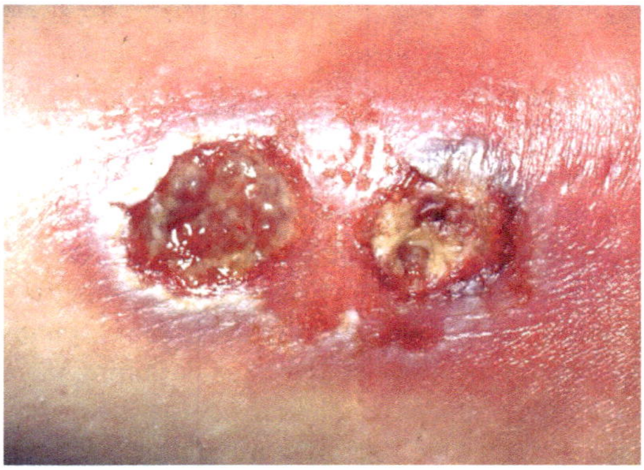

Fig. 5.24 Typical streptococcal 'school sores' with some cellulitis, although the body is controlling this somewhat. Systemic antibiotics are needed and will be immediately effective

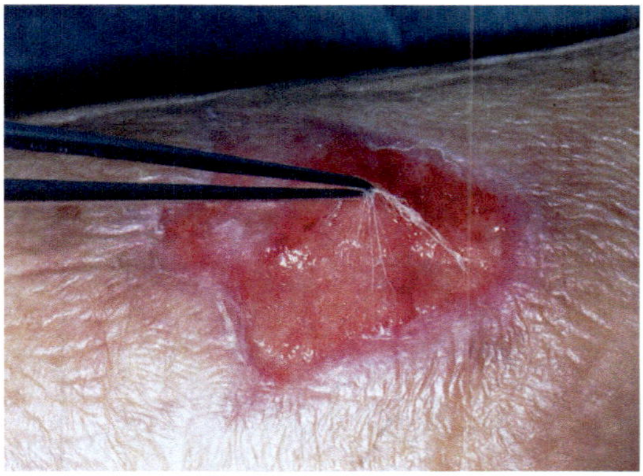

Fig. 5.28 This raw surface is not healing because of incorporated cotton wool fibres, which must be removed

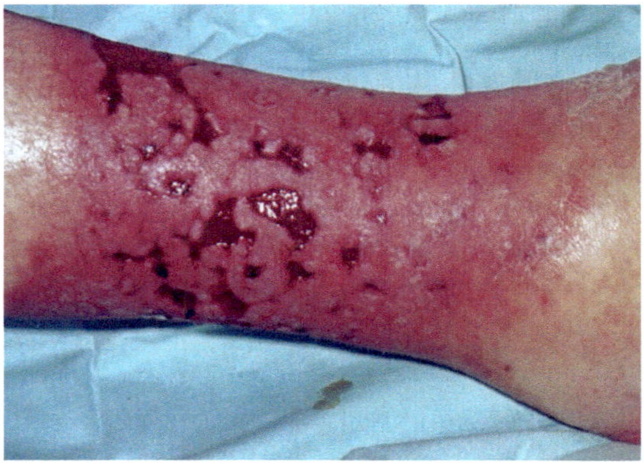

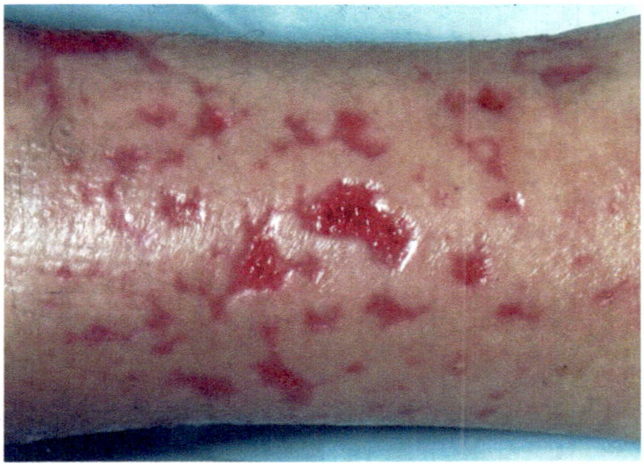

Figs. 5.25 and 5.26 Multiple painful ulcers have been unhealed for 3 months and are being packed 6 hourly with Elase™-soaked gauze. They were initially caused by streptococcal infection in varicose eczema. Changing to saline washing and tulle/gauze dressings reduced the pain and inflammation immediately and allowed rapid healing. Appearance 5 days later

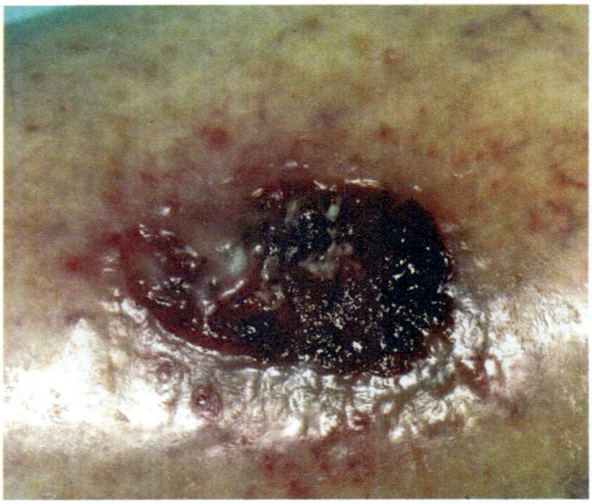

Fig. 5.29 Three year duration leg ulcer, which was diagnosed as a basal cell carcinoma by a small biopsy after excluding other causes of non-healing. It was treated successfully by excision and split skin graft repair

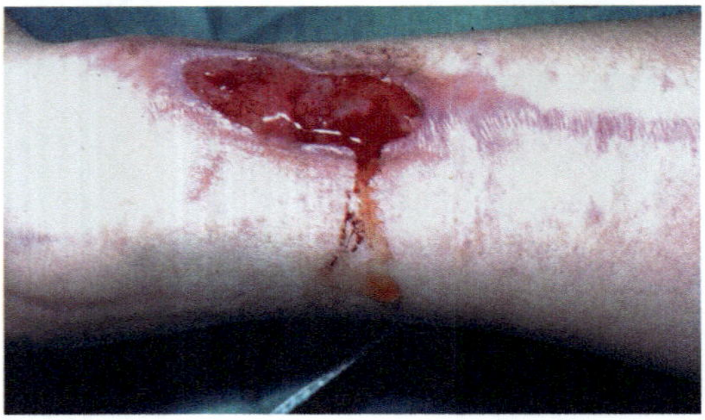

Fig. 5.30 Three month delay of healing caused by a streptococcal wound infection after surgery. Systemic antibiotics were rapidly effective

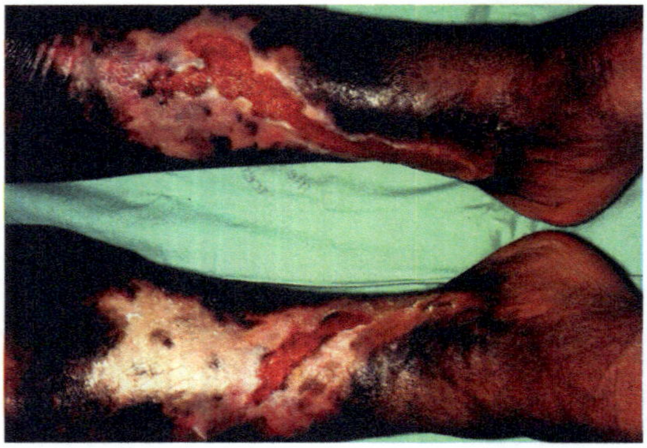

Fig. 5.31 Ten year duration streptococcal ulcers in skin damaged by football injuries. The problem was not recognised because although the ulcers were painful, there was no obvious cellulitis or malaise

Toxic Applications

In the course of treating or preventing infection, the patient or the professional may be regularly applying something that is toxic enough to completely discourage epithelialisation. Doctors are not immune from the 'if some is good, more is better, more often and stronger for longer' approach to antibacterial chemicals. Most antiseptics are capable of discouraging healing, and it is sometimes only a matter of stopping them to see if healing will resume. ELASE™ [an enzyme slough digester] is a particularly harmful chemical as it can further disadvantage the adjacent debilitated tissue (Figs. 5.25 and 5.26).

Desiccation

All open wounds tend to leak, with those which are poorly nourished and those which have got rid of dead tissue producing the least discharge. If dry dressings are used or if someone or other has decided that it is better to dry up seeping wounds by leaving them out of dressings or putting them in the sun or under lamps or oxygen, the new surface slough which forms will continually postpone the production of healthy granulation tissue. In the case of lower leg ulcers, regular drying can discourage healing continually and permanently. Dry surfaces cannot support the migration of, or sustain, epithelial cells. Allowing a healthy granulating surface to dry beneath a guard even for 20 min can prevent a skin graft from taking on it. This environment is different for a healing wound beneath a serosanguinous scab where the skin cells are able to migrate on a moist living layer. The protective scab flakes off as soon as the epithelial surface is reconstituted. Whenever living cells are exposed, they must be protected from drying by a moist occlusive dressing of some sort.

A Foreign-Body Reaction

Foreign material embedded in granulation or a raw surface will sometimes discourage healing.

This can be cotton-wool or lint fibres, occasionally threads of tulle-gras, or a non-absorbable suture. Particulate matter from the original injury is also implicated. Any deep dead tissue gives rise to a discharging sinus and causes non-healing behaviour. It may eventually be worthwhile taking an X-Ray or exploring wounds to exclude buried causes of non-healing. The body is quite sensible about not healing in all these situations because it needs to get rid of something before it does so.

Neoplastic Granulations

Just occasionally, after infection, toxic and foreign substances, interference and drying have all been excluded, a small incisional biopsy is indicated to exclude malignancy [low grade basal cell carcinoma or squamous dysplasia]. Incisional biopsy is, of course, quite inappropriate if a solid neoplasm is present.

Interference with the Wound

Very occasionally, factitious wounding by the patient may require a clever dressing designed to exclude this together with some frank discussion and encouragement towards facilitating healing.

Chronic Ulcers of the Lower Leg

In chronic ulcers, circulation is always one of the issues, and there is usually associated infection. It is important to try to elucidate the circulatory problems in case something specific can be done for them.

Symptoms and signs of localised arterial insufficiency may need further investigation, particularly if they are unusual, markedly unilateral, or in a young patient. Claudication with exercise is symptomatic of arterial insufficiency to muscles. This is often bilateral and associated with atrophy of skin and subcutaneous tissues. Such patients usually have skinny legs with tight dry skin and poor pulses. Nail and hair growth is reduced. The toes are often scaly and may show signs of clawing/atrophy. Pain is often prominent, and this may or may not be associated with infection. Patients may report needing to hang their legs over the side of the bed at night. They may be more comfortable in bed with their legs housed in a cardboard box taking the weight of the bedclothes. Pressure dressings are completely inappropriate for ulcer patients with any element of arterial deficiency.

Venous insufficiency has a common association with leg ulcers. There may be a family history of vein problems and ulcers, a past history of thrombosis during pregnancy, injury, or vein surgery. There may be evidence of raised venous pressure, obvious varicosities, local perforators from deep veins or chronic dermatitis, and venous pigmentation in areas of severely compromised skin. Standing or sitting with the legs passively down will worsen congestion and contribute to aching and tiredness. Pain is usually otherwise associated with infection. These patients often have bulky 'juicy' legs. When there is excessive leakage and the condition is bilateral, it is worth considering whether or not there is any congestive heart failure, renal disease, or lymphoedema which needs treatment. If the congestion is largely venous and the patient leads an active ambulant life, the use of an appropriate elastic pressure bandage or Class II compression stocking may facilitate healing, relieving the venous congestion by muscular activity. It is however important to counteract excessive focal pressure on the ulcer surface and also combine this regime with intermittent rest intervals where the legs are elevated rather than pressed on to assist venous drainage.

Elastic pressure is particularly helpful in ulcers related to incompetent venous perforators. Some of these patients also benefit greatly from surgery to tie off specific perforators. Perforators can be diagnosed by palpating for the opening in the deep fascia with the patient on a couch, holding a finger on this while they stand, then removing the pressure and watching the rapid filling of veins in the vicinity.

Editors' Note *This is not a definitive test, and these days, a duplex ultrasound scan would be more diagnostic.*

In many older patients, when ulceration is recurrent or long-standing, there is very likely to be both arterial and venous insufficiency related to the non-healing. Their veins may not be especially prominent, and they may have had one or more operations for them. There may also be chronic scarring, from previous injury, operations, ulceration, or infection. They often have pain associated with their ulcers, even when no pathogenic infection can be found and usually find pressure dressings extremely painful. These patients do not benefit by incorporating pressure into their regime and may benefit distinctly from stopping it.

Chronic ulcers may be slow or stationary but it is usually possible to devise a dressing regime combined with pain management and intermittent antibiotics, which will enable most patients to manage surprisingly well. Once infection is controlled, one of the most helpful pieces of advice is to remind patients to remain physically active. Arterial input is assisted with the legs dependent, but the venous drainage will be assisted by elevation. Patients should therefore alternate intervals of walking around with periods of leg elevation for 10 min or so to help drain away venous blood. Patients can in fact lead a surprisingly active life like this, providing a kind of additional 'circulation' for their tissues by using the assistance of gravity. They should arrange to sit and sleep with their legs neither elevated nor dependent unless they are more comfortable in one particular position.

Overgrown Granulations/Granuloma/Proud Flesh

Granulations only over-proliferate if there is a problem with the second stage of healing, namely epithelialisation. All of the causes for non-healing need to be carefully considered. The most usual problem is pathogenic bacteria, and topical antibiotics may be all that is needed. Granulomas form sometimes in the presence of a foreign body, where the message going out is not to heal because the body still needs to get rid of something (Figs. 5.32 and 5.33).

Sometimes ingrown toenails or pieces of disrupted nail can act as a foreign body and need excision under local anaesthetic. Fibres of cotton wool or road dirt can usually be picked out. Sometimes it is necessary to remove the prominent granulations and start again. Granulation tissue is very vascular but insensitive, and it can usually be snipped or sliced away without anaesthesia. It is however important to elevate the wound after doing this, applying pressure to the area, preferably with adrenaline local on a swab for 5 min or so. After this, bleeding is rarely a problem. A simple dressing routine is then recommended until the wound heals. Prominent granulations flatten out miraculously once epithelialisation occurs.

Most traditional treatments for overgrown granulations are historic, barbaric, and quite inappropriate. They consist of some form of cautery, and all of them create dead tissue (Fig. 5.34). Copper sulphate, Podophyllin resin, Silver nitrate, Liquid nitrogen, carbon dioxide snow, or

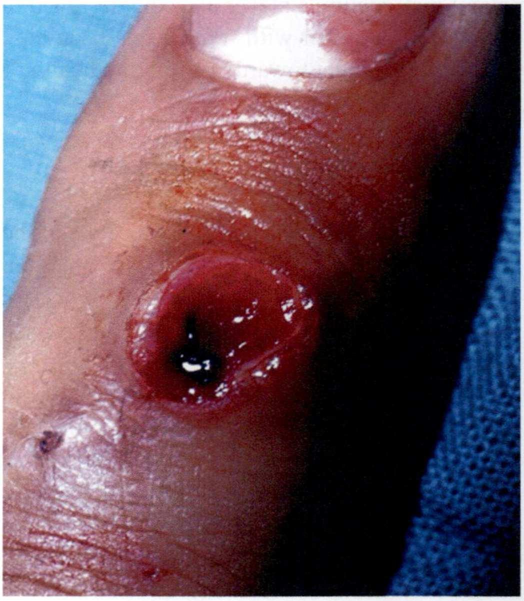

Fig. 5.32 This discharging wound 6 weeks after tendon repair is clearly related to a non-absorbable tendon suture

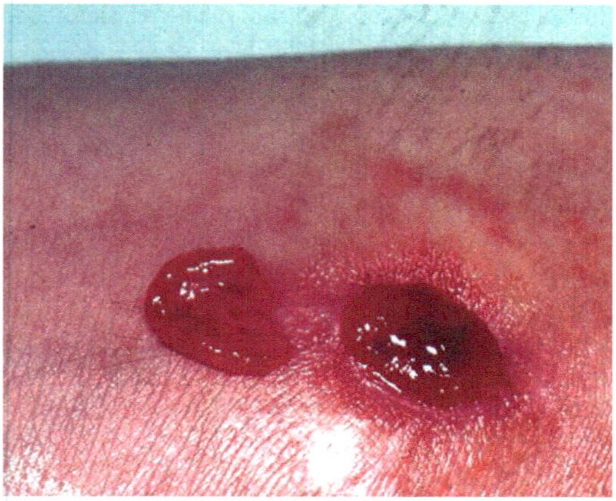

Fig. 5.33 Granulomatous discharging forearm wounds related to non-absorbable deep sutures after a laceration. Healing cannot now occur until these sutures are removed

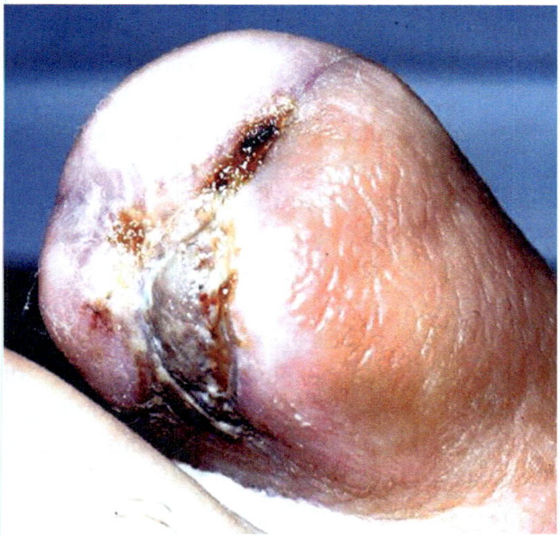

Fig. 5.34 The unhealthy granulations after toenail surgery further discouraged from healing by application of silver nitrate. All cauterisation actually discourages healing by creating new slough

heat cautery are all still used. The new slough they produce then has to separate from adjacent tissue, which is nearly but not quite dead—a process that is bound to be slow, after which the wound has to try again to produce granulations and epithelialise. Most wounds treated in this way heal eventually not because of their treatment but because living tissues remain resourceful. Such treatments may of course have killed off the pathogenic bacteria that might have been the original basis for the delayed healing, but there are much more appropriate ways to treat infection.

Commentary by Mark Thomas FRACP MD

Following injury, it is essential that all wounds be adequately cleaned and devitalised tissue removed to reduce the level of contamination and tetanus toxin release. Further treatment depends on the circumstances of each case.

If the injury is considered to be tetanus-prone and there is any doubt about the adequacy of previous tetanus immunisation, the individual must have tetanus immunoglobulin (TIG) and commence or complete the recommended primary course of three doses of a tetanus toxoid-containing vaccine (depending on age and other antigens required: DTaP-containing vaccine or Tdap).

The definition of a tetanus-prone injury is not straightforward, because tetanus can occur after apparently trivial injury, such as from a rose thorn, or with no history of injury. However, there are certain types of wounds likely to favour the growth of tetanus organisms. These include:

Compound fractures, bite wounds, deep penetrating wounds, wounds containing foreign bodies [especially wood splinters], wounds complicated by pyogenic [pus-forming] infections, wounds with extensive tissue damage [e.g. crush injuries, avulsions, contusions or burns], wounds associated with vascular insufficiency [e.g. leg of foot ulcers in the elderly], any superficial wound obviously contaminated with soil, dust or horse manure [especially if topical disinfection is delayed more than 4 h] and finally; re-implantation of an avulsed tooth [in this case, minimal washing and cleaning of the tooth is conducted to increase the likelihood of successful re-implantation] (See [4], Table 5.1).

Table 5.1 Tetanus prophylaxis in wound management ([NZ Immunization Handbook 2020]—with permission)

History of tetanus vaccination[a]	Time since last dose	Type of wound	Tdap[b]	TIG[c]
≥3 doses	<5 years	Tetanus-prone wounds	No	No
≥3 doses	>5 years	Clean minor wounds	No	No
≥3 doses	>5 years	Tetanus-prone wounds	Booster dose[d]	No
≥3 doses	>10 years	Clean minor wounds	Booster dose[d]	No
<3 doses or uncertain		Clean minor wounds	Complete the course[e]	No
<3 doses or uncertain		Tetanus-prone wounds	Complete the course[e]	Yes

[a]People who have experienced Arthus-type hypersensitivity reactions (see 20.7.2) after a previous dose of a tetanus toxoid-containing preparation should not receive tetanus toxoid-containing preparation more frequently than every 10 years, even if they have a wound that is neither clean nor minor

[b]See Appendix 2 for catch-up schedules for previously unimmunised children. DTaP-containing vaccine may be used in children aged under 10 years

[c]*TIG* tetanus immunoglobulin. The recommended dose is 250 IU given by IM injection as soon as practicable after injury. If more than 24 h has elapsed, 500 IU is recommended. A dose of TIG can be given for up to 3 weeks after injury

[d]If appropriate, this may count as the booster dose at age 45 or 65 years.

[e]To complete the 3-dose primary immunisation course, give 1–3 doses at not less than 4-weekly intervals

Commentary by Mr Ian Burton FRACS

In this chapter Dr Chapple makes some very important points on avoiding surgical complications that are as relevant today as they were when she wrote the chapter.

Make sure a wound is clean before closing. One cannot sterilise a wound, but one must take time to clean it. In a large or particularly 'dirty' wound, pulsed lavage is very valuable. Consider a short course of a narrow spectrum oral antibiotic (such as Flucloxacillin) after excising a lesion in which there is superficial ulceration, however small, as such wounds have a higher risk of becoming infected. Remove any devitalised tissue before closing a wound and if in doubt, a second look one or more days later may determine whether one needs to excise more. Avoiding tension when closing a wound is paramount.

Be very careful when opting to remove a skin lesion larger than 1 cm diameter on the shin where tension along with the poor blood supply to the subcutaneous border of the tibia can result in wound breakdown that can be difficult to treat, particularly in diabetics and those with other vascular impairment. Oedema should be treated before elective surgery.

Dr Chapple's dislike of pressure dressings in general contrasts with the usual practice for breast biopsy surgery, where the risk of haematoma is quite high and pressure dressings are combined with suction drains. A 2008 trial [5] did show a reduction in seroma formation after mastectomies when pressure dressings were applied.

Dr Chapple's clinical experience also predates the introduction of calcium alginate dressings for packing wounds or abscesses after drainage, which has been shown to aid haemostasis, is easily washed out painlessly with gentle irrigation and may be very valuable [6]. Many abscesses are currently treated with ultrasound and antibiotics.

Other modern innovations in wound care include negative pressure wound devices which have become a game-changer in providing physiological conditions for delayed or problematic wound healing. Prior to this innovation silastic foam stents were useful for temporary control of deep and complex wounds.

The addition of nanocrystalline silver products to dressings, conferring antimicrobial actions, is another modern development.

Natural dermal templates with extracellular matrix also contain silver which aids wound healing.

References

1. Flint MH. The development of the circle technique for determining the optimum. Line of tumour excision. ANZ J Surg. 1979;49(6):690–6. https://doi.org/10.1111/j.1445-2197.tb0649.x.
2. Auersvald A, Auersvald LA, De Lourdes M, Biondo-Simões P. Haemostatic net: an alternative for the prevention of hematoma in rhytidoplasty. Rev Bras Cir Plást. 2012;27(1):22–30.
3. Farrow S, Toth B. The place of EUSOL in wound management. Nurs Stand. 1991;[22]:25–7. https://doi.org/10.7748/ns.522.25.s39.
4. New Zealand Handbook of Immunisation. 2020.
5. Kontos M, et al. Pressure dressing in breast surgery: is this the solution for seroma formation? J BUON. 2008;13(1):65–7.
6. Sega HC, Hunt BJ, Gilding K. The effects of alginate and non-alginate wound dressings on blood coagulation and platelet activation. J Biomater Appl. 1998;12(3):249–57. https://doi.org/10.1177/088532829801200305.

First-Aid, Assessment, and Treatment of Acute Wounds

6

Summary
After attending to the patient's airway, breathing, and circulation [ABC of Emergency First Aid Measures], the first aid for wounds is mostly a matter of elevating the bleeding part, applying focal pressure to stop the bleeding, and otherwise resting the patient as flat as possible.

The history and mechanism of injury supplies information necessary to evaluate the full extent of injury and the expected reaction to it. A detailed assessment of circulatory status of injured tissue in conjunction with an accurate anatomical diagnosis is then necessary to arrive at the most appropriate primary treatment.

After anaesthesia, meticulous cleansing and haemostasis, accurate repositioning of displaced tissues is often safer for the circulation than a standard sutured closure. Where areas of skin are dislodged or flaps are non-viable, replacement of the skin as a graft can provide it with a second chance to achieve primary healing.

First Aid

Treat the whole patient first, making sure they can breathe and don't need cardiopulmonary resuscitation [CPR]. Put patients at rest, and there is nothing like friendly communication to reassure them. Stop the bleeding with accurate local focal pressure. When injuries of the face or scalp are bleeding, it is better to rest the patient against something rather than lying them flat, but with most other injuries and especially if the patient is faint or nauseated, they should be lying down with the bleeding part elevated. Do not give patients anything to eat or drink if they may require a general anaesthetic.

> Elevation and accurate local pressure is always the most effective way to stop bleeding.

If other things need to be done, accurate local pressure can be maintained by a bystander or the patient themselves, or by something elastic bandaged on over a pad (a folded up piece of clean cotton material or a clean handkerchief), followed by a crepe bandage (or the sleeve of a jersey).

Steady pressure is tolerated better than fluctuating pressure from a hand. Leg wounds often bleed particularly freely, especially if a vein is

P. Charlesworth, M. F. Klaassen, *Chapple's Principles of Wound Care and Healing*,
https://doi.org/10.1007/978-3-031-53104-0_6

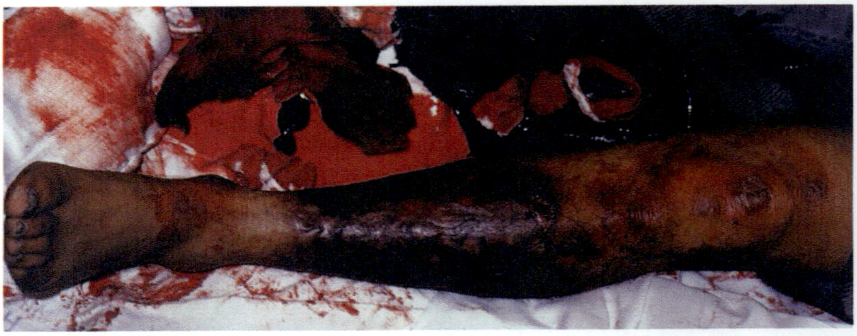

Fig. 6.1 Serious venous bleeding from a scraped vein after misguided and inadequate use of a tourniquet. Elevation and local pressure would have stopped the bleeding immediately. This patient unfortunately required a blood transfusion

punctured (Fig. 6.1). It is urgent to put the leg up and press accurately on the bleeding point. Accurate local focal pressure and elevation is quick, effective, much easier and much safer than applying a tourniquet. Never attempt to apply an amateur tourniquet for first aid, no matter how many times you have seen it at the movies!

Four Reasons Not to Use a First-Aid Tourniquet

1. It can sometimes be quite difficult to completely stop bleeding with a tourniquet.
2. All the while you are looking around for something to use as a tourniquet and endeavouring to apply it successfully, unnecessary blood is being lost.
3. Without a proper pneumatic BP cuff, there is no idea what the patient's BP is, or whether the cuff is above arterial pressure. If it isn't, the tourniquet will make bleeding many times worse by congesting the limb (Fig. 6.1).
4. The circulation to a digit or a limb is immediately stopped by a successful tourniquet, usually without any idea as to when and where the tourniquet is going to be removed again, and who is going to be sure to do this. This can itself constitute another emergency, because there is no circulation at all in the meantime.

First-Aid Dressings

If you have some greasy tulle dressings, these should be put on first. If this type of dressing is not available, cover open wounds with something clean and cotton-based, so that fluffy stuff does not adhere to them and dressings can then be soaked off with saline. What follows rather depends on the complexity of the wound and whether the first-aid dressing is going to also be the definitive one. If wounds continue to bleed, a temporary firm bandage, or local pressure for 15–20 min, usually ensures that it stops. After this, with elevation maintained, the pressure from bandaging can usually be reduced. It is especially important to reduce pressure as soon as it is safe to do so. The tissues will benefit from the improved circulation, and patients will be much more comfortable while they are waiting for treatment or to be transferred.

First-Aid for Burns

The first-aid for burns is immediate cooling, preferably with running water, putting out flames by smothering and/or water. Immediate and rapid cooling provides the only chance to do anything to reduce the depth and extent of burn damage (Figs. 6.2 and 6.3).

The faster the cooling, the less the damage will be, and it needs to be continued for at least 15–20 min. Continued cooling will effectively relieve pain, so it is also worthwhile doing this in

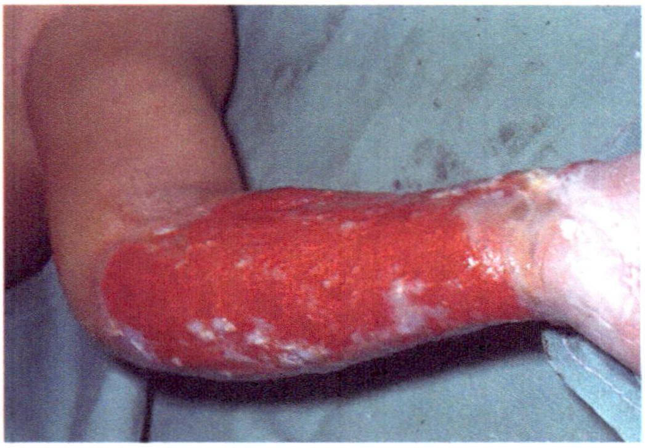

Fig. 6.2 Full-thickness scald burn at 4 weeks, in a child whose clothing was not removed, nor the burn wound cooled

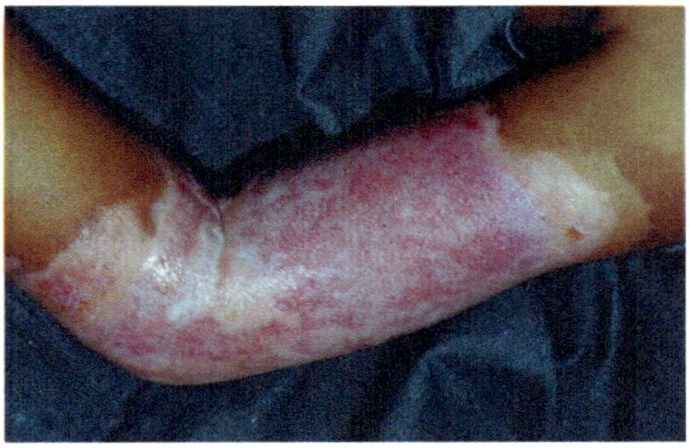

Fig. 6.3 Partial-thickness burn 3 weeks after scald burn, where prompt cooling made a huge difference to burn depth

smaller burns. While cooling cannot retrieve cells already dead, it probably temporarily reduces the metabolic needs of injured cell, thereby assisting their recovery. Continuing to cool extensively burned patients, however risks inducing hypothermia. Large burns are best covered in wet dressings after initial cooling. Seriously burned patients need to be transferred to hospital as soon as possible for monitoring and intravenous therapy. Oral fluids should be encouraged freely in all burned patients from the beginning.

Burned areas can be covered with Vaseline gauze and cotton dressings, which soak off readily with saline. Small dry burns do not necessarily need dressing initially, although they are often deep and inevitably discharge. They then require dressings within a week or so.

Assessment and Evaluation of Acute Wounds

History

An accurate history is essential to a full and accurate diagnosis. The nature of wounds sets the stage for the evaluation of both the structural and cellular damage. The subsequent behaviour of tissue depends largely on the mechanism of injury and the forces involved. Major tissue reaction can be predicted where heavy weights, momentum or heat are present, as in crush and gunshot wounds or injuries from power tools (Figs. 6.4, 6.5, 6.6, 6.7, 6.8 and 6.9), in addition to high velocity accidents, frictional injuries which rapidly generate heat (Fig. 6.10) and all burns. Evaluating total injury, as against just describing physical disruption, is especially relevant to the design of treatments which will most safely accommodate swelling during the first 48 h.

Anatomical Assessment of Function

Specific injuries will often elicit useful information from the patient or bystanders. Careful testing for nerve and tendon function needs to be undertaken before anaesthesia is induced. While it is exceedingly unlikely that tendons, nerves, or important vessels will be severed if there is no

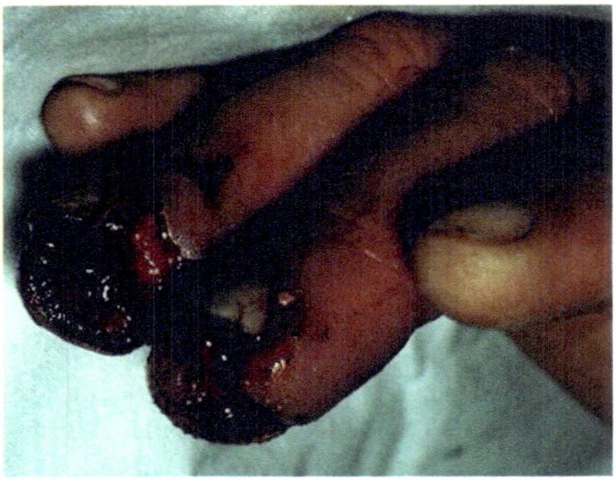

Fig. 6.4 A typical motor mower injury to finger tips

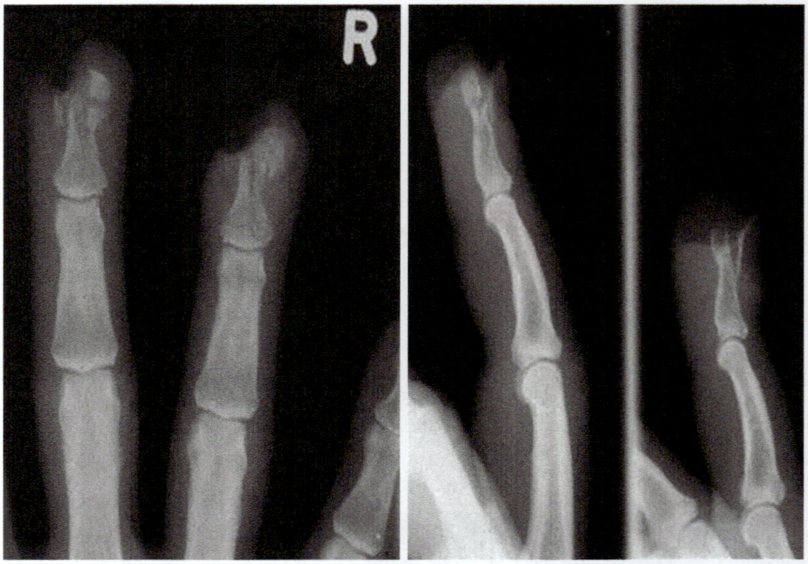

Fig. 6.5 X-Ray of the two fingers, showing damaged phalangeal tufts

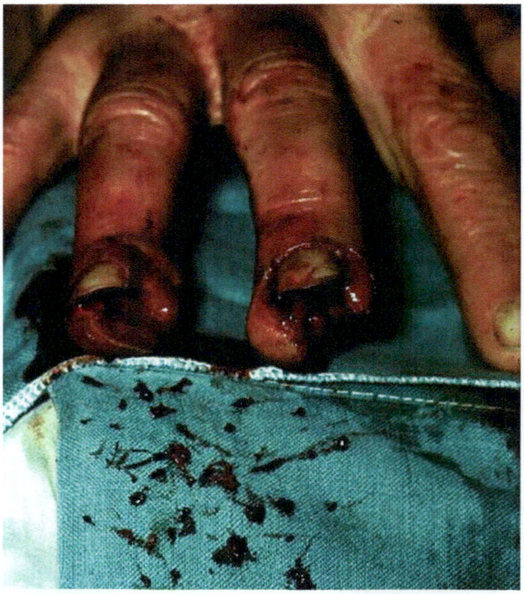

Fig. 6.6 After local anaesthesia, dirt, grass, and bone chips were cleaned out from the crushed finger tips, which were then moulded with tulle and both healed comfortably and uneventfully

skin wound, nevertheless, nerve conduction may be affected and ligaments, joints, and bones may be damaged. X-Rays may be indicated (Fig. 6.5).

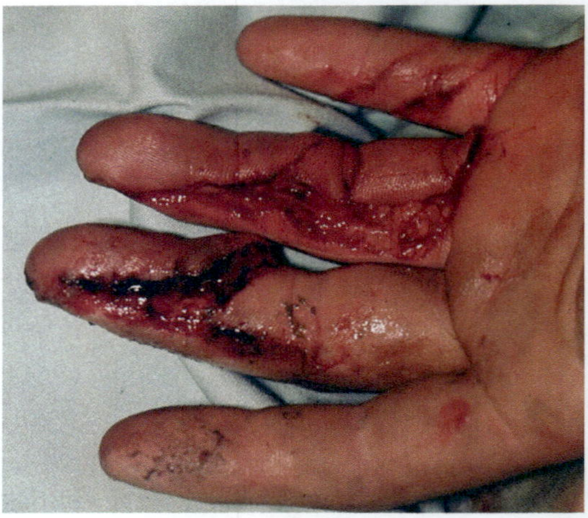

Fig. 6.7 Initial appearance of a hand caught in pastry rollers. The flaps look viable, but these fingers are burst fingers which will swell

Conversely, if there is a skin wound, however small, spikes of glass or knives can sever or penetrate anything underlying, and all such wounds should be regarded as potentially serious until serious effects have been specifically excluded, sometimes by open surgery.

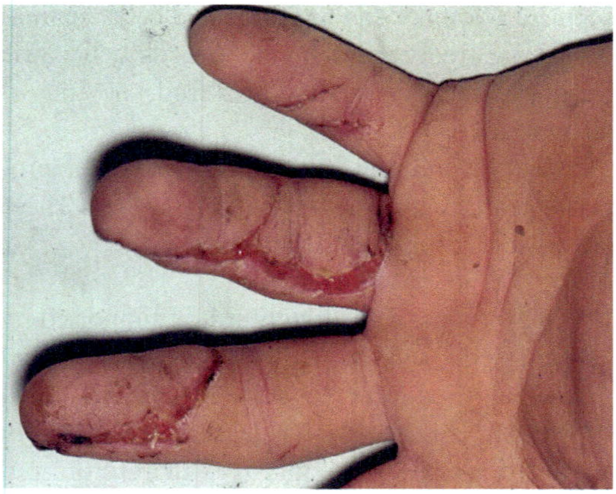

Fig. 6.8 The 10-day appearance after tulle gras stabilisation, gauze bandages, and splintage. All tissues are healthy and most of the swelling is gone. The hand has been remarkably comfortable, and all wounds are almost healed

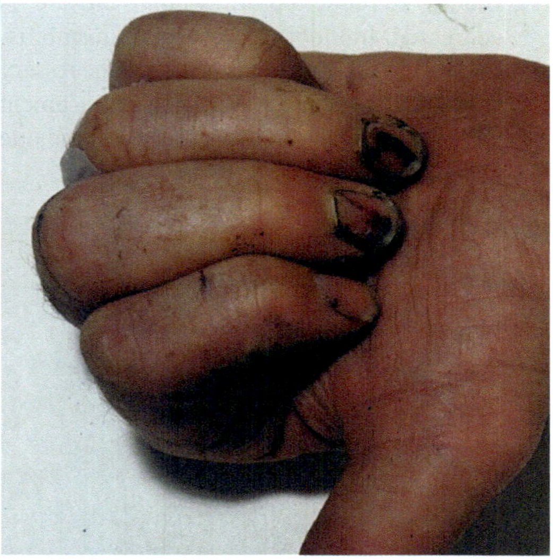

Fig. 6.9 At 3 weeks, the healed fingers flex comfortably into the palm already. This patient made a complete recovery from a very serious injury

Wound Inspection and Exploration

This is often best deferred until full facilities for dealing with bleeding are available and the definitive treatment can be undertaken. In most wounds, anaesthesia is needed for cleansing, surgical debridement, haemostasis, exploration, and treatment, which are all going on more or less simultaneously. Occasionally, when the diagnosis indicates that specialised treatment is required, it may be best to deal with bleeding before redressing the wound, leaving full exploration to the later operator.

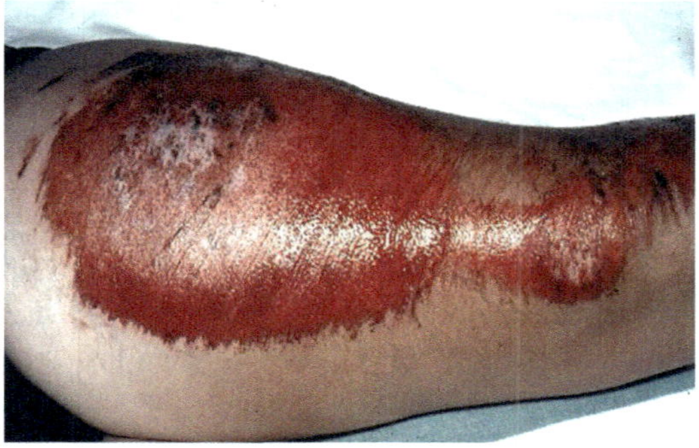

Fig. 6.10 This extensive road graze is a friction burn, with its central area showing the deepest destruction. It took about 6 weeks to heal

Circulatory Assessment

The circulation to tissues may be affected by direct injury to blood vessels, the wound site, the geographic predicament of tissue, or less specifically by concussion or bruising, and circulatory distress may be indicated by either pallor or congestion. A precise circulatory assessment of all parts of the wound should always form the basis of primary treatment. The important issues are whether tissues are alive and capable of surviving by means of their attachments, whether they can be restored to health by microvascular surgery, or whether they can be helped to pick up additional circulation to survive as a graft. These diagnostic differences are not just interesting theoretical distinctions but are absolutely fundamental to designing appropriate treatment.

Acute Treatment

The initial treatment for all wounds, after taking a careful history and thereby establishing the mechanism of injury, is to stop the bleeding, clean them thoroughly and after the assessment period is complete, consider the following treatment options:

1. What is the likely outcome of cleansing, stopping the bleeding, and accurately re-positioning the wounded tissues? Only if more treatment will improve this is it helpful to pursue additional procedures of any kind.
2. Are there specialised structures other than skin requiring specific repair? Patients with tendon and nerve injuries often require referral to specialists for treatment. Most patients with fractures and joint injuries also need to be X-Rayed and referred.
3. Is there skin missing or displaced—where is it and can it be retrieved and used? Unattached pieces of skin need to be kept moist and very often can and should be re-applied. This type of skin grafting will almost always be successful; the techniques are simple and should be part of everyone's skill base. However, if a new skin graft is required, the operator should have had some tuition and experience, as well as the equipment to do this properly.
4. Most flaps need special consideration. Circulatory requirements must always be translated into treatment responses that are appropriate. Skin from non-viable flaps can be used as a graft. Deeper non-viable tissue is best removed.
5. Does the extent and quality of the damage mean that circulatory problems could arise during the period of swelling? Treatment always needs to allow for this possibility.
6. Haemostasis is always a specific goal of treatment so that pressure can be avoided in the definitive dressings. Lower limb wounds need a particularly detailed bandaging regime. [See Appendix].

Only after considering all these things is it possible to decide which form of wound closure is most appropriate. Accurate re-positioning, rather than replacement at all costs is always the best approach, because the 'costs' are always circulatory. Watertight closure should never be an objective, because local tension is reduced by seepage. Wounds don't get infected because fluid is draining freely **out** of them, but usually because they are unclean, poorly perfused, or full of haematoma.

Arising from these concepts, the most appropriate primary treatment begins to emerge. There are always several possibilities:

(a) Will tissue sit accurately if it is supported by tulle-gras and dressed, rested, and protected while it recovers (Figs. 6.11, 6.12, 6.13, and 6.14]? This approach is least likely to focally restrict circulation, and it is therefore especially appropriate for crush and burst injuries, complex and multiple lacerations, and many flaps. Both venous circulation and ease of closure can be improved if posturing or long tapes are able to reduce tension in the wound vicinity. Any posturing of joints should be done before wound closure is addressed. Immobilisation assists in stabilising the circulation and is generally necessary to maintain accuracy of tissue replacement when sutures are not used. Local anaesthetic

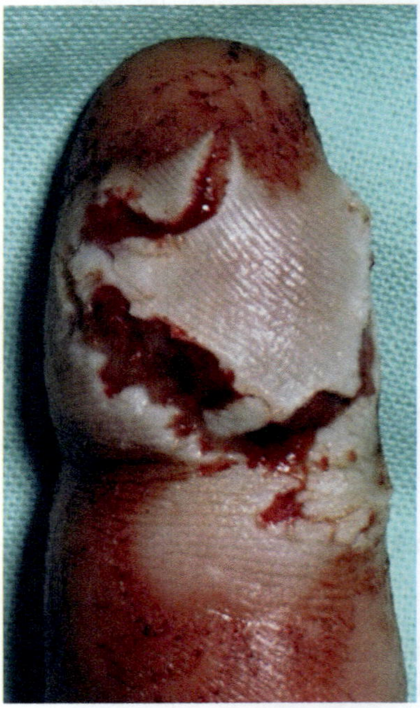

Fig. 6.11 Crushed fingertip, treated without sutures, at day 05 showing white but not unhealthy skin flaps. Healing progressed well

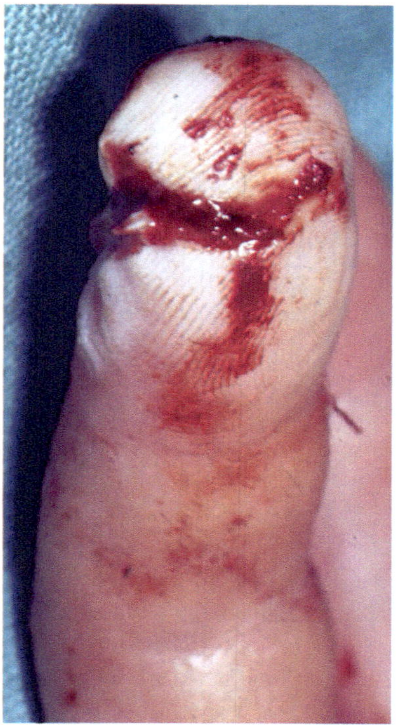

Fig. 6.12 White wet skin adjacent to crush lacerations, also at day 05. Unsutured fingertip healed

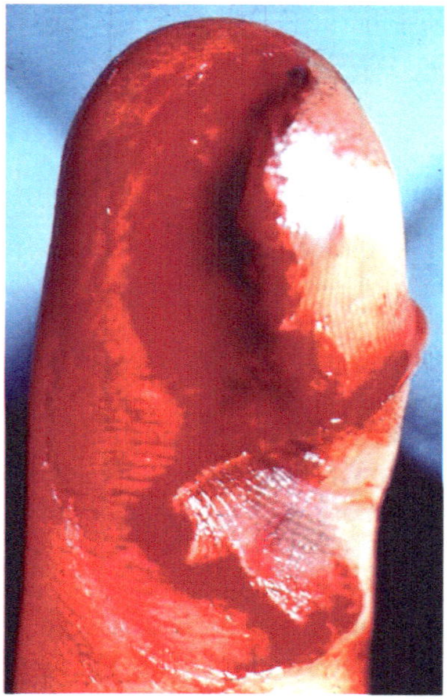

Fig. 6.13 Severely traumatised fingertip, best treated by tulle moulding, NOT suturing

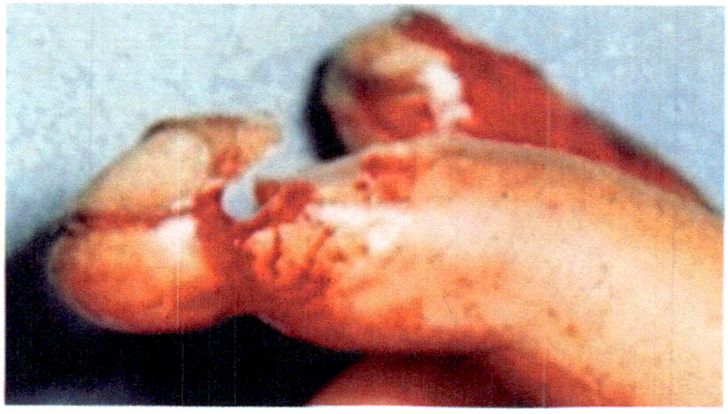

Fig. 6.14 Unstable but very healthy fingertip, best held by accurate tulle moulding and without sutures. Splintage and protection is important in this scenario for about a week

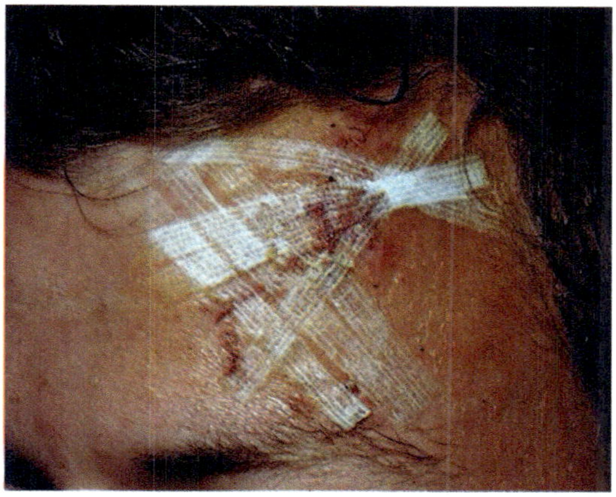

Fig. 6.15 A complicated laceration from a blow with a bottle has been very successfully treated with tapes

is often needed for cleansing and replacement, even when there is going to be no suturing.

(b) Can the wound be held accurately and securely with tapes [Steristrips™]? Taping is particularly suitable for multiple or complex lacerations and for flaps (Figs. 6.15, 6.16 and 6.17). The skin must be clean and dry. It helps to paint the skin with Tincture of Benzoin before applying the tapes. Medical tape off a roll [Micropore™] can be used if longer tapes are needed. Gaps should always be left between the tapes for seepage. Skin glue is equivalent to surface tapes and can be used in a similar way. It should not be used to

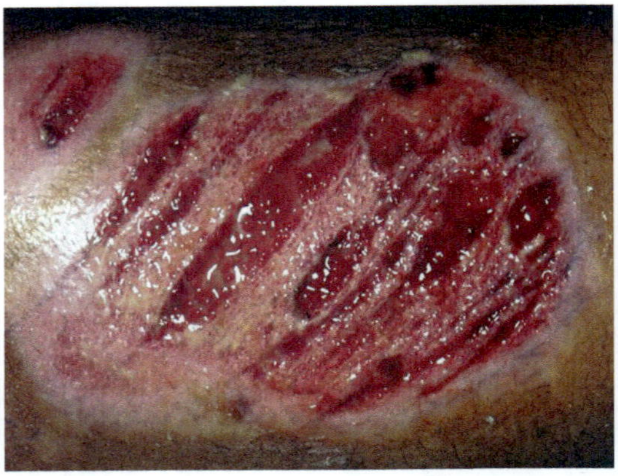

Fig. 6.16 Clean linear raw surfaces 3 weeks after initially sutured lacerations broke down and became infected. Raw surfaces are now healthy

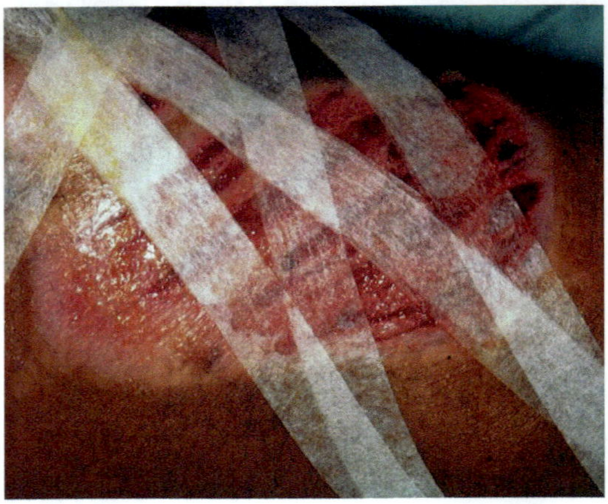

Fig. 6.17 Long tapes were able to reduce the gaps on the same day as Fig. 6.16 and rapid uneventful healing followed

completely seal wounds, but to tack the skin edges accurately together intermittently. Tulle can be applied over tapes or glued wounds so that outer dressings do not stick.

(c) Is it best to suture the wound? Suturing is the most traditional method of closure and can be both secure and accurate. However, each suture does alter the circulation to the wound somewhat and should therefore be inserted with discretion and expertise. Suturing may be safe and appropriate for facial and scalp lacerations where the circulation is very robust, but it is always more dangerous for flaps, particularly on the front of the shin, where perfusion is notoriously poorest (Figs. 6.18, 6.19 and 6.20). Deeper repairs are best restricted to a few accurate sutures to fibrous layers. Large subcutaneous sutures have a considerable potential to interrupt circulation and are best avoided [1]. Planes of separation and dead spaces are best obliterated by dressings, bandages and/or suction drainage, rather than by suturing. The reduction of tension in the vicinity of sutured wounds achieved by posturing and/or long tapes not only assists closure but also confers an additional margin of venous safety to the wound, as swelling occurs.

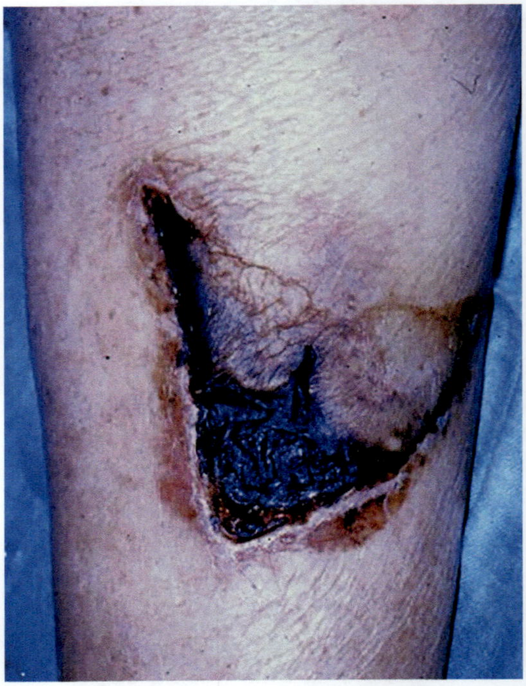

Fig. 6.18 Typical venous necrosis following suturing of a triangular flap. Note further zone of partial-thickness loss

(d) Is there any tissue needing consideration for a particular flap or graft? All tissue requires circulation in order to survive. However, there are quite specific techniques that will help tissues with a sluggish flap circulation,

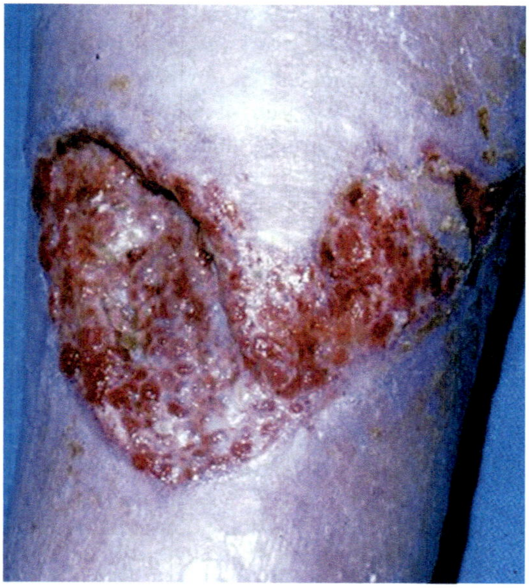

Fig. 6.19 Ragged, raw surfaces on the lower leg a month after proximally-based flap had been sutured back and died

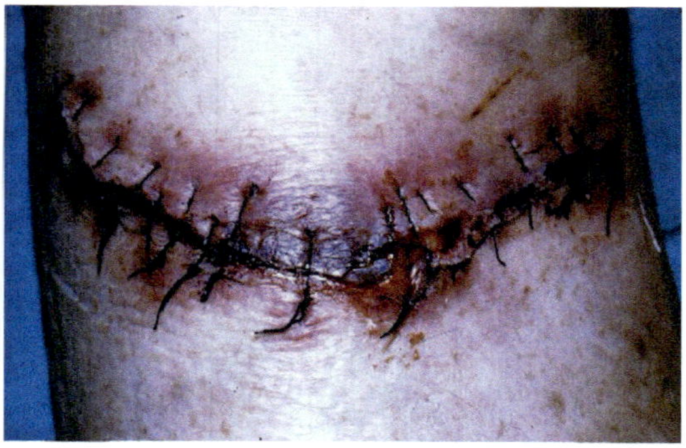

Fig. 6.20 Broad proximally based knee flap showing circulatory problems caused by sutures. Infection is already present. Taping this traumatic flap would have been a much safer option and the knee would have needed splinting

and for grafted tissue that has none, a different set of techniques which are aimed at assisting with the rapid re-establishment of capillary perfusion. See Chap. 4. These two scenarios can exist within the same wound and treatment needs to accommodate both of them. See Chap. 10.

(e) Dressings and bandages complete all these treatment procedures and are so important that they are dealt with in a separate chapter. See Chap. 11. Immobilisation for the first few days maintains the best conditions for the recovery of both flaps and grafts.

The appropriateness or otherwise of any treatment can only strictly be assessed in retrospect, ideally by the original operator, who knows what was done initially and why- and can then correlate the outcome with this knowledge. This is the only way of accumulating reliable personal expertise.

Editors' Note *While the logic of these aspirations is undeniable, unfortunately the logistics of Dr Chapple's style of practice were markedly different from those widely prevailing today. Nevertheless, a philosophy of meticulous personal follow-up of cases can only result in improved education and better outcomes.*

Commentary by Dr James Klaassen MBChB [Auckland]

A review of this succinct and brilliant chapter on Dr Chapple's approach to Acute Wounds demonstrates how little has changed over the decades, and this is a recognition of her clinical foresight.

Triage nurses today understand that steady pressure is superior to hand pressure, and they will apply a simple dressing and crepe bandage pressure to avoid the fluctuations in local capillary perfusion that occur when holding an improvised dressing with a hand. Broad arm slings are also popular in the ED treatment of upper limb injuries. Head injury patients are advised to sit up, and patients with lower limb injuries are advised to elevate the foot on waiting room chairs or pillows, wherever and whenever physical space allows.

Dr Chapple's conscious bias for the superiority of non-suture closure was well explained, with interesting examples, and is a good reminder that "less is sometimes more". A Cochrane review in 2014 confirmed this in terms of: minimising dehiscence, infection, patients' assessment of cosmetic appearance, patient satisfaction or surgeon satisfaction [2]. Often, the application of products like tulle is faster, less painful, and thus especially useful in uncooperative children or patients with dementia.

Dr Chapple's warnings about allowing gaps for wound seepage with the use of tissue glues, and not sealing wounds along their entirety are key points. An interesting modification in modern practice is a combination of cyanoacrylate glue and Steristrips™. Glue is applied to the end of the Steristrips™ well away from the wound, so as to discourage/prevent premature uplifting of the tape by moisture, or indeed a frustrated child's fingernails.

Finally, her concern in regard to the importance of continuity of care by the initial treating doctor is a reality, but the aspiration is failed by many modern health systems today. In large Emergency Departments this concept is a challenge and has implications for both the patient and the clinician. The patient is subjected to multiple healthcare professionals, all with their idiosyncratic personalities. The clinician misses out on objective feedback of their management decisions and actions. One solution is to teach the patient how to digitally photograph their wound on their smart phone, when a dressing change is done. This provides a visual record/history for future (potentially multiple) service providers.

References

1. De Holl D, Rodeheaver GT, Edgerton MT. Potential of infection by suture closure of dead space. Am J Surg. 1974;127:716.
2. Dumville JC, Coulthard P, Worthington HV, Riley P, Patel N, Darcey J, Esposito M, van der Elst M, van Waes OJ. Tissue adhesives for closure of surgical incisions. Cochrane Database Syst Rev. 2014(11):CD004287. https://doi.org/10.1002/14651858.CD004287.pub4.

7 Cleansing

Summary
The thorough cleansing of wounds is a mechanical process. Dirt is best syringed or washed out with saline, picked out, and/or excised with a layer of tissue. Potentially dead or severely damaged non-specific tissue, as well as discoloured grimy tissue, is often best excised to prevent it from becoming a focus for discharge or infection. The use of anything other than saline solutions within wounds is unhelpful as other agents can potentially damage cells.

The body surfaces are covered by skin or mucous membranes, with cell division replacing the dead cells which are continually flaking off the surface. After open injury living cells are vulnerable to desiccation and toxic substances, as well as the interior of the body being open to bacterial invasion. Dirt may not only carry bacteria more deeply into a wound, but it also acts as a foreign body irritant, giving rise to persistent discharge and delayed healing.

The use of antiseptics within wounds is unhelpful. If they are sufficiently concentrated to kill bacteria, they then damage cells. If solutions are diluted so as not to do this, they are no longer effective against bacteria. Alexander Fleming [1881–1955], as long ago as 1919, commented that all antiseptics instilled into wounds probably did more harm to the tissues than to the bacteria. During WWI, when he was in the Medical Corps, antiseptics were the primary means to combat infection [1]. All solutions with a spirit base denature cell proteins and hydrogen peroxide produces a chemical slough.

Intact skin can be washed with soap and water. Dried blood is readily removed by leaving saline-soaked swabs applied to it for several minutes, before cleaning it with wrung-out swabs. Cleaning wounds has two aspects: washing and active debridement. Normal saline is best for washing wounds. This can be dripped or poured into the wound or used even more effectively in a syringe with a large needle. It is often advisable to prepare a set-up that will collect the fluid run-off, so that washing can be really generous. Irrigation is the best way of diluting bacterial contamination and flushing out dirt. Some washing does not need anaesthesia at all, e.g., minor injuries to fingertips crushed in clean doors can simply be washed and dressed, so long as tissue is not displaced or disrupted by haematoma. Using saline swabs to sponge dirt out of wounds, or any sharp dissection, usually requires prior anaesthesia. Irrigation may need to be followed by picking out any retained particulate dirt with instruments. Scrubbing of wounds is unspeakably traumatic, although it is a very widespread practice observed and copied by generations of professionals. Grazes are going to get rid of their surface grime into the early dressings with the 'burn' slough and can be left to do just that. Sharp

P. Charlesworth, M. F. Klaassen, *Chapple's Principles of Wound Care and Healing*,
https://doi.org/10.1007/978-3-031-53104-0_7

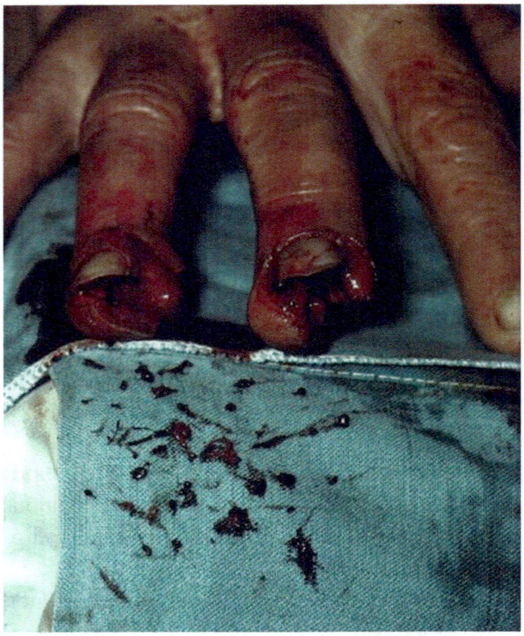

Fig. 7.1 Typical motor-mower fingertip injuries with dirt, grass, and bone chips cleaned out from compound crush wounds under local anaesthetic. Tulle moulding then applied and uneventful healing ensued

dissection of deeper, dirty tissue is sometimes necessary. Motor-mower injuries (Fig. 7.1) or injuries with paint or grease injected under pressure always require full exploration under anaesthetic to clean out all foreign material (Figs. 7.2, 7.3, and 7.4).

The important consequence of not properly removing dirt/dead material from a wound is that it then has to clean itself by producing a discharge, and frequently becomes further complicated by invasive sepsis. Healing will be delayed until problems in the depths, and any associated infection, have both been resolved. Another long-term effect of such complications is increased and often unsightly scarring. Occasionally, a persistently discharging wound may need re-exploration to remove retained foreign material or dead tissue.

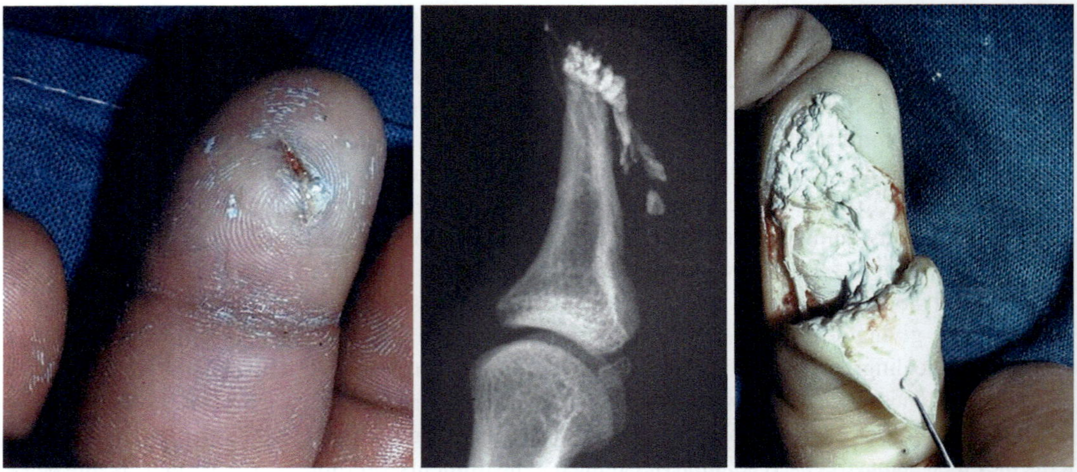

Figs. 7.2–7.4 Injury from paint injected under pressure while spray painting. Pulp of fingertip was pale and extremely painful. X-ray of another patient injected with material under pressure. (Note – a negative X-Ray does not exclude foreign material. The same fingertip as Fig. 7.2, at exploration. This finger eventually required amputation)

Commentary by Dr Michael F. Klaassen FRACS

My practise over 35 years differs slightly from what Dr Joan Chapple has boldly stated above, with respect to the cleansing of dirty wounds. These have included a scope of civilian maxillofacial, hand, upper and lower extremity injuries, trunk wounds, and the broad range of burn trauma. During my decade working at Waikato Hospital, we dealt with many farming injuries due to industrial machinery and contaminated with soil and farm-based toxins. Over many years, I have used saline mixed with Gentamicin, half strength Betadine, and Hydrogen Peroxide to wash out wounds with good effect. The pulse lavage system used commonly in orthopaedic trauma scenarios is also very useful. In addition, and in contrast to Dr Chapple's principles, I have commonly used antiseptics if they are diluted or washed out with saline after use. I favour McIndoe's non-toothed dissection forceps for picking out foreign bodies and grit from dirty wounds. Although I completed only a year of advanced training in orthopaedic surgery, the common practice of scrubbing contaminated and very dirty, traumatic wounds with a soft hand brush, of the type used when scrubbing-up, is indeed extremely helpful. Cleansing of a contaminated and dirty wound with damaged tissues is really the start of proper wound debridement. It is often necessary to combine generous saline pulse-lavage irrigation with sharp scalpel debridement to transform an untidy wound into a tidy one, ready for the next phase of repair/reconstruction.

Reference

1. Tan SY, Tatsumura Y. Alexander Fleming (1881-1955): discoverer of penicillin. Singapore Med J. 2015;56(7):366–7.

8 Local Anaesthesia

Summary

Modern local anaesthetics are generally safe, but it is very important to remember that they can have significant cardiovascular and central nervous system side effects. While these are rare, they are dose-related, and more likely to occur with the use of plain local anaesthetic without the vasoconstrictor adrenaline. It is helpful to consult a standard chart of weight-related maximum doses, and extra care is necessary with local anaesthetic use in children.

Local anaesthetic is best regarded as a kind of contract between the operator and the patient. It works best if everything is clearly and honestly explained. Saying, 'This isn't going to hurt', just before the patient is hit with the exquisitely sharp first jab is not likely to engender confidence. Ice, or a topical agent, such as EMLA cream, can be used on the skin before the first injection, and are especially useful in children. Injections through an open wound are much less painful than those through intact skin. Subsequent injections should, if possible, always be made through already anaesthetised tissue. The actual injection of local anaesthetic causes intense pain like a wasp sting. It is fortunately short-lived but will be tolerated much better if patients are told what to expect and

Table 8.1 Local anaesthetics

LA	Onset of action (min)	Duration of action (min)	Max dose (mg/kg)
Lignocaine	5	60–90 (intermediate)	3
Lignocaine + adrenaline	5	120–360	7
Prilocaine	5	60–120	6
Bupivacaine, levobupivacaine	10–15	200+ (long)	2
Ropivacaine-benefit of intrinsic vasoconstrictor activity, less cardiotoxic and less motor blockade compared with bupivacaine	5–15	200+	3

Duration of effective analgesia depends on type, volume and concentration of injected local anaesthetic
This Table 8.1 is from Chapter 18 of Atlas Of Extreme Facial Cancer [editors Ian Burton & Michael F. Klaassen], by Dr. Su Thon [FANZCA] and titled Perioperative & Anaesthetic Care in Head and Neck Cancer [Springer 2022].

P. Charlesworth, M. F. Klaassen, *Chapple's Principles of Wound Care and Healing*, https://doi.org/10.1007/978-3-031-53104-0_8

if the injection rate is very slow. Never say 'this is going to stop you feeling anything', because local anaesthetic doesn't obliterate pressure, pulling, or the awareness of something going on, which the patient will feel, and then interpret as pain. Patients will be reassured by something like, 'you shouldn't feel any sharp pain or cutting but you will be aware I'm doing something to you'. Post-injection, gentle massage of the area will help to distribute the local and improve its effect.

The operator is dependent on the patient's confidence to ensure that the anaesthetic is maximally effective and that the operating conditions are ideal. Once credibility and trust are lost, these are hard to rebuild. Invite the patient to comment or indicate if they feel anything uncomfortable at any time during the procedure so they never feel trapped. Never ever cover the patient's face with guards. Heat and CO_2 build up uncomfortably and the overall effect is to create acute anxiety and panic. Avoid skin preparations anywhere near the eyes, nose, or mouth as many of these contain spirit or other chemical irritants. The usual skin bacteria are unlikely to cause infection, and it is impossible to sterilise skin without damaging it.

Use 1% Lignocaine and a 25-or 26-gauge needle (or the even smaller one on the integrated 1 mL insulin syringe) for the initial skin injection, to make a skin bleb. A longer and larger needle may be needed subsequently. After the injection, tell the patient that it is necessary to wait for 10 min before checking to make sure that it is working properly, so that they are not lying there wondering and anxious. *It is useful to spend this time engaging the patient while setting up necessary instruments and resources.* Patients' physical relaxation and confidence always potentiates the effectiveness of local anaesthesia. Make sure they are lying as comfortably as possible, especially relaxed about the head and neck and with their legs uncrossed. Talk to them. 'Concentrate on feeling your full weight being supported. Breathe quietly and slowly with your abdomen, and relax your arms and legs and all your muscles. Start thinking of something nice, a long, long way from here'. Reassure them in particular that they will be well able to cope with everything you will be doing. Patients often get really worried that they are not going to behave well.

Editors' Note *MFK has found that asking the patient to breathe out slowly during the initial LA injection helps their skin relax and reduces resistance and therefore makes the initial LA infiltration more bearable.*

After 10 min, check the effect of the anaesthetic with a series of very small pricks from a 25 or 26 needle (these should not draw blood), starting from the numb skin and going out onto normal skin saying, 'I am testing now and I will go out onto your normal skin sometimes, so I need to know whenever you feel a small prick'. Any inconsistencies or gaps are immediately apparent and will sometimes require a bit more anaesthetic injected, after which a further wait or starting in another place may be best. It is simply not worth commencing any operation if the patient is going to feel sharp pain from the procedure. Be on the lookout for the slightest indication of pain from the patient. It can be a catch in the breath, a wince, a restlessness or involuntary movement, a tensing of jaw muscles, or a screwing up of the eyes. Either wait a bit longer or put a bit more local in. Keep talking to the patient to maintain accurate communication.

There is not any other stage in the whole procedure when it is so necessary to be tuned in to patients' reactions as at the beginning. Local anaesthetic is after all the beginning of a calculated 'attack' on their person. Restrain others (such as assisting nurses) from asking leading questions like, 'does that hurt', because patients will be talked into feeling pain if they think anyone is nervous about whether the anaesthetic is working. If they obviously have not felt anything unpleasant as the operation starts, it is immensely reassuring to them to simply say, 'we're well under way here, it seems to be quite numb already, but let me know at any time if you do feel anything unpleasant'. Let them know as you are progressing, especially towards the end of a procedure. Patients last much better as soon as they know that there is a definite end in sight. Remember, it otherwise feels to them that the whole scenario may go on forever. Poor communicators don't usually like operating under local anaesthetic, but it is a very safe and extremely useful technique to learn to do well.

Failure of Local Anaesthetic

The most common failures with local anaesthetic result from not having the injection in the right layer or place and/or commencing the operation before it has taken effect properly, without testing. Having a patient who from then on 'feels' everything because their pain threshold and morale has been reduced to zero is likely to be an ordeal for everyone. Patients who have previously had a bad experience need patience and special care. Try to ascertain that this was neither an allergic response nor a convincing failure of local anaesthesia. In most cases it is worth another try, saying that it may have been a different anaesthetic, or the previous doctor may not have waited long enough for it to work and that you certainly won't be proceeding until you are sure that it is working properly this time. A very occasional patient never gets adequate anaesthesia from Xylocaine, and other alternatives then need to be worked out. The very first of these must always be to consider how 'nature' will deal with the particular current problem if left to do so. Never ever blame patients for local anaesthetic failure. In selected cases, combining local anaesthesia with intravenous sedation is a very helpful approach for the nervous patient.

Adrenaline in Local Anaesthesia

The use of local anaesthetic with adrenaline is especially useful about the head and neck where bleeding can be a nuisance. It is usually more effective than plain local because it lasts about twice as long than plain local and also blanches the anaesthetised area. The total amount of anaesthetic solution that can be safely used may be doubled if the adrenaline version is used because the absorption is slowed. As there will however be a rebound phase after the adrenaline effect wears off, it is wise to apply some form of dressing for a few hours whenever local containing adrenaline has been used.

Do Not Use Adrenaline Solutions for Digital Blocks (Fig. 8.1)

Editors' Note *This admonition has very frequently been given to medical students and residents over the years, and it has been repeated in numerous reputable surgical texts for decades. However, there is no substantive evidence to suggest that modern local anaesthetics containing adrenaline have caused digital necrosis. In a comprehensive literature review of cases of presumptive digital necrosis following vasoconstrictor-containing local anaesthetic[1] a total of only 48 cases were found over the past 120 years, none of which were in the period after the introduction of commercial local anaesthetic with adrenaline in 1948. Of the cases of digital necrosis reported, none of these involved the use of lignocaine and only half the use of adrenaline. Many had co-morbid conditions or external factors that may have been responsible or contributory, such as perhaps the case in Fig. 8.1 below.*

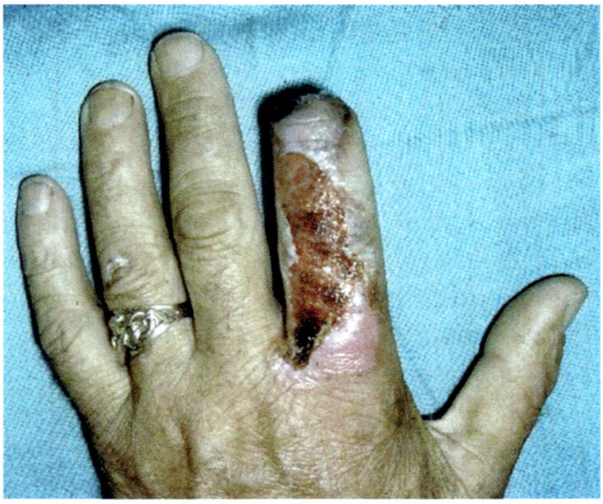

Fig. 8.1 Unfortunately, the digital block for the partial amputation had adrenaline in it. The cold ischaemic finger sustained deep burns when it was warmed up under a heat lamp while it was still anaesthetised.

Ischaemic Blocks

Ischaemic blocks are a specialist anaesthetic procedure, not without risks, and are unsuitable for children. The appropriate anaesthetic solution is administered intravenously into a limb exsanguinated by a tourniquet. The tourniquet cannot be tolerated on un-anaesthetised skin, so two tourniquets are needed, with the proximal one used for the administration of the block and removed after a second one has been applied and inflated on the anaesthetised skin below it. Perhaps the biggest drawback is the total dependence of the anaesthesia on the tourniquet. Tourniquet removal is followed rapidly by return of sensation and a hyperaemia lasting as long as 40 min, making the achievement of absolute haemostasis extremely difficult if not impossible without pressure bandages. Additional unseen bleeding into fractures and other injured tissues can occur during the hyperaemic phase and can sometimes give rise to complications. The firm bandaging required to control bleeding always produces throbbing pain, which indicates a degree of circulatory impairment, and worsens as tissue swells.

Editors' Note *In this chapter, and elsewhere in the book, Dr Chapple expresses very negative opinions about the use of ischaemic local anaesthetic blocks, but the strength of her antipathy may well have been influenced by the relatively restricted range of her clinical practice. While the majority of her specific criticisms of the technique cannot be denied in principle, the fact remains that it has a valuable selective role in modern surgery and trauma treatment. Purpose-designed newer cuff devices and new local anaesthetic agents have essentially eliminated the issues that Dr Chapple found unacceptable.*

Increasingly, haematoma blocks with 10 mL plain Lignocaine are used in the Emergency department scenario for reduction/manipulation of displaced Colles' fractures of the wrist. [Personal communication: Dr Cheatan Patel, Advanced trainee in Orthopaedics].

Digital Nerve Blocks

These are extremely useful. ***USE PLAIN LIGNOCAINE 1%, WITHOUT ADRENALINE.*** (See Editors' Note, above) Using the finest possible needle, inject about 0.5 mL subcutaneously on the dorsal aspect of the finger, about 1 cm distal to the level of the metacarpo-phalangeal joint. Wait at least 30 s, and then inject another 0.5 mL down each side towards the web. Wait again and aiming towards the angle between web and digit, inject a further 0.5 mL on each side through numbed skin, feeling and watching this expand the subcutaneous tissue towards the front of the digit in the vicinity of the digital nerve. On the outer side of both the index and little fingers it is usually necessary to make one further injection around towards the front of the digit to arrive at the actual course of the nerve. Wait and test, and if necessary, use a little more local distal to the original injections. Wait again and test carefully. It is also alright to use a little more local through the edges of an open wound if it seems to be not quite numb enough.

In the thumb both nerves lie close together, running in the subcutaneous tissue around the distal edge of the thenar muscle bulge. They start to separate opposite the MC/P joint. It is possible to infiltrate around both nerves with a 1 mL. injection put in from the dorsum of the thumb web, watching it accumulate in the palmar tissue along the basal thumb crease. Lastly, inject a further 1 mL. subcutaneously across the dorsum. It is an easier block than that for fingers.

Topical Anaesthesia

Topical local anaesthesia is not particularly useful in wound care, although techniques may be evolved to improve this situation. The gels presently available are quite strong and absorption cannot be reliably assessed. The use of Ethyl Chloride spray, which acts by freezing, is ineffective unless the circulation can be excluded by a tourniquet. It can be very useful in digits for the removal of a visible fishhook, needle or subungual splinter etc., where the tourniquet on non-anaesthetised skin can be tolerated for a short time. Ethyl Chloride is useless in the drainage of infections, because the inflammatory heat continuously inactivates the cooling and accordingly, the anaesthetic effect.

Commentary by Dr Sophie Klaassen BBiomedSc [Hons], MBBS [ANU], FANZCA

The clinical use of local anaesthesia combines the elements of both art and science. The scientific aspect demands a comprehensive understanding of the various types of local anaesthetics including short-acting, long-acting, with and without adrenaline. It is crucial for professionals to be well versed in their potential toxicities, side-effects, and protocols for managing an overdose. No professional should administer local anaesthesia without a thorough knowledge of the **safe** dosage limits (See Table 8.1). On the other hand, the art of administering local anaesthesia involves not only technical proficiency but also the ability to establish a connection with your patients, fostering trust and confidence. While some individuals may possess a natural inclination for establishing rapport, this skill can also be learned and developed. It is essential to observe your patient's verbal communication and body language to gauge their comfort levels and adjust accordingly.

To establish a comfortable atmosphere, I often share a simple joke especially with my younger patients as an icebreaker. For instance:

QUESTION: How do you put a baby astronaut to sleep?

ANSWER: Rocket!

Regional anaesthesia is a specialist skill set that requires the necessary training and practical experience to become proficient. Since its first experimentation in Europe by Koller and others in 1884, the clinical applications of local anaesthesia have evolved to become safer and more universal. Dr Su S. Thon considers the brief history of anaesthesia in the Western World in her chapter published by Springer in 2022 [2]. In the modern sense, the role of the anaesthetist encompasses comprehensive care throughout the perioperative period, spanning preoperative, intraoperative and postoperative stages.

References

1. Denkler K. A comprehensive review of epinephrine in the finger: to do or not to do. Plast Reconstr Surg. 2001;108(1):114–24.
2. Burton I, Klaassen MF. Atlas of extreme facial cancer: challenges and solutions. Switzerland: Springer Nature; 2022. https://doi.org/10.1007/978-3-030-88,334-8.

9 Suturing Versus Non-suturing Methods

Summary
While suturing wounds makes them look better immediately, sutures often interfere with the skin circulation. When injuries are severe and/or affect the circulation significantly, alternative approaches to closure are likely to be much safer. Although almost anyone can learn how to suture, with living tissue the art is in the judgement of whether and when to suture, and in particular, *when not* to stitch tissue which has been injured acutely and is yet to swell. Several adaptable and useful techniques are described in this chapter.

Evolution of the New Approach

I became increasingly aware in my clinical encounters with all sorts and sizes of wounds that most complications were circulatory in origin, and were frequently related to surgical technique, very often to the effects of individual sutures (Figs. 9.1, 9.2, 9.3).

While a good-looking immediate result could usually be achieved by suturing, there were too frequently also some serious effects on the circulation (Figs. 9.4, 9.5, 9.6, 9.7, 9.8, 9.9, 9.10, 9.11, and 9.12). Approaching wounds in a physiological way obviously needed a different approach from simply restoring the anatomy as soon as possible.

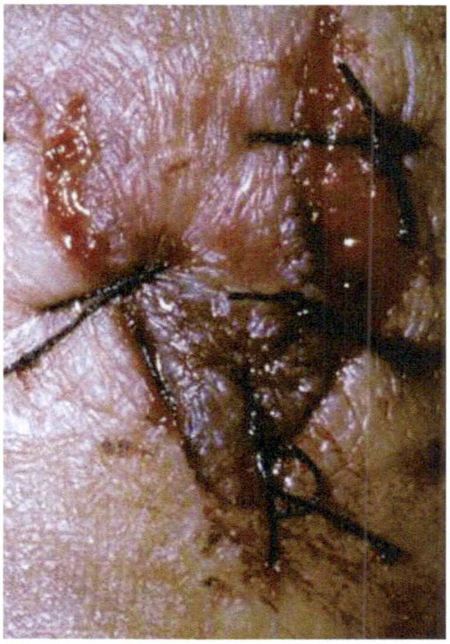

Fig. 9.1 Classic triangular flap with bands of tension between sutures, restricting the venous circulation

It became very important to figure out how to use sutures more safely and to learn how to combine them with other methods of closure in order to reduce their disadvantages (Figs. 9.13, 9.14, and 9.15).

Crucially, it was necessary to learn when to avoid sutures altogether and how to use alternative methods of closure (Figs. 9.16, 9.17, 9.18, 9.19, and 9.20).

P. Charlesworth, M. F. Klaassen, *Chapple's Principles of Wound Care and Healing*,
https://doi.org/10.1007/978-3-031-53104-0_9

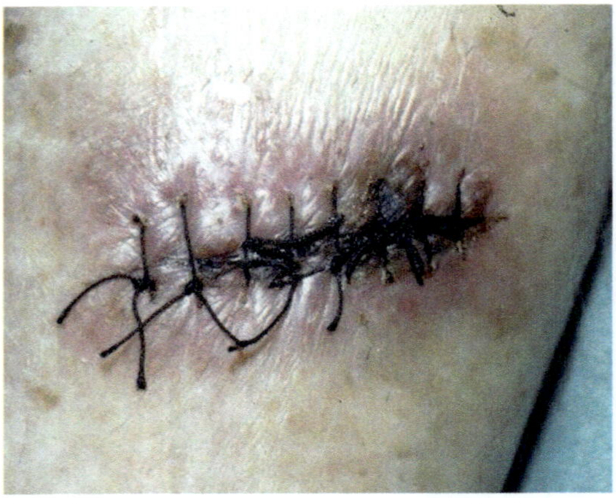

Fig. 9.2 Circulatory problems along both edges created by the sutures with infection becoming established. This was a surgical wound post lesion excision at 10 days

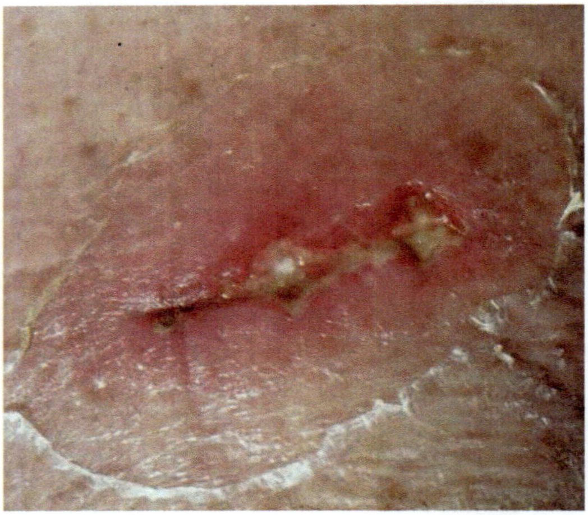

Fig. 9.3 The loss of edge circulation related to the initial sutures. Associated infection required antibiotics and is now settling

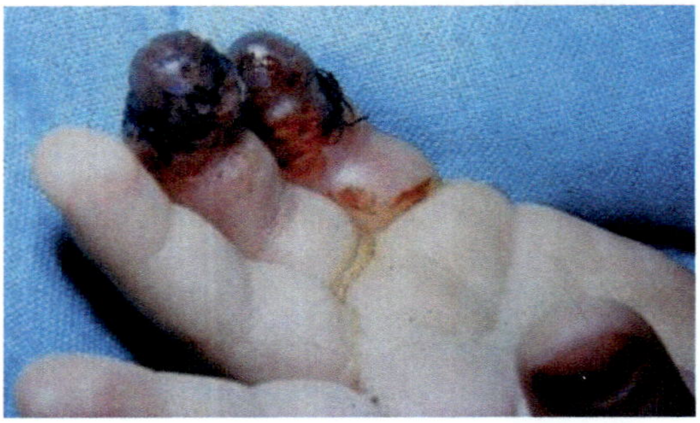

Fig. 9.4 Venous stasis in crushed fingertips leading to their death. Although the suturing is accurate, it has in fact worsened the venous return problems

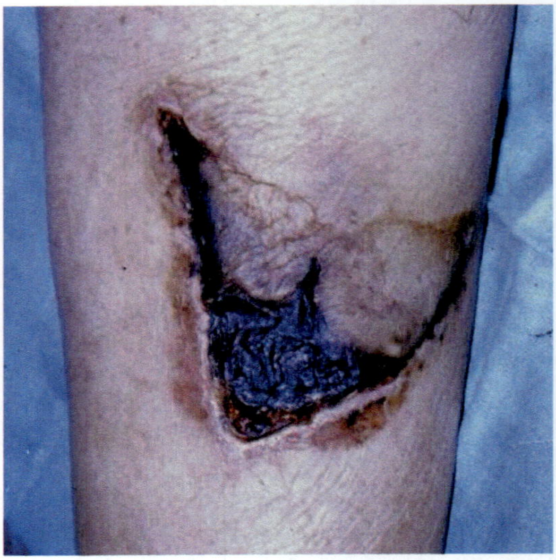

Fig. 9.5 Typical venous necrosis following the suturing of a triangular flap. Note the further zone of partial thickness loss

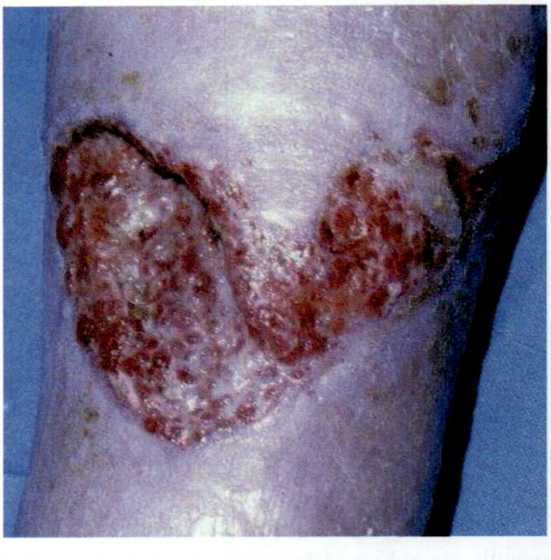

Fig. 9.6 Ragged, raw surface on the lower leg a month after a proximally based flap had been sutured back and died

The primary commitment to all wounds had to be safeguarding the existing circulation throughout the period of reactive swelling, replacing the concept of immediate coercive closure by one of accurate disposition, with or without sutures.

Encouraging free drainage of oedema from the wound vicinity had to be beneficial in terms

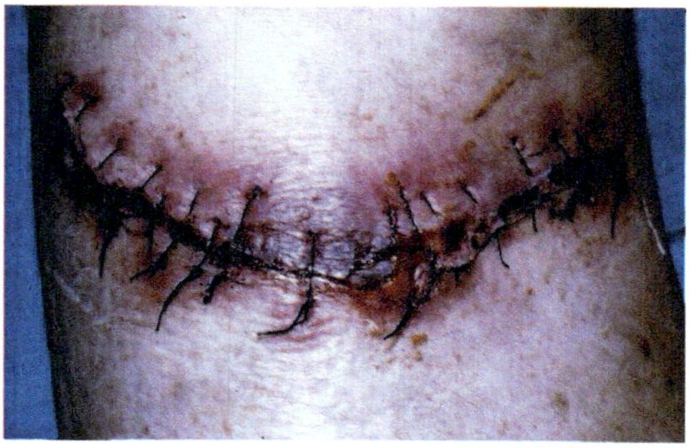

Fig. 9.7 Broad proximally based knee flap showing circulatory problems caused by sutures. Infection is already present. Taping this flap would have been a much safer option and additionally, the knee would have needed splinting

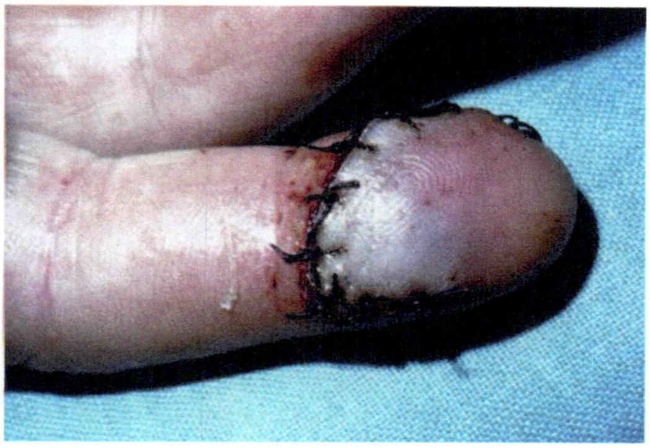

Fig. 9.8 Impending necrosis of a pulp flap on the day of injury. The patient returned with severe pain later the same day

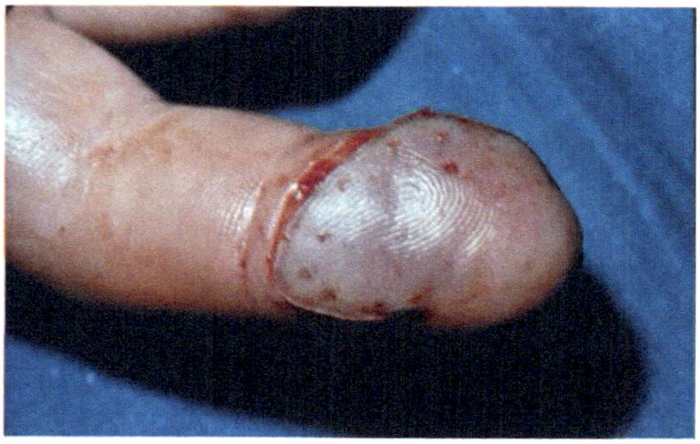

Fig. 9.9 Immediate relief of pain and recovery of the circulation followed the removal of sutures. Same day as Fig. 9.8. The finger proceeded to heal well with tulle dressings

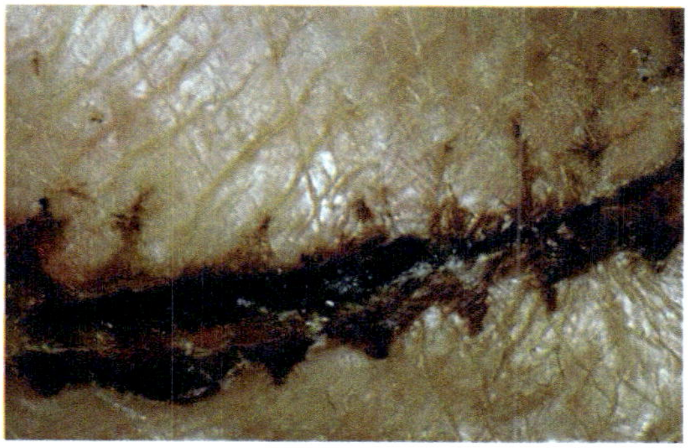

Fig. 9.10 Ten-day-old operation wound. The circulatory effects are clearly related to the sutures. They are worse in the distal flap. This loss of circulation is caused by venous stasis

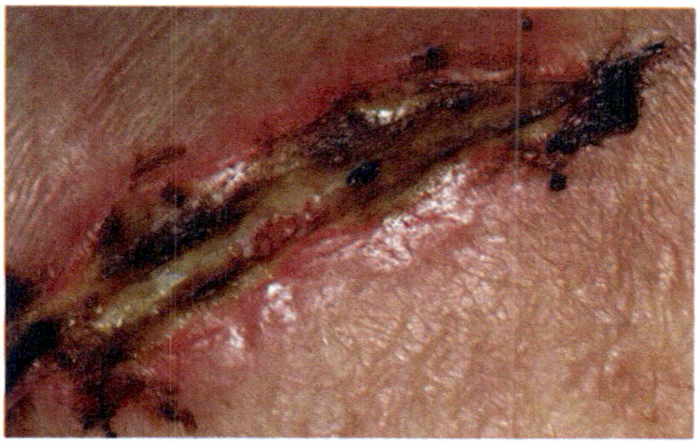

Fig. 9.11 Another part of the same wound as Fig. 9.10 shows suture-related slough separating slowly. This image is at 3 weeks post-surgery. Luckily no infection has occurred yet

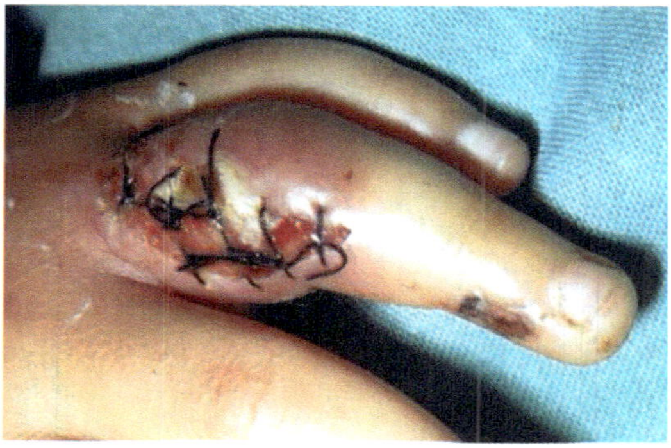

Fig. 9.12 This unhealthy infected wound has followed the inappropriate suturing of a crushed finger. The underlying fracture became infected. The eventual result was poor

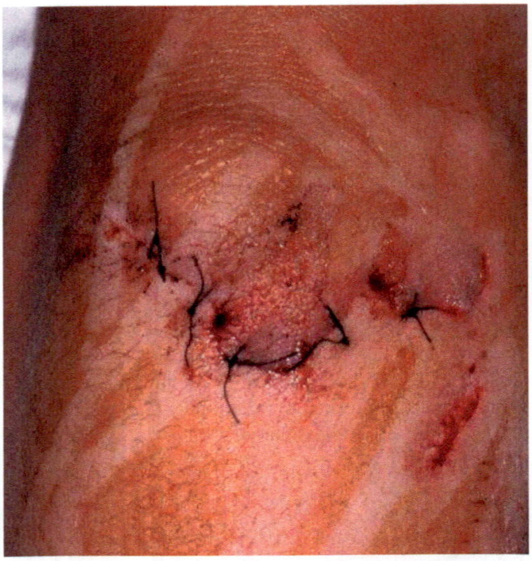

Fig. 9.13 A 5-day result where both tapes and sutures have been used. Minor congestion relates more particularly to the sutures

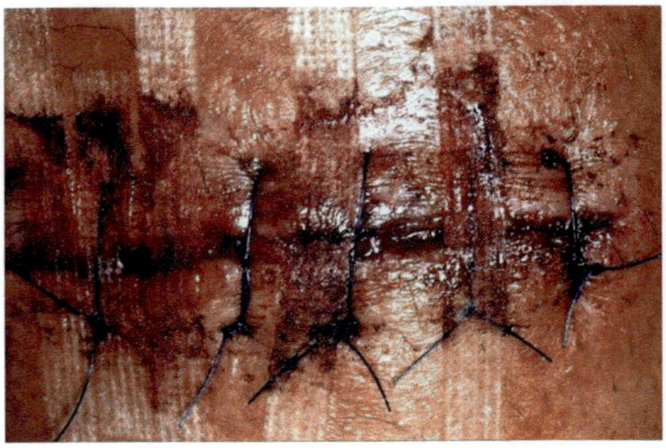

Fig. 9.14 A combination of sutures and tapes are providing fairly safe closure at 3 days. Note the slight oedema of the edges

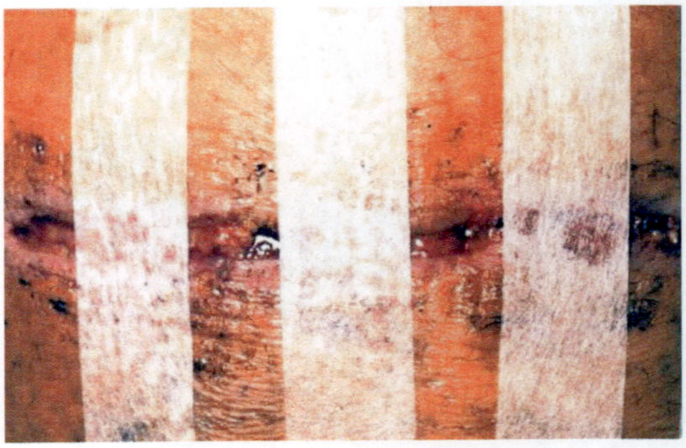

Fig. 9.15 Sutures were replaced by tapes, with a much quieter wound 3 days later

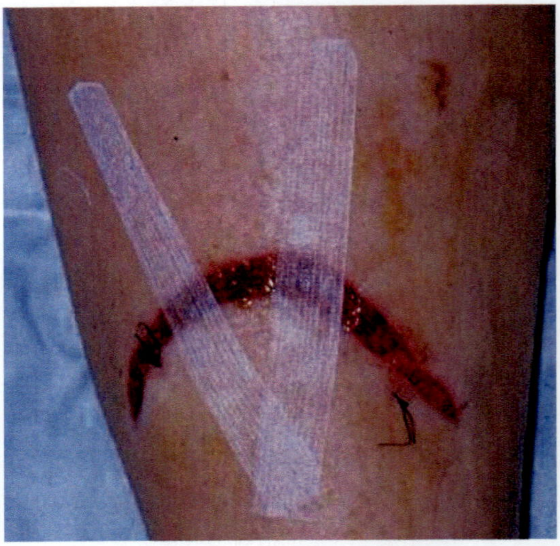

Fig. 9.16 A distally based flap has been taped on day 01. Full closure can be achieved by revising the taping in 3 days' time

of reducing tension. Wound infection seemed to be much more closely related to circulatory insufficiency rather than whether the closure was watertight or not, and free drainage **out** of a clean wound seemed a particularly unlikely basis for infection getting in.

Suturing is the standard way of accurately replacing and holding disrupted tissues back together. The public and many doctors expect wounds to be sutured, and indeed the number of skin sutures inserted is customarily used by lay people to convey the presumptive seriousness of their wounds. Managing acute wounds without sutures might in these terms be taken to indicate lesser injuries or more minor procedures. However, it can take more expertise to devise optimal wound care without sutures than it does to stitch everything up and instantly make it look deceptively good again.

Whenever tissues are not going to be held by traditional sutures, it is necessary to carefully explain the reasons for the alternative regime to

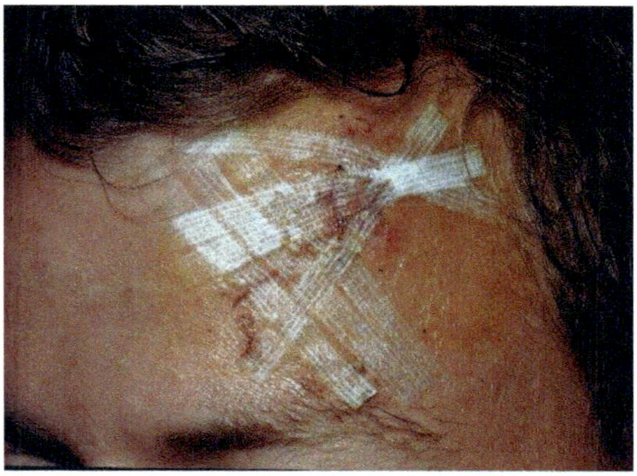

Fig. 9.17 A complicated laceration from a blow with a bottle has been very successfully treated with tapes. Uncomplicated result shown at 5 days

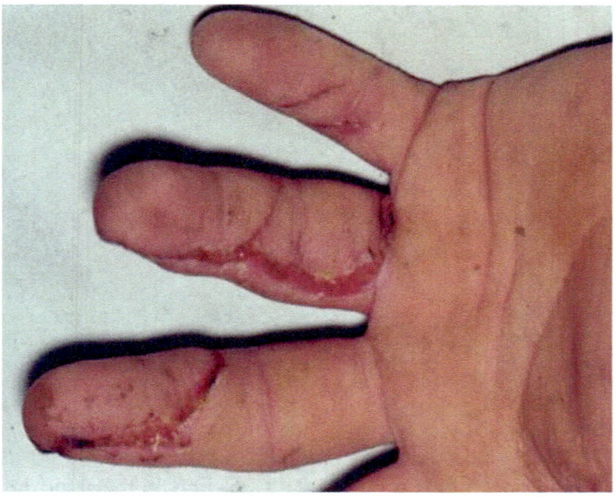

Fig. 9.19 The 10-day appearance after tulle gras stabilisation, gauze bandage, and splintage. The flaps are healthy, the swelling has resolved, and the hand is remarkably comfortable

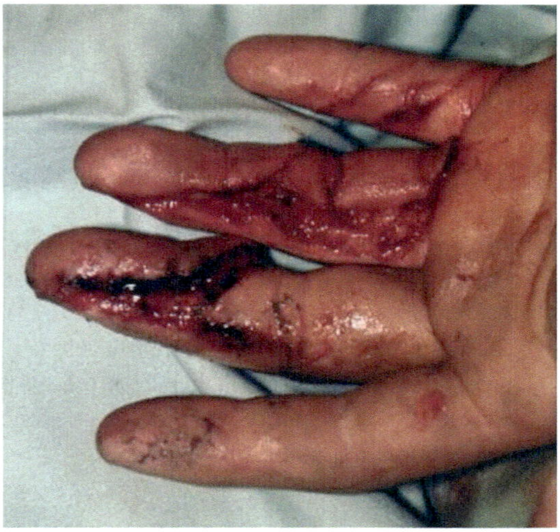

Fig. 9.18 Burst fingers from a pastry roller crush injury and the early appearance. The flaps look viable but swelling will develop

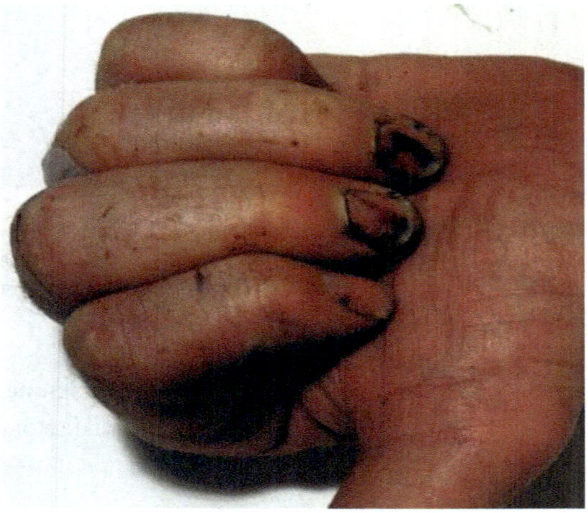

Fig. 9.20 At 3 weeks, the healed fingers flex comfortably into the palm already. The patient made a complete functional recovery

the patient, their relatives, and sometimes even their doctors. They are all otherwise liable to think that they and their wounds have been poorly treated. They may even go off in disgust to another clinic to get the wound 'stitched up properly'. My approach became simply to tell patients that much less suturing was being done these days, in order to safeguard the circulation. Not only was this the most modern, the very latest technique, but it also significantly reduced the level of post-operative pain. Patients invariably found these arguments compelling. Doctors were sometimes harder to convince, unless they were also the patient!

Removing early the clearly disadvantageous sutures that other doctors had inserted required a particularly diplomatic explanation (Figs. 9.21 and 9.22). '*Why would the doctor have put them all in then, if they weren't helpful?*', I remember being asked on a number of occasions. An excel-

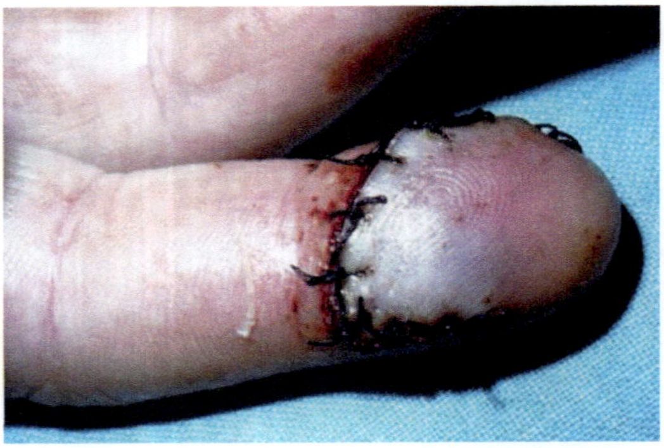

Fig. 9.21 Impending necrosis of a pulp flap sutured as shown. The patient returned with severe pain the same day

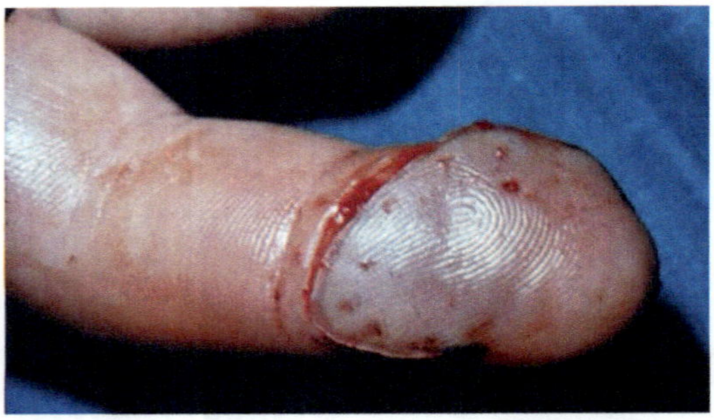

Fig. 9.22 With removal of the sutures, there was immediate relief of pain and the circulation to the pulp flap recovered. This is the same day as Fig. 9.21 and the finger healed well with tulle dressings

lent question indeed, the 64-million-dollar one, and one to which I did not have a satisfactory answer.

The Rationale for the Use of Sutures (to Be Always Weighed Against Their Disadvantages)

1. They hold tissue well, immediately restore the appearance, and clearly reassure most people, including most operators, that everything has been put right.
2. They are particularly useful in scalp wounds, and in eyebrows where perfusion is excellent and other methods of closure are inapplicable, or where dressings are difficult.
3. They allow early movement without disruption of the wound.

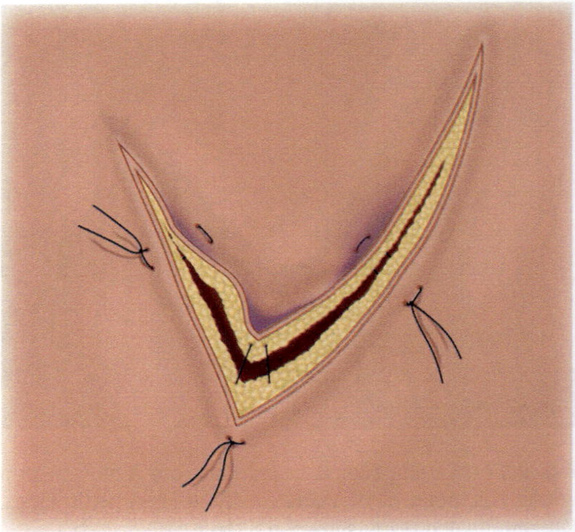

Fig. 9.23 'Guy-rope' tethering. Small mattress sutures are being used to evert rolling edges. Stretching this flap out to size will only worsen the already obvious venous congestion

4. After a day or two, a sutured wound can be left without dressings.
5. Small accurate tacking sutures may at times be useful adjuncts to other treatments.
6. Small mattress sutures can be used as 'guy-ropes' to evert the edges or points of tissue where these are rolling under (Fig. 9.23). These tethering sutures do not necessarily have to be pulled up to achieve perfect closure, unless it is safe to do this. Tapes alone cannot control such thin rolled edges.

Summary of the Adverse Effects of Sutures

1. Each suture encloses a **plane** of tissue (Fig. 9.24) across which there is reduced or obstructed venous flow, and this effect worsens with swelling. Other effects arising from this phenomenon then depend on suture patterns and relationships.
2. Each stitch across a laceration also creates **four triangular flaps,** which tend to develop venous congestion especially at their tips (Figs. 9.25 and 9.26).
3. Every two adjacent sutures along a laceration create a rectangular 'flap' on each side of the

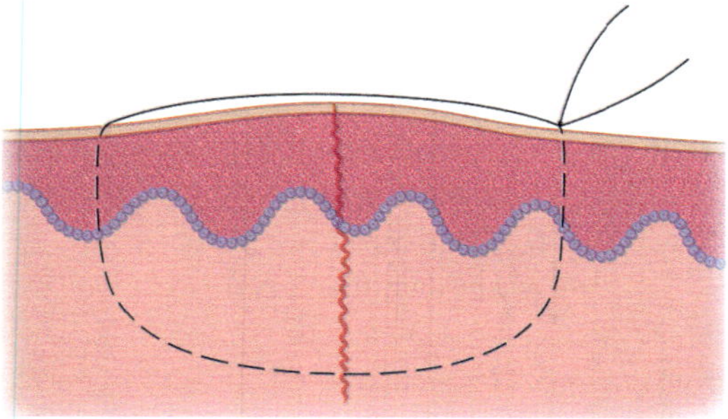

Fig. 9.24 Each suture encloses a plane of tissue capable of obstructing the venous flow across it

wound between them (Figs. 9.27, 9.28 and 9.29). It therefore makes a huge difference whether these 'flaps' created by the suture pattern are broad and shallow or long and narrow. If similar 'flaps' had been created by a series of scalpel cuts, the operator's sanity would have to be seriously in doubt.

4. When a laceration is transverse, the adverse effects of suturing will always be worse along the distal edge, which has an interrupted venous and lymphatic return, as well as a reduced arterial input (Figs. 9.30, 9.31, and 9.32).

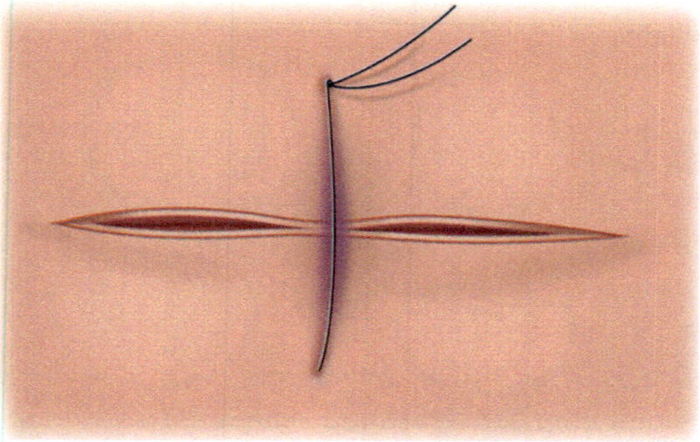

Fig. 9.25 Sutures across wound edges create subsidiary triangular flaps. Each suture creates congestion towards the tips of the four triangular flaps it forms with the wound edges

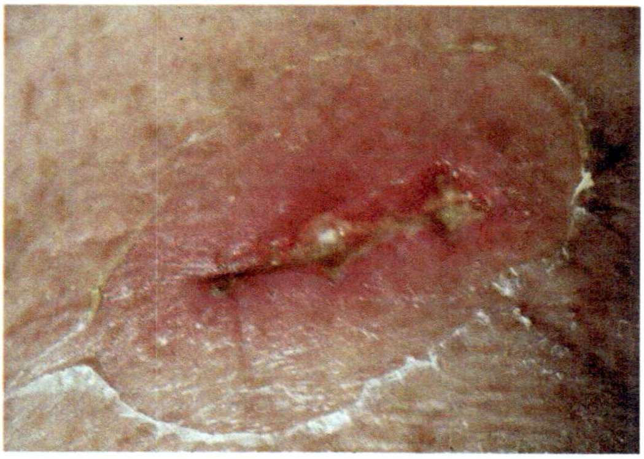

Fig. 9.26 The loss of edge circulation here is clearly related to the initial sutures. The associated infection has required antibiotic treatment and is now settling

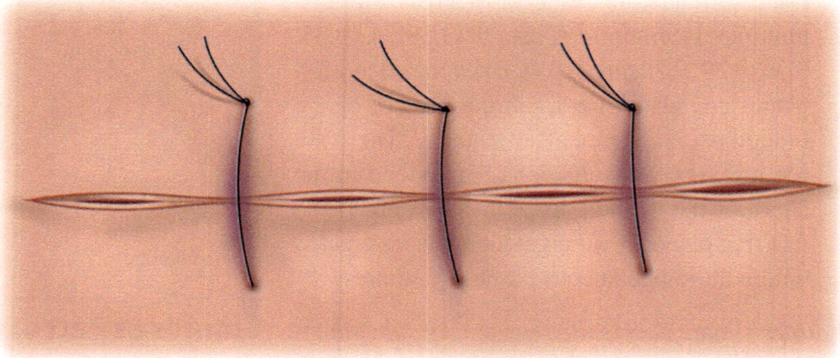

Fig. 9.27 Every two sutures create flaps between them. Rectangular flaps along each side of the wound are showing venous congestion related to the sutures

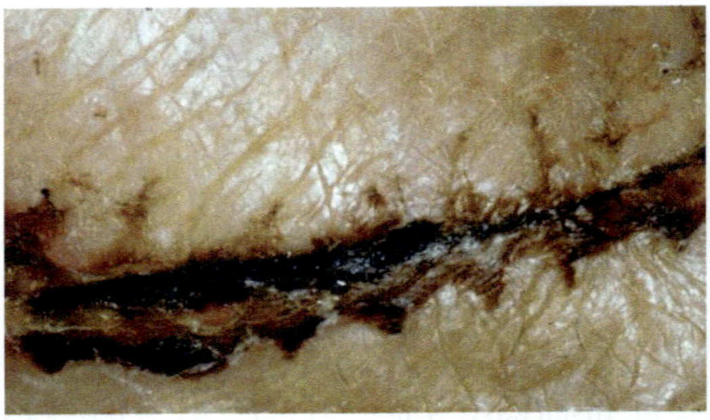

Fig. 9.28 Ten-day-old operation wound. The circulatory effects are clearly related to the sutures. They are worse in the distal flap. This loss of circulation is from venous stasis

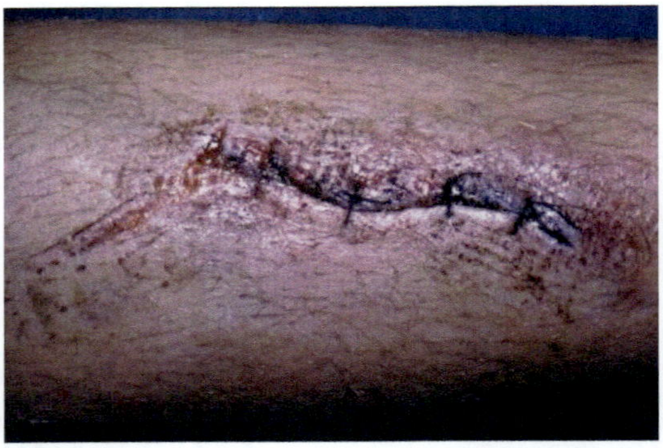

Fig. 9.29 Five days after suturing of a scrape to the front of the shin. This loss of circulation is from venous stasis of the flap. The shelving flap shows some edge congestion. This wound would have been much more safely helped with tulle or tapes

5. Sutures can create **tension planes between them** within tissues, especially across flaps and multiple lacerations (Figs. 9.33, 9.34, 9.35, 9.36, 9.37, 9.38, and 9.39). Unexpected tension planes can also arise when the posture of the injured part is altered **after** suturing. These are not just surface phenomena, but extend to the depth of the sutures. Equally important is the fact that planes of strangulation can be created within the subcutaneous tissues by sutures.

Editors' Note *This is the reason why subcutaneous or deep sutures are never used in the Keystone Perforator Island local flap technique of Felix Behan.*

6. **Circumferential bands of tension** around digits or limbs can also be created by sutures (Fig. 9.40)

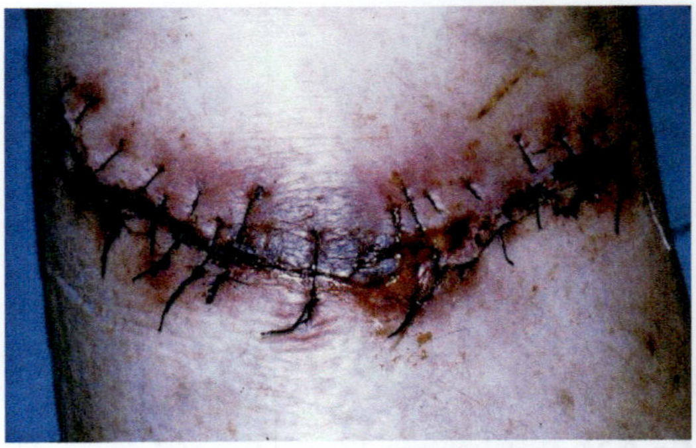

Fig. 9.30 Broad proximally based knee flap showing circulatory problems caused by sutures. Infection is already present. Taping this flap would have been a much safer option and additionally, the knee would have needed splinting

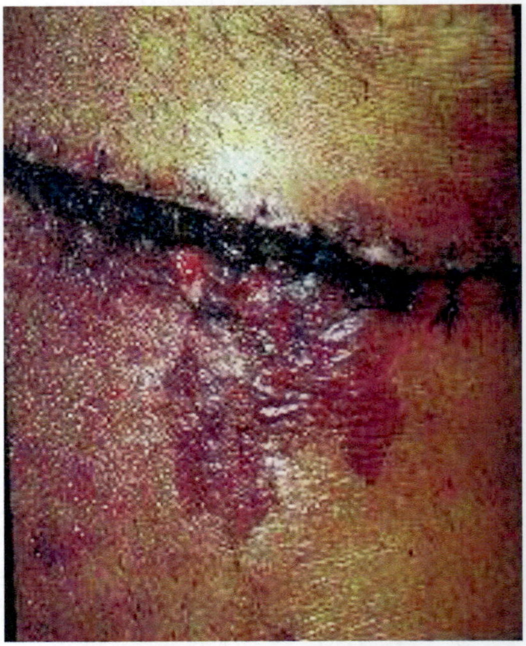

Fig. 9.31 Ten-day result of suturing a transverse knee flap. The venous insufficiency is typically more marked in the distal edge

Sutures as Part of a Closure Concept

In general, the smaller the sutures and the further apart they are, the less they affect the circulation to the wound edge. Focal dragging tension is sometimes created by individual stitches, and this effect is reduced by using tapes between the

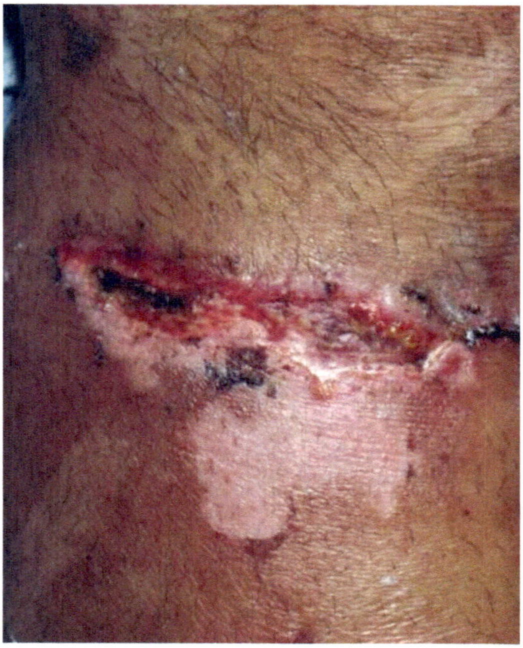

Fig. 9.32 The full effects of the suturing in Fig. 9.31 were clearly evident 6 weeks later, showing both partial and full thickness skin destruction

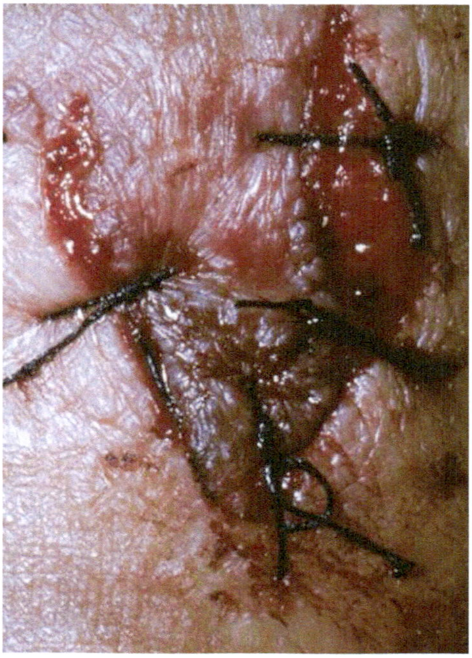

Fig. 9.34 Classic triangular flap showing the bands of tension between sutures, which are restricting the venous circulation

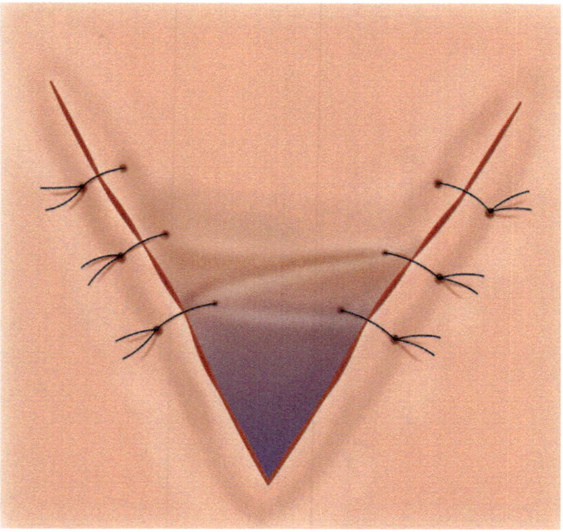

Fig. 9.33 Suturing flaps can create tension bands which worsen venous drainage. Venous congestion is increased towards the tip of this replaced flap, and tension bands across the flap created by the sutures are worsening this problem

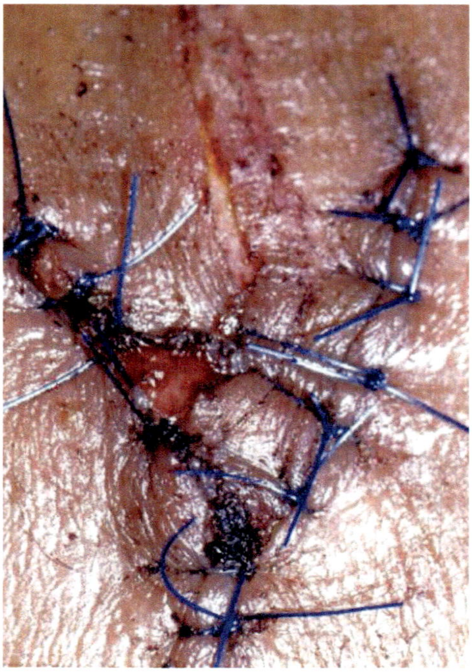

Fig. 9.35 Y-shaped laceration 3 days after routine suturing. Apart from oedema, it is almost looking alright

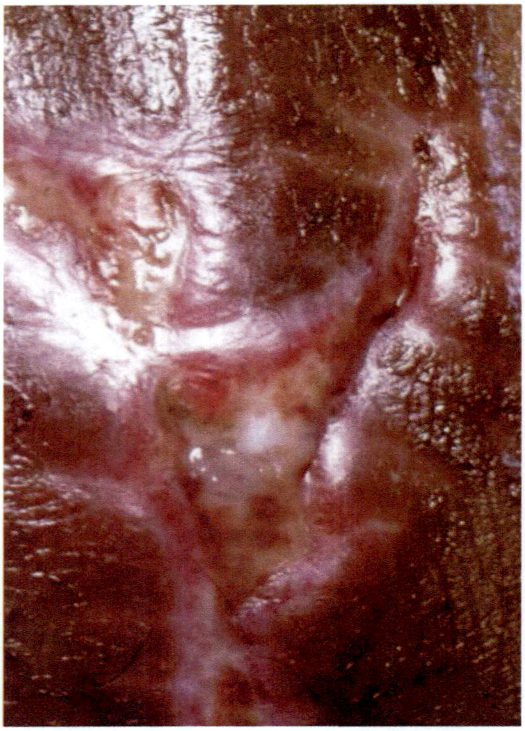

Fig. 9.36 The destructive effects of the suturing shown in Fig. 9.35 are more clearly reflected in the poor result at 6 weeks

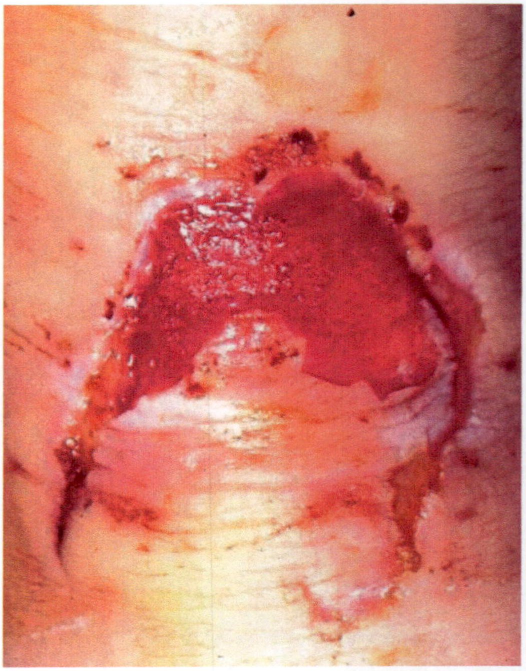

Fig. 9.38 The partial-thickness damage was apparent 5 days later. Plantar flexion and tulle would have been safer. Necrosis of this flap would have been disastrous

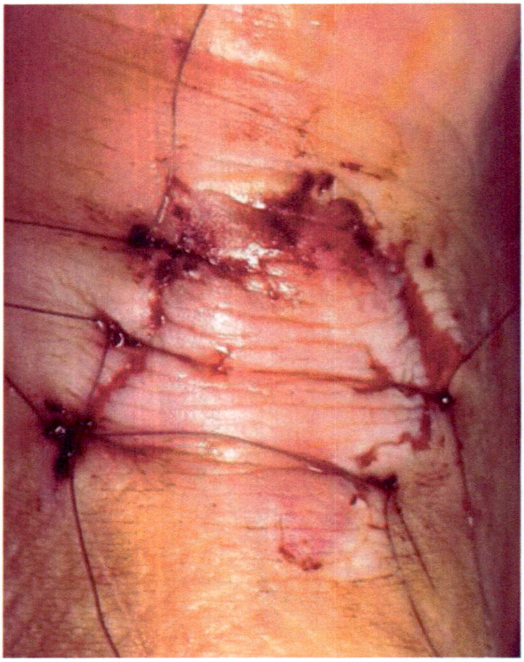

Fig. 9.37 Three-day-old heel flap showing transverse bands of tension caused by the ill-advised suturing

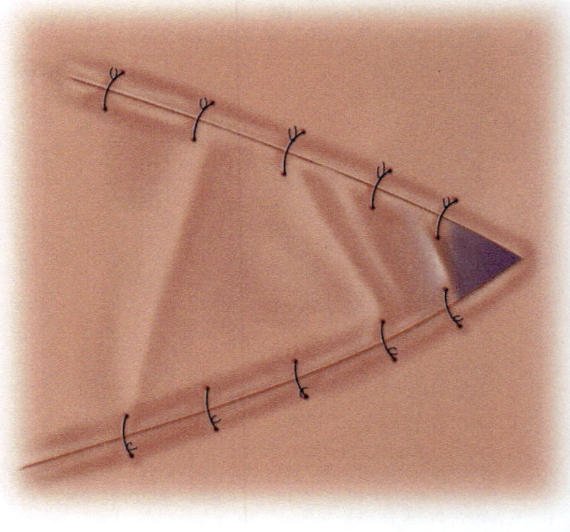

Fig. 9.39 This diagram replicates a physical paper model that Dr Chapple used to teach the dangers of flap closure. Tension bands interrupting the flap circulation are demonstrated. Most of the flap will die unless it is allowed to relax. If it does not recover a reasonable circulation, some of it may need to be turned into a graft [see details of this surgical technique in Chap. 10 Flaps and Grafts]

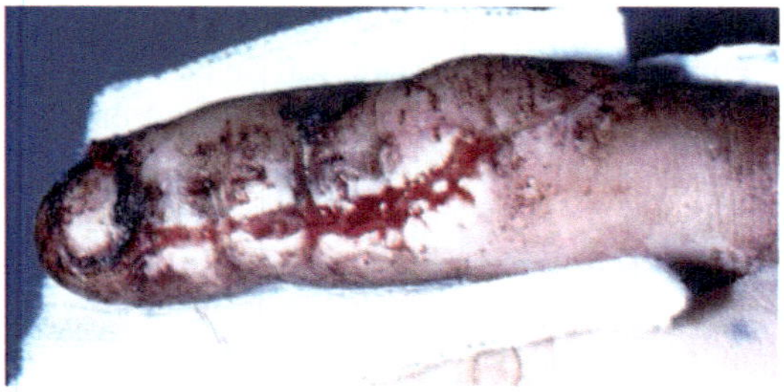

Fig. 9.40 The 7-day result of suturing a burst finger. Sutures have caused circumferential constriction and oedema. White skin is just wet

sutures, rather than inserting more and more sutures (Figs. 9.41, 9.42, 9.43, and 9.44).

The safety of sutures is enhanced by considering the effect of each one before it is inserted, being aware of its relationship to others, and if possible, incorporating measures to reduce general tension in the wound vicinity by the use of long tapes and/or by posturing adjacent joints. It is important that posturing for this purpose, or to protect joint function, be done **before** any type of closure, because tissue tensions are always radi-

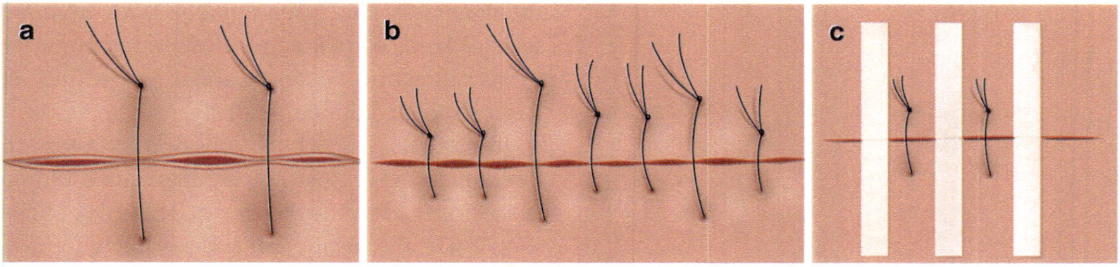

Fig. 9.41 (**a**–**c**) Additional sutures can be counterproductive. (**a**) The two sutures are producing some venous congestion and there is some gaping. (**b**) The insertion of more sutures accentuates the venous difficulties along the edge. (**c**) using tapes to close the gaping actually improves the situation by relieving the focal tension

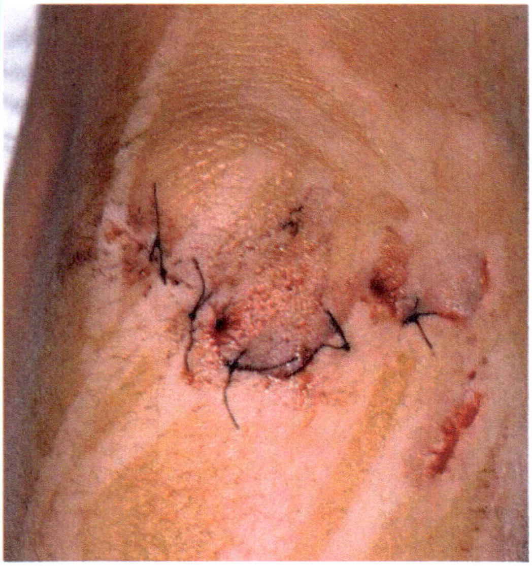

Fig. 9.42 A 5-day result where both tapes and sutures have been used. Minor congestion relates more particularly to the sutures

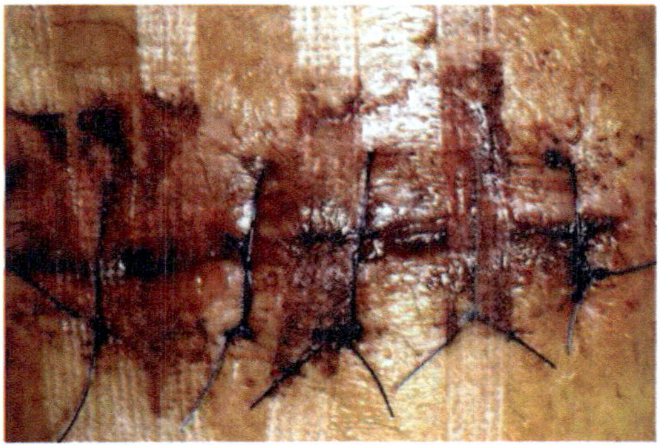

Fig. 9.43 A combination of sutures and tapes are providing fairly safe closure at 3 days. Note the slight oedema of the edges

cally altered by changing joint position. The soft tissues of the body are differentially mobile as adjacent bones and joints are moved about.

Nowhere is it written on stone tablets, ***'Thou shalt pull up all sutures fully'.*** The first consideration when there is a simple open wound with no tissue missing is to see how safely the edges can be brought together, without necessarily being committed to full elimination of the gap. Small guy-rope mattress sutures may be helpful to evert rolled edges, but do not have to be pulled up tightly unless this is safe for the circulation.

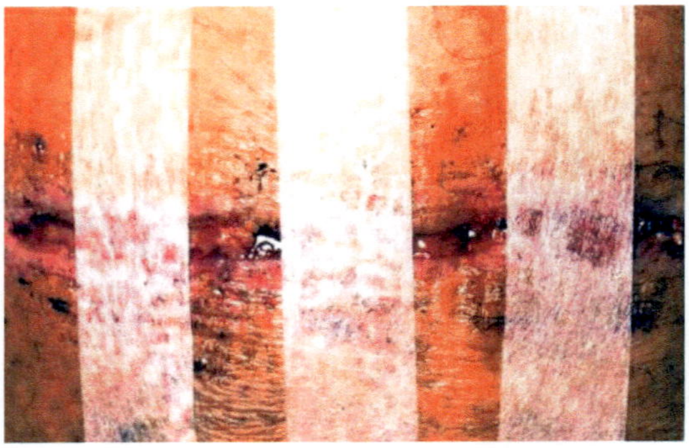

Fig. 9.44 Sutures were replaced by tapes, with a much quieter wound 3 days later

Sutures can also be either tightened or loosened if they are tied in the 'half hitch' manner, and then locked off eventually by knots tied in a running configuration (Fig. 9.45: Keystone flap suture method). Sutures must be loosened, removed, or replaced whenever they are noticed to be restricting the circulation. Gaps between sutures often diminish or disappear during the phase of post-injury tissue swelling, but if still present at the first dressing change can usually be closed by serial re-taping. Healthy gaps heal spontaneously and very quickly, with minimal scar. When wound edges lose circulation or wound infection delays healing, this results in considerable additional scarring.

In injuries caused by crushing or bursting mechanisms (Fig. 9.46) where there are multiple lacerations close together, or complex flaps (Fig. 9.47), the local circulation is likely to have been affected so significantly by the injury that the added imposition of suturing is particularly inappropriate.

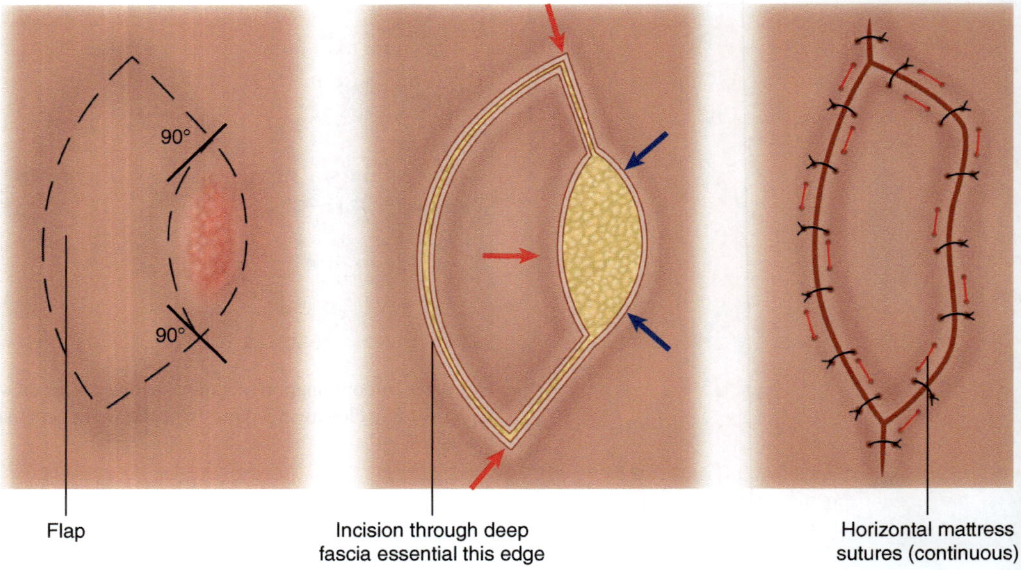

Fig. 9.45 Keystone Flap suture method using interrupted 'half hitch' tacking sutures (black) to locate the flap in the defect followed by horizontal mattress running continuous sutures (red). With permission from Springer Nature, *Simply Local Flaps [Springer International Publishing 2018]*

Repositioning of such disrupted wounds accurately with tulle, tapes, and dressings, after selecting the optimal posture, will give the tissues the best chance of avoiding circulatory complications. The loss of viability of flaps overlying important structures, especially about the hand, can be particularly disastrous (Figs. 9.48 and 9.49).

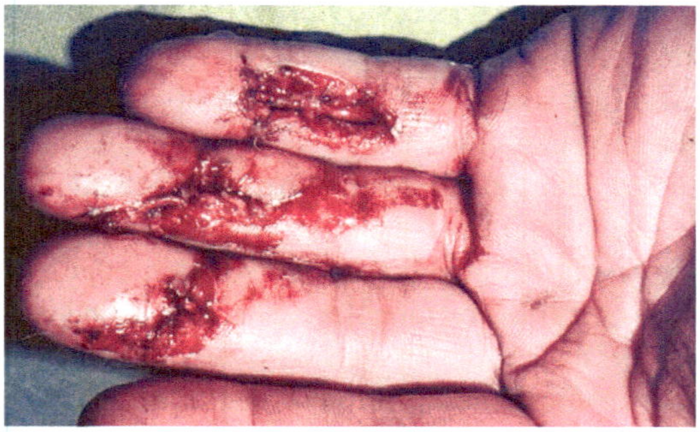

Fig. 9.46 Early appearance of crushed fingers, particularly unsuitable for suturing

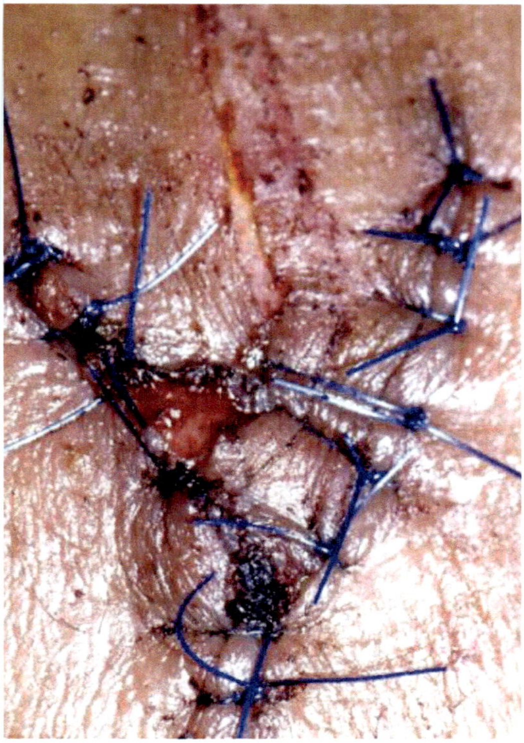

Fig. 9.47 Y-shaped flap laceration 3-days after suturing

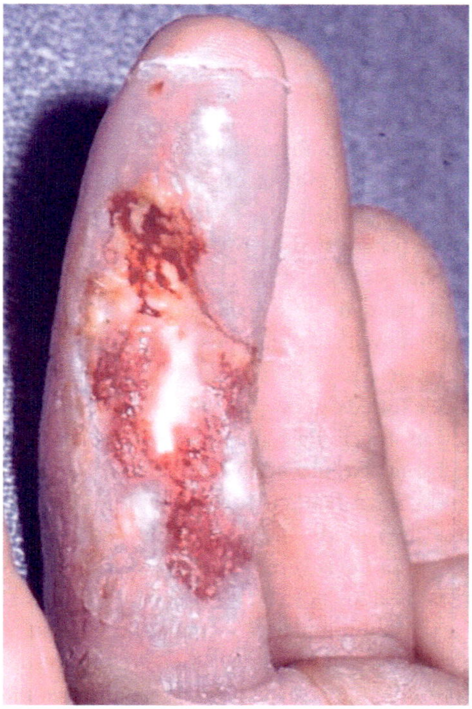

Fig. 9.48 Deep destruction down to tendon followed the suturing of a burst finger

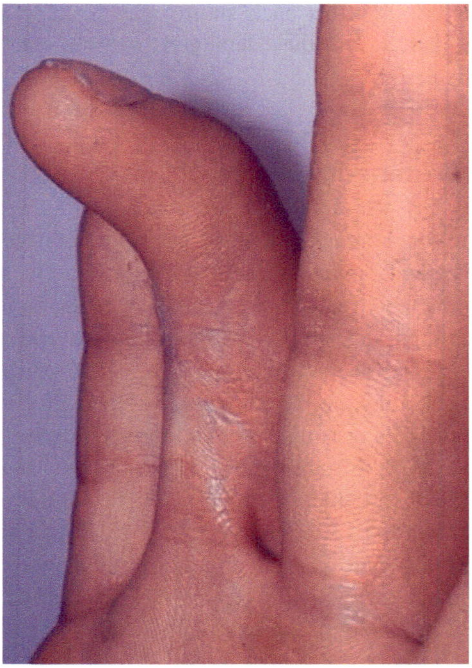

Fig. 9.49 Permanent and severe flexion contracture of the same finger inevitably followed healing and was untreatable

Suture Materials

Skin Sutures

Interrupted non-absorbable sutures are best for skin. Although 3-0 is often used in sites other than hands and faces, 5-0 is more than strong enough for most skin. Monofilament sutures are technically more difficult to use than braided thread, but cause less irritation. There are several excellent synthetic varieties. **Silk should no longer be used**. The concept of absorbable skin sutures sounds good, but often they cause more reaction for longer than non-absorbable ones, which can be replaced by tapes within a few days. Continuous subcuticular absorbable sutures often cause low-grade irritation and inflammation throughout the several weeks they take to absorb. The body does not particularly like the intrusion of any foreign material so the fewer and smaller the stitches, and the sooner they are removed, the less trouble they cause. It is a great pity that many doctors get so distracted by the variety and qualities of the different suture materials now available that the more vital question of what deleterious effect each suture may have on the circulation of the damaged skin is rarely considered.

Subcutaneous Sutures

Flaps or separated planes of tissue do not need to be tacked down, as they will more safely and comfortably reattach themselves once the wound dressings and supportive bandages are applied. Injuries to deep structures, such as tendons and nerves, may need treatment by specialist surgeons. Ties or sutures applied to bleeders should always be of absorbable material and small. Small absorbable 3-0 or 4-0 synthetic sutures can be helpful to accurately align fascial layers or dermis. Sutures enclosing larger quantities of subcutaneous fat are particularly dangerous as they are liable to interfere markedly with circulation. Not surprisingly, there is evidence that wound infection can be related to overzealous subcutaneous suturing. In the face, where circulation is good, accurate approximation of subcutaneous layers by absorbable sutures is needed because important muscles of expression in this layer are often divided. The sutures can be inserted upside down if they are close to skin, with the knots buried deeply, to avoid them poking through the wound.

Technical Aspects of Skin Suturing

Accurate suturing of a wound involves aligning the two sides correctly. This may sometimes be a matter of trial and error. When the laceration is vertical, that is, not shelving, the ideal is to insert the needle vertically into the first skin edge and take up a small rectangular block of skin and dermis with a little fat and in a second separate movement come up through a similar block on the opposite edge, to exit the skin vertically the same distance out from the second wound edge as the initial entry. The thread is then pulled through until only a short length remains to tie with. This will produce a stitch that will oppose and evert the edges very accurately with minimum tension (Fig. 9.50a–c).

Pushing a curved needle through both edges in one manoeuvre often inverts the skin edges, requiring an additional vertical mattress suture to correct this (Fig. 9.51a–c).

It is better not to do a mattress stitch unless it is absolutely necessary, as it interferes more with the circulation and also leaves more buried foreign material, possibly causing more inflammation.

Excessive use of forceps is also damaging to skin edges. Using non-toothed forceps simply crushes tissue. The use of the needle alone or with a small-toothed pair of forceps, used as a hook, is the least traumatic technique.

The first part of the knot should be tied with one turn only, turning the long, needle end of the thread into a half-hitch around the short end at the original entry, forming the beginning of the knot on one side of the wound. Instead of pulling on both threads evenly and tying a running knot across the wound, the half-hitch is created by pulling vertically on the tail of the thread at the initial entry point, which turns the long thread from lying as a running knot into a half-hitch across the short end (Fig. 9.52).

The second turn can be done in the same or the reverse direction, with one turn only, tying it on top of the first as another half-hitch, so that eventually the thread entering the skin passes through two half-hitches (Fig. 9.53).

At this point, the suture can be drawn up with the main tension retained in the vertical thread and the half-hitches being slid down it against the skin, on one side of the wound. If this doesn't hold, a third half-hitch can be added, but at this point it is worthwhile pausing to re-evaluate the total tension and the circulatory effect which is being developed by the suture. It is not necessary to be committed to complete approximation of the edges unless that is safe. At this stage, the whole suture can still be either tightened, and also loosened, until the optimum tension and degree of closure is achieved. The knot can then finally be locked off with two or three ordinary running knots (Fig. 9.54). Monofilament nylon may need several more locking knots than a braided thread.

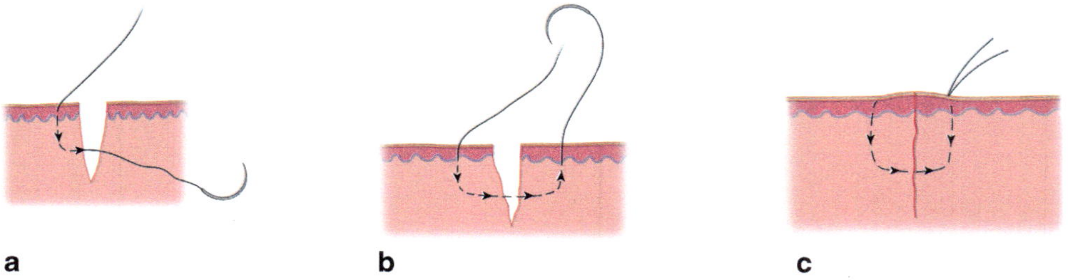

Fig. 9.50 (**a**–**c**) The insertion of a standard suture. (**a**) Each side of the wound is secured in a separate manoeuvre taking up a roughly right-angled block of tissue. (**b**) The needle should exit from the skin on the opposite side of the wound the same distance from the edge as the initial entry. (**c**) The suture is more accurate in everting if tied against one or other side of the wound

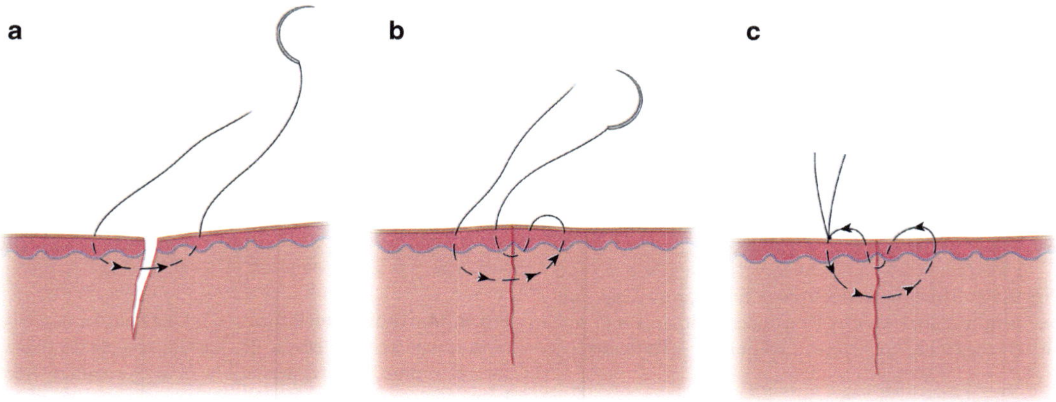

Fig. 9.51 (**a**–**c**) One manoeuvre suture requiring a vertical mattress: (**a**) The needle has been pushed through both edges of the wound and these are likely to invert. (**b**) A second manoeuvre returning through both edges as a mattress stitch will be required. (**c**) The mattress suture is then tied on the original side. A simple accurate suture is less intrusive and much easier to remove

Once this technique is mastered, suturing becomes very easy. Tension can then be carefully selected, as distinct from the situation where running knots may either lock or slip. The use of several running turns on the initial knot in a desperate attempt to get the wound to stay closed initially makes for an excessively wide first knot, which often bunches up when the second running knot is tied on top of it. It is not reliably adjustable.

If the wound is shelving, it is best to start on the thicker side and to come back beneath the thin edge **[subdermally]** and finally back through the original edge as a small vertical mattress stitch (Fig. 9.55a–c). This is also known as the Gillies' 3-point suture.

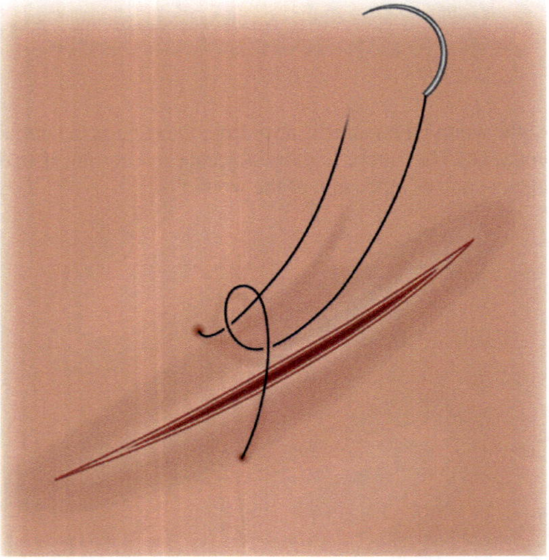

Fig. 9.52 The first manoeuvre in tying knots. Using only one turn, the first knot is tensioned to lie as a half hitch around the initial entry thread by pulling it vertically

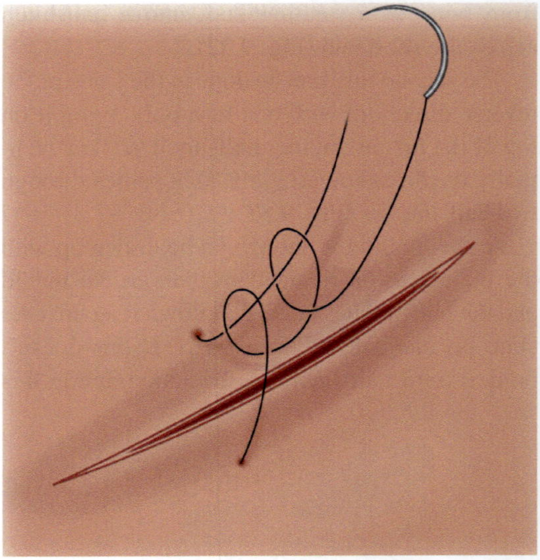

Fig. 9.53 Tying the second half-hitch to create the adjustable knot

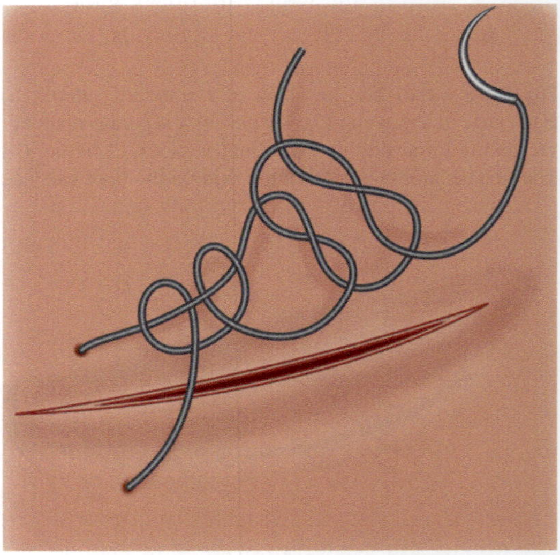

Fig. 9.54 The completed locked knot. Once the degree of closure has been selected, the knot is completed by two further running knots, preferably tied as a square [reef] knot

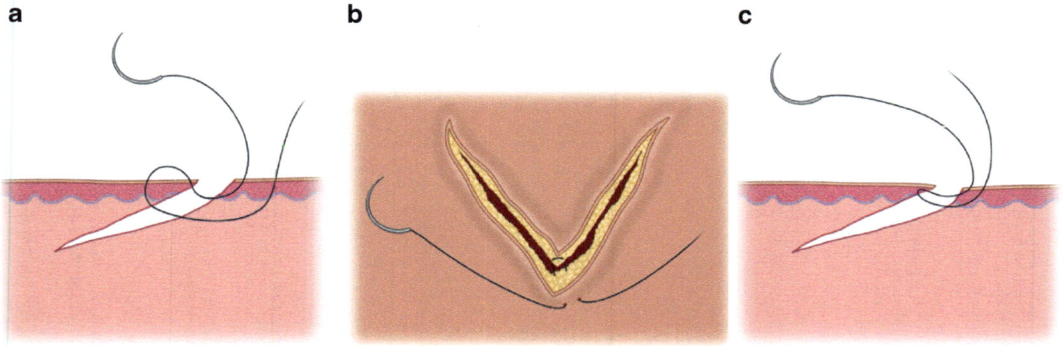

Fig. 9.55 (**a–c**) Suturing a shelving edge. A subdermal mattress suture is best for a shelving laceration or the tip of a flap, but it is often unwise to attempt to replace flaps fully with sutures

Mattress Sutures

Mattress sutures all take a return course through each edge of the wound and can be executed as a ***vertical mattress***, which may be useful for everting a rolled edge or approximating edges in a concavity or a ***horizontal mattress*** which raises and affects the circulation of the wound edge even more, if too tight! (Fig. 9.56 and 9.57).

All mattress sutures affect the circulation more than simple ones and are rarely necessary except in concavities. They are much more complicated to remove. *MFK strongly believes all sutures affect the circulation and it is a matter of surgical skill/judgement in application.*

Editors' Note *Subcuticular or intradermal suturing using absorbable materials. While this suturing technique is perhaps more suited to use in elective surgical wounds, it should not be excluded for selected clean traumatic wounds with little tissue damage. Joan Chapple probably would not have approved of the method, since the common absorbable suture materials available during most of her career, such as various forms of 'catgut', were absorbed by phagocytosis, associated with marked tissue inflammation. In contrast, modern monofilament materials highly suited to this technique (for example, polydioxanone) are degraded by hydrolysis and cause very minimal foreign body reaction in tissue.*

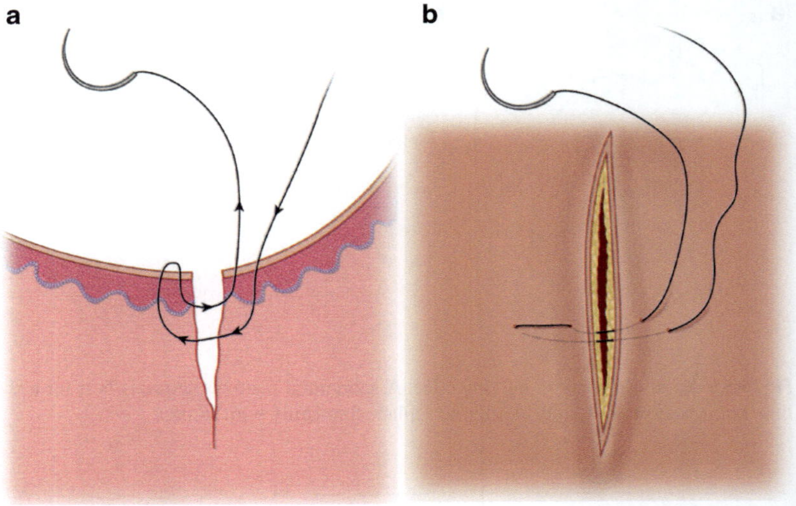

Fig. 9.56 (**a**, **b**) Vertical mattress suture. Following the initial bites through both edges, the needle is returned taking a tiny piece from each edge again

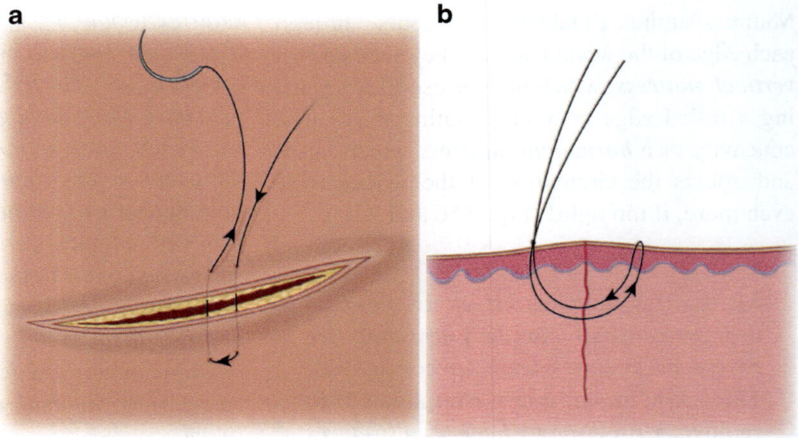

Fig. 9.57 (**a**, **b**) Horizontal mattress suture. The return stitch is the same size as the original and lies beside it. This suture interferes quite markedly with the circulation of the block of tissue enclosed within it

Removal of Sutures

Sutures can and should be snipped whenever they are tight or removed altogether if they become the focus of inflammation. The wound and the patient will both benefit dramatically. Tight sutures snipped within a day or two of insertion are best not actually removed immediately. They are still of some use in a splinting function, are no longer doing harm, and their early removal may be unnecessarily painful or cause bleeding. Removal of cut sutures can be left until the wound is quieter when it then needs to be securely supported with tapes. Wound inflammation and sepsis are often associated with the circulatory effect of individual sutures (Fig. 9.58a, b).

Established wound infection will settle much more quickly if all the sutures or at least the offending tight sutures are replaced with tapes.

If sutures become involved with craggy blood clot, it may be helpful to apply very greasy tulle and send the patients away for a few days to shower and apply cream or Vaseline™, before attempting suture removal. This technique is especially worthwhile for scalp lacerations.

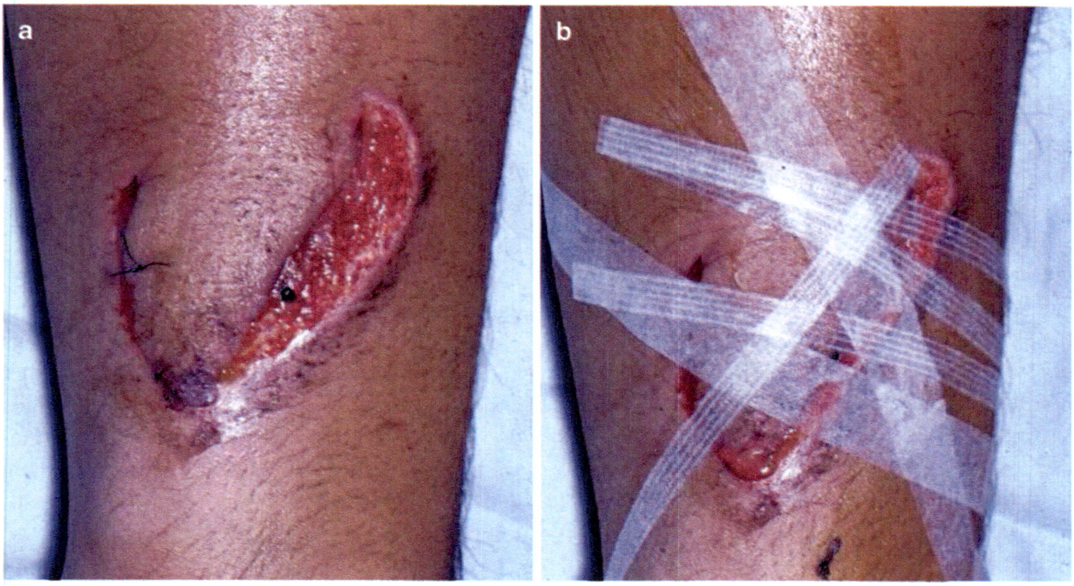

Fig. 9.58 (**a**, **b**) A large healthy traumatic flap 5 days after one suture was inserted and a simple dressing applied. At this time, the suture was removed and the flap then redistributed by skin tapes

When sutures have not been used or where suture closure has been only partially achieved because of tension, a review at 3-5 days usually presents an ideal opportunity to bring about a more complete closure with tapes as swelling is subsiding. To apply tapes properly, the skin first needs to be shaved, cleaned, and dried, then painted with Tincture of Benzoin, which is left to dry. Local anaesthesia is necessary if formal secondary suturing is to be undertaken.

A healthy wound has usually developed enough strength by 5–6 days to withstand the replacement of sutures by tapes. Using tape support for all wounds for several days following suture removal is always a good policy. Some wounds may look well-healed but on close inspection after suture removal have obviously not done much healing. It is particularly important that such wounds are well taped for a further week or two to prevent them bursting open. Patients can keep tape support on for longer than this if they lead a particularly active life, especially with wounds on the back, which are rather slow to heal. Taping wounds for several weeks (or months) may discourage scars from widening.

The Technique of Suture Removal

Snip all sutures selected for removal before removing any of them, especially in children. Once suture removal has become an ordeal, the patient is unlikely to be able to stay still enough for accurate snipping of the remainder. Snipped sutures can and will then come out with dressings or in the shower if formal removal becomes difficult. Sutures are best snipped with fine sharp iris scissors, inserting the lower blade under the visible thread before cutting it. It may be useful to hold onto the knot, but it is not usually necessary to pull on it at this stage. Lifting knots may be necessary in the removal of mattress sutures when no suture material can be located on the side opposite the knot. It is important to isolate and cut only one thread in order not to leave suture material buried within the tissues where it can give rise to an abscess or discharging sinus.

When sutures are being lifted out, it is very much less painful if the skin doesn't get pulled. The slightly open points of the scissors laid on the skin on each side of the thread work admirably to prevent skin distortion. A quick pluck holding onto a thread or the knot is better than a slow pull. Some sutures will cause more pain than others and the main thing is to keep talking to patients and reassuring them how well they and you are getting on. It is often helpful to take a short pause intermittently for everyone to recollect their composure. Sutures that are neither inflamed nor tight can always be left for another occasion. ***This does risk the complication of suture scarring*** [Fig. 9.59]. If this happens along the length of a wound, it results in 'railroad' scarring, which is all too common, and usually blamed on the patient's skin. Like any other surgical procedure, suture removal depends on meticulous attention to detail and it can be done well or badly.

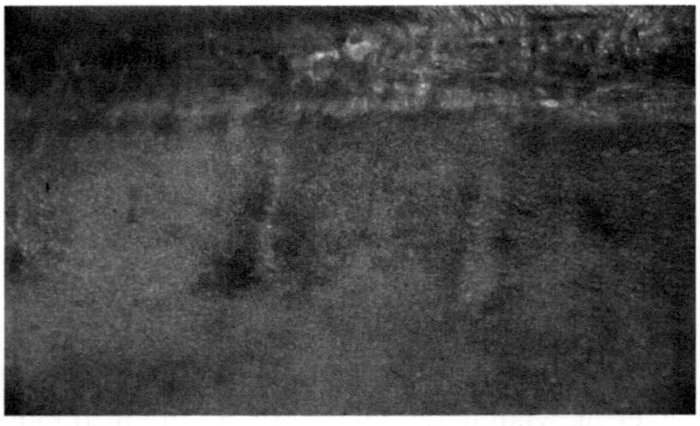

Fig. 9.59 Unacceptable 'railroad' scar markings caused by tissue death in the planes enclosed by tight sutures, which have become planes of permanent scar tissue. ***This can also be the result of sutures being left in too long!***

Alternative Closures

For many simple wounds, it is acceptable to use other means of closure rather than sutures. It is important that the use of tapes is not used as an excuse to not fully diagnose or clean wounds. Sterile skin tapes are easy to use and effective once the skin is clean and dry. If longer tapes are needed, 1 cm medical tape [such as Micropore™] can be used off a roll. If this is not available, clean tape of any kind may be used. Dressings and the elasticity of crepe bandages further assists closure, especially in the limbs. If wounds do need exploration and cleansing and anaesthesia is unavailable, it is better to leave them open and simply cover them in a surgically clean fashion until they can be adequately treated.

When suturing compromises the skin circulation, taping may provide safer closure. It is necessary to use careful judgement even with tapes, as to the amount of tension that can be applied to an acute wound, because maximum swelling is yet to come. Broad support by means of tulle gras is the safest technique of all for crushed tissue and complex injuries. ***The relaxation of injured tissue by posturing adjacent joints always improves the circulation and safely assists closure.***

It is especially important not to apply tapes across acute flaps or circumferentially around newly injured digits.

Taping between sutures is preferable to the option of closing gaps with additional sutures. The application of a transverse tape across the ends of the longitudinal ones on each side of the wound will confer further security to a tape closure. The reattachment of deeper layers is best allowed to happen spontaneously.

When closure has not been fully achieved at the primary procedure, tapes or secondary suture can improve on it, particularly at 3–4 days, just as there is some tissue slack returning to the system. It can be seen that wound closure is sometimes more appropriately regarded as a progressive process, which can be assisted by on-going professional attention.

Commentary by Dr Peter J Bovey MBBS (Hons) FRACS

Suturing wounds remains the most common way of closing them. Reading this chapter made me realise that it's become a bit dated. Accurately apposing well-vascularised tissues without undue tension has always been an underlying principle of all surgery. Dr Joan Chapple is focused on principally traumatic wounds rather than elective incisions and as such the basic surgical principles remain unchanged.

Modern surgical tools now exist to help us assess the vascularity of soft tissues including Indocyanine green fluorescence, tissue oxygen saturation, and infrared spectroscopy with handheld devices.

Tissue glues are now being used more frequently for wounds in children and in elective keyhole surgery.

Negative pressure dressing systems add much to the armamentarium of the surgeon in both trauma and elective surgery. They prevent wound edge retraction, apply uniform force across the wound acting somewhat as a splint, and remove exudate. The patients find them to be more comfortable, allow for more mobility and decreased frequency of dressings.

A new generation of barbed sutures allow us to close wounds without knots which have always been the commonest point of suture failure either in the knot or immediately adjacent to it. Barbed sutures tend to be either bidirectional or unidirectional with a loop at the start. They are usually used in elective surgery particularly in laparoscopic and robotic surgery and can be used to make anastomoses and bridge facial defects. They can be used to precisely place sutures in a parachute technique or be tightened as you go but are difficult to undo. They also retain some wound strength if cut. Many plastic surgeons and gynaecologists use them in elective surgery such as in body contouring and Caesarian sections. Though they are much more expensive than traditional non-barbed sutures, the time saved is usually considerable.

In trauma surgery, I'd agree with Dr Joan Chapple that interrupted monofilament non-absorbable sutures remain the gold standard. For elective surgery, absorbable dermal sutures and continuous skin sutures with small bites is what most of us today practice. This results in more even tension on the wound, less vascular compromise to the wound edges and closure speed. For those patients wanting the best scar, I've always thought a subcuticular non-absorbable suture left in 3–4 weeks before removal followed by taping with Steristrips™ for 6 weeks gave the best result. Dr Chapple's method of removing sutures is excellent and I would add good lighting and some form of magnification.

10 Flaps and Grafts

Summary
Making the distinction between flaps and grafts is a circulatory matter. It is not only essential for appropriate initial treatment but it is also highly relevant to the proper understanding of the outcomes. Correlating assessments and treatments with outcomes provides the only reliable way of accumulating technical expertise.

The distinction between flaps and grafts is not just a theoretical exercise, but underpins all acute wound care. Most wounds manage to heal fairly well, while others inexplicably do badly. The understanding of this variability, and the improvement of our wound management skills, requires rigorous attention to the circulatory details. By setting out to tailor treatment specifically to the different circulatory requirements of flaps and grafts, and diligently reviewing the results, it is possible to accumulate reliable expertise, which translates into consistently better outcomes. A comparison of the characteristics of Flaps and Grafts is summarised in Table 10.1.

> **Immobilisation is helpful** for both flaps and grafts. For flaps, it assists the stabilisation of the circulation, and for grafts, it facilitates capillary attachment and graft survival. The **double-bandage regime** is also necessary for both flaps and grafts in lower limb situations [See Appendix].

Table 10.1 A Comparison of the distinctive clinical characteristics of flaps and grafts

Flaps	Grafts
1. Are still attached to the body but have reduced perfusion	May be attached to or separated from the body but have insufficient circulation for survival
2. Are expected to survive by means of the continuity of existing blood vessels	The tissue cannot survive from any existing attachment
3. Commonly suffer from venous congestion and are blue	Circulation is absent and the tissue is either congested or pale
4. Will survive if circulation can be maintained or improved	Grafts will only survive if they can pick up a new capillary circulation from adjacent tissue
5. Any trimming of fat will reduce the chances of survival as a flap	Trimming of all subcutaneous fat will allow bed circulation to reach the skin

(continued)

P. Charlesworth, M. F. Klaassen, *Chapple's Principles of Wound Care and Healing*,
https://doi.org/10.1007/978-3-031-53104-0_10

Table 10.1 (continued)

Flaps	Grafts
6. Haematomas affect the circulation by causing pressure. Fenestrating flaps is not helpful to the circulation	Every tiny haematoma will prevent bed circulation from reaching the graft. Fenestrating the graft is an insurance against the development of haematomas
7. Even when there is no tissue missing, stretching or spreading will worsen venous drainage	Stretching a graft out to size will assist its survival not only by thinning it but also by giving the skin access to a greater circulation from the larger area of bed
8. Sutures can endanger the circulation in several ways as reactive swelling occurs. Small sutures can be used to prevent edges rolling under	Sutures can be useful to hold grafts accurately and do not reduce their circulation. Tapes and tulle will also do this and do not risk causing bleeding
9. Posturing and positioning to assist venous drainage will assist flap survival	Posturing and positioning makes no significant difference to the circulation
10. External pressure is dangerous as it impacts on the low-pressure venous circulation which is often already precarious	A little accurate pressure is an insurance against haematomas and is relatively safe for grafts because bed circulation is normal

Flaps

A flap is any piece of tissue which has had its circulation reduced by injury, operation or treatment.

The word 'flap' originated allegedly from the sixteenth-century Dutch word FLAPPE, which referred to anything that hung broad and loose, fastened only by one side [1] *Simply Local Flaps—Springer 2018].*

The anatomical and physiological definitions of a flap are in contrast, but equally applicable to many situations where there is no tissue missing and after excisions, where there is always additional tension involved in wound closure tending to reduce the circulation to the edges (Fig. 10.1).

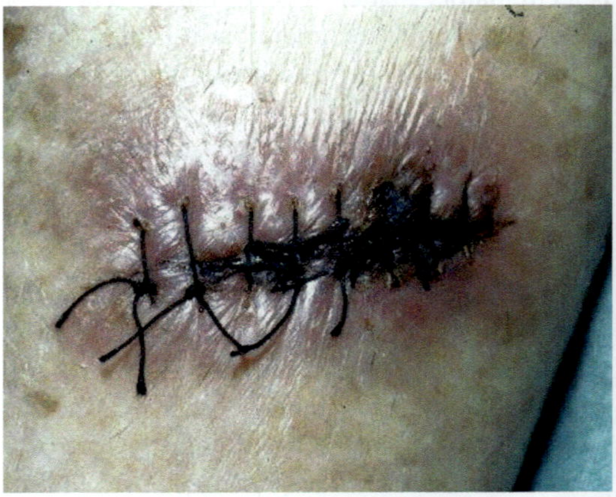

Fig. 10.1 Circulatory problems along both edges have been created by the sutures and infection is becoming established. This was a surgical wound for excision of a lesion. Appearance at 10 days

In vascular sites such as the head and neck, suturing flaps may be quite safe. In other sites, the outcome may be uncertain unless tension can be reduced by posturing and/or with tapes. In many cases, finger-tip injuries are best regarded as flaps and like the front of the shin may be best handled by avoiding sutures altogether (Figs. 10.2, 10.3, 10.4, and 10.5).

Most people's concept of a flap is a lifted-up or pulled-back piece of surface tissue still attached to the body. If no tissue seems to be missing, the conventional response is to assume that whether or not it looks alive, it can be replaced forthwith. The actual reality is that many flaps without missing tissue do not have enough circulatory throughput to be safely replaced. Infection very often follows the death of tissue (Figs. 10.6, 10.7, 10.8, 10.9, and 10.10).

In the classic triangular flap scenario, the continuity of subcutaneous tissue has been interrupted along two of the three sides, and the tissue is usually undermined (Fig. 10.9).

This means that such flaps retain only about a quarter of their original vascular attachment, so it

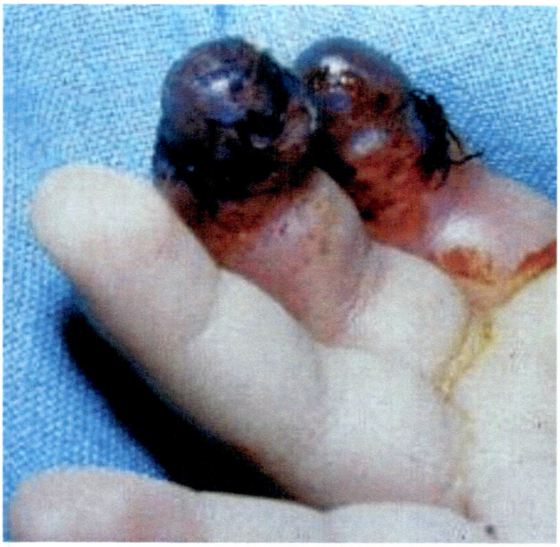

Fig. 10.2 Venous stasis in crushed fingertips, where sutures have worsened the situation

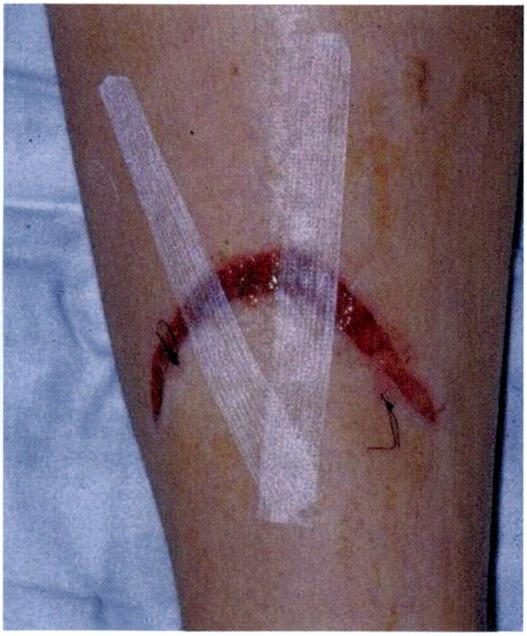

Fig. 10.3 A distally based flap has been taped on day 1. Full closure achieved by revising the taping at day 3

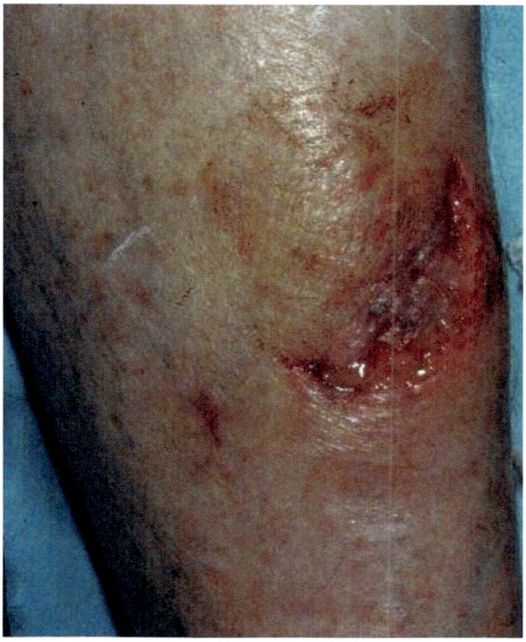

Fig. 10.4 A ragged leg flap which had been held with tulle and dressed accurately shown at 5 days

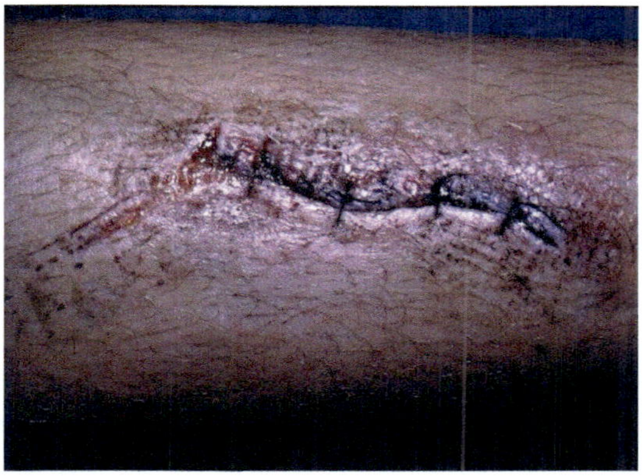

Fig. 10.5 5 days after suturing of a scrape to the front of a shin. The shelving flap shows some edge congestion. Tulle or tapes would have been a better option

is hardly surprising that most of them require special circulatory consideration. Longer flaps are more precarious and distally based flaps will swell more because they always have both venous and lymphatic return interrupted. When there is blunt trauma to the vicinity, all tissues will be worse off because of swelling and there can also be complex and multiple flaps. The treatment of all these less favourable flaps by conventional suturing is particularly hazardous (Figs. 10.11 and 10.12).

There are alternatives (Figs. 10.13 and 10.14).

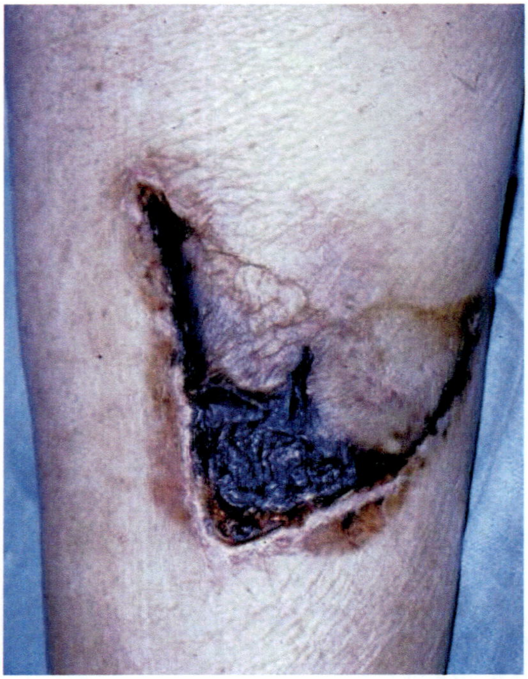

Fig. 10.6 Typical venous necrosis, following the suturing of a triangular flap. Note further zone of partial-thickness loss

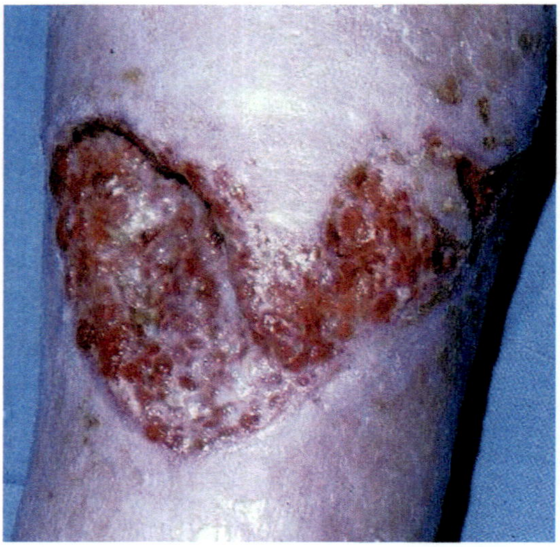

Fig. 10.7 Ragged, raw surface on the lower leg a month after a proximally based flap had been sutured back and died

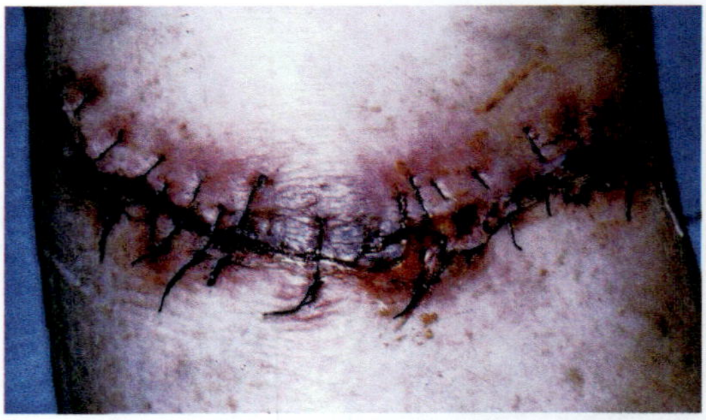

Fig. 10.8 Broad proximally based knee flap showing circulatory problems caused by sutures. Infection is already present. Taping, combined with splinting, would have been safer

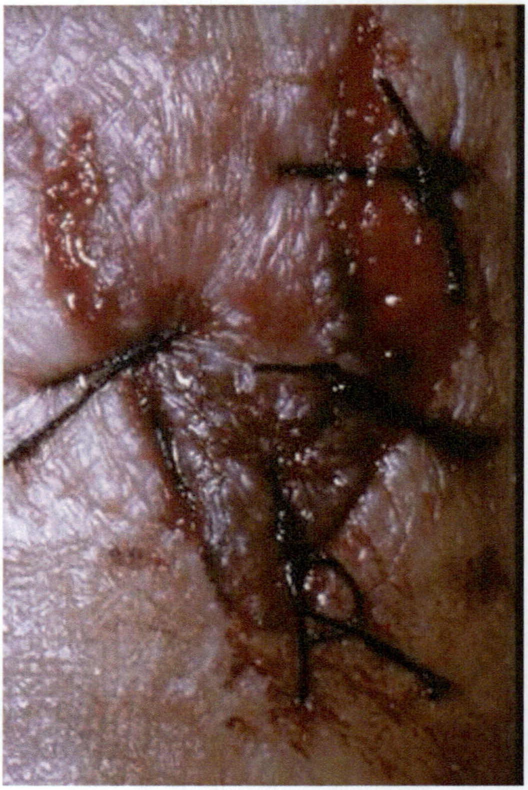

Fig. 10.9 Bands of tension shown in a classic triangular flap, which are restricting venous circulation

Necrosis is usually blamed on everything except technique. Bad luck or statistical excuses are common scapegoats. For some reason, modern professionals seem reluctant to take personal responsibility for assisting tissue that is distressed or prepared to take simple technical measures to assist venous return even when venous congestion is the obvious problem. Giving the skin of

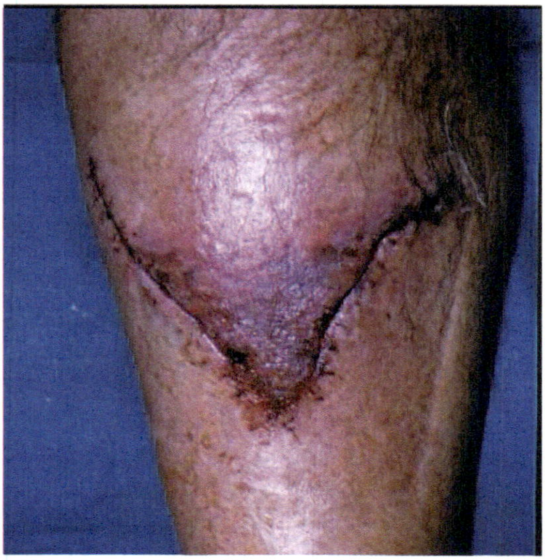

Fig. 10.10 Venous problem 10 days after a shin flap was sutured back. The skin would have survived more securely as a graft

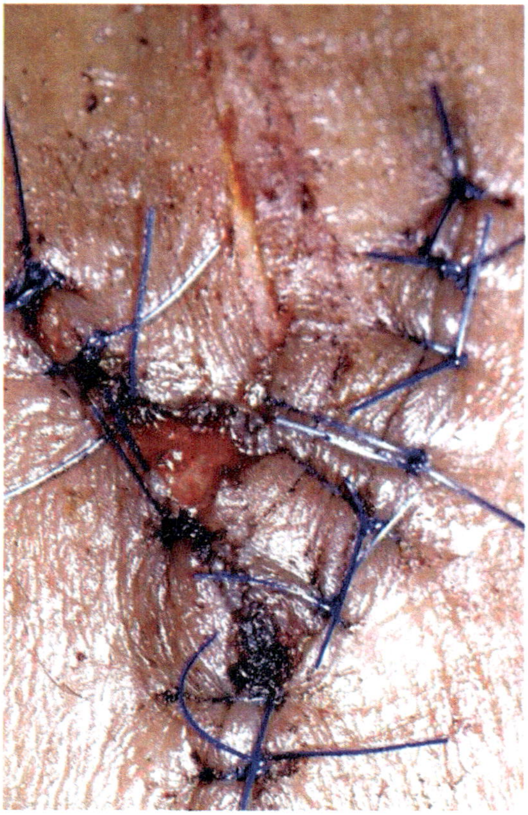

Fig. 10.11 Y-shaped laceration 3 days after routine suturing. Apart from oedema, it is almost looking alright

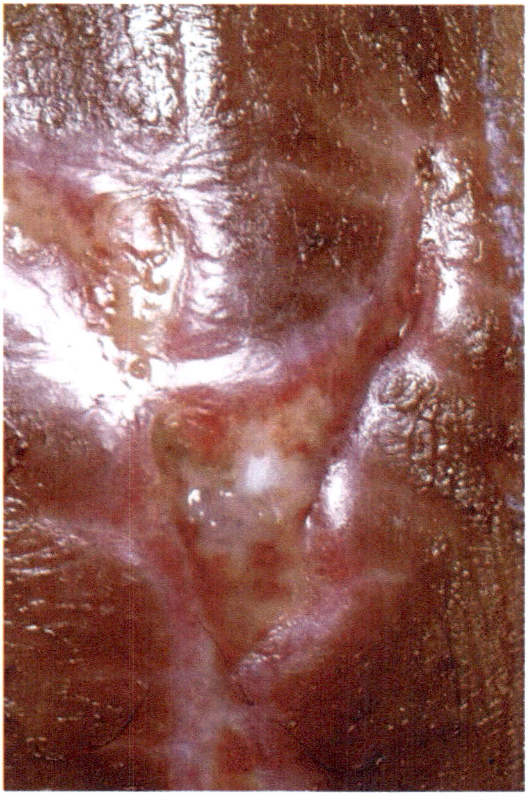

Fig. 10.12 The destructive effects of the suturing are more clearly reflected in the poor result at 6 weeks

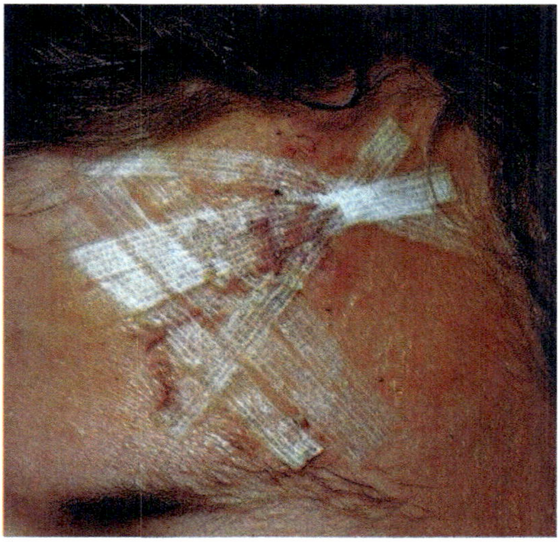

Fig. 10.13 A complex forehead laceration from a blow with a bottle has been very successfully treated with tapes—result at 5 days

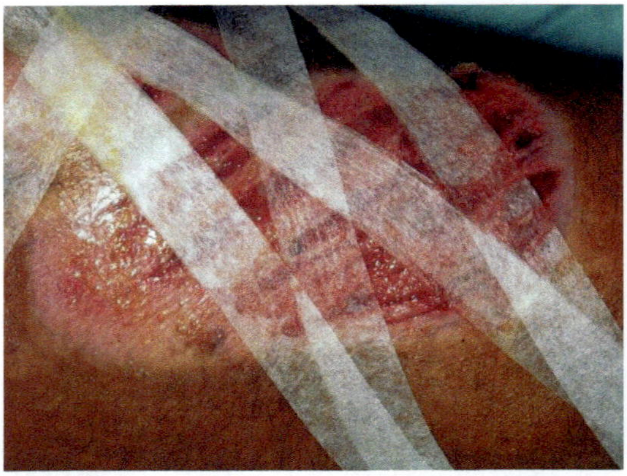

Fig. 10.14 Linear lacerations held together with long tapes

potentially dead flaps a second chance to survive as a graft is a realistic possibility which is readily achieved and should always be considered.

The Clinical Management of Flaps

The important decision initially is to determine whether or not a flap has enough circulation to survive as it lies, not whether any tissue is missing! If it is folded back or rumpled, this should obviously be corrected first. If it recovers circulation, the next question is can it be more adequately replaced without adverse circulatory effects, by reducing tension by taping and/or posturing adjacent joints. This is a judgement call, determined sometimes only by trial and error. Stretching flaps always worsens their venous drainage and conversely, relaxing them always improves their prospects. Suturing flaps back into place, in addition to attenuating veins, can also produce tension bands, capable of physically obstructing venous drainage (Figs. 10.15 and 10.16).

Initial control of flaps can always be much more safely achieved with tapes or tulle, followed 3 or 4 days later by re-taping or even secondary suture to assist closure just as swelling is subsiding. Tulle support and dressings, with the avoidance of all suturing and splintage provides the safest initial treatment for the most precarious flaps (Figs. 10.17 and 10.18).

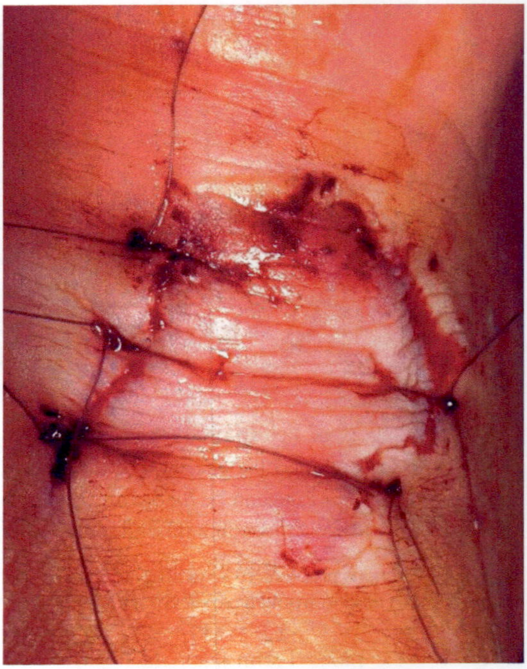

Fig. 10.15 Three day-old heel flap showing transverse bands of tension caused by ill-advised suturing

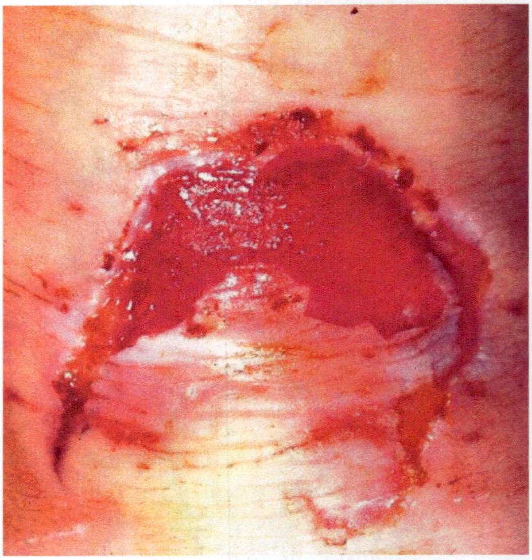

Fig. 10.16 The partial thickness damage was apparent 5 days later. Plantar flexion and tulle would have been safer

Patients with leg flaps all need the two-bandage technique described in Appendix.

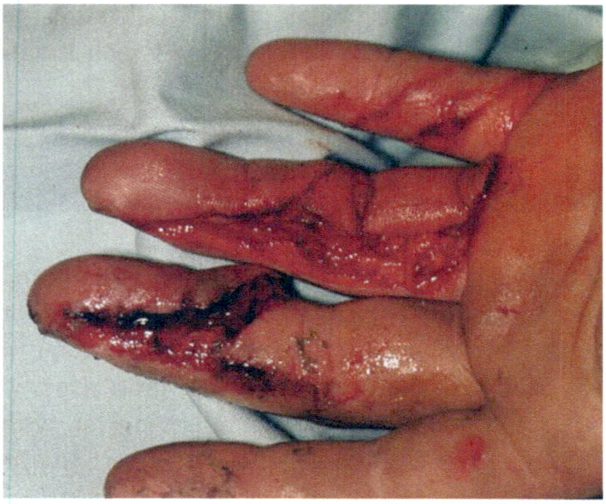

Fig. 10.17 Initial appearance of a hand caught in pastry rollers. The flaps look viable but these are burst fingers which will swell

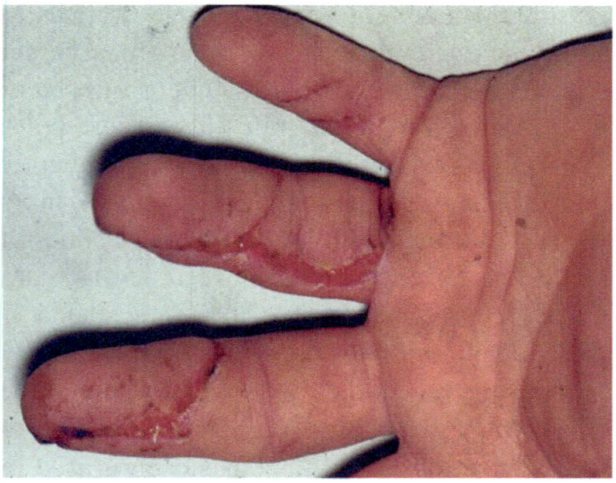

Fig. 10.18 The 10-day appearance after tulle gras stabilisation, gauze bandages, and splintage. All tissue is healthy and most of the swelling is gone. The hand has been comfortable and healing almost achieved

Grafts

A graft is a piece of tissue which has no circulation at all until it picks up a new capillary attachment from adjacent tissue.

When a piece of tissue is totally deprived of its perfusion, the only two ways it can possibly survive are: by surgically reconnecting sizeable vessels (which is rarely applicable) or (much more commonly) by picking up a new capillary circulation from an adjacent vascular bed. Skin is the most usual tissue needing graft consideration. The most common presentation of skin for grafting back occurs when old people or those on long-term steroids shear fragile skin off the subcutaneous layers (Fig. 10.19).

Such skin may or may not be still attached but it has no intrinsic circulation. If attached, it is frequently described as a 'flap', but for treatment purposes, it must be regarded as a 'graft'. Every professional should be able to do this (Figs. 10.20, 10.21, and 10.22).

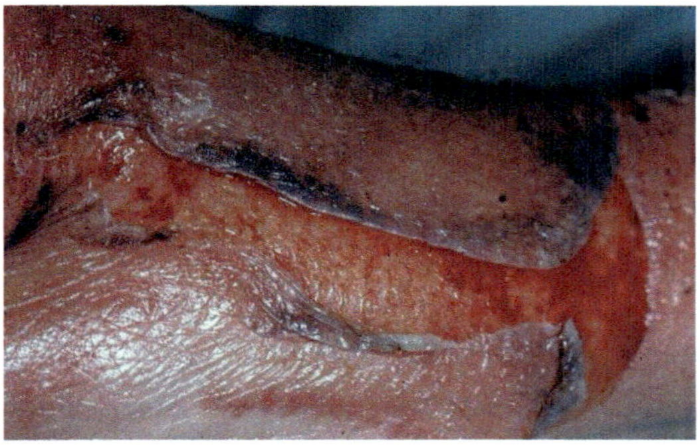

Fig. 10.19 Extensive dislodgement of skin in patient on long-term steroid treatment for asthma. Such skin needs accurate replacement and holding with tulle. It will take as a graft if carefully replaced

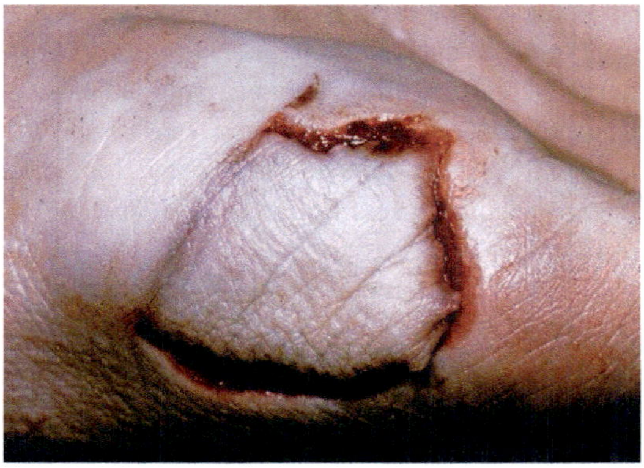

Fig. 10.20 This thickish flap has insufficient arterial input. It will therefore die as a flap, but will survive if it can be given a second chance reapplied as a graft

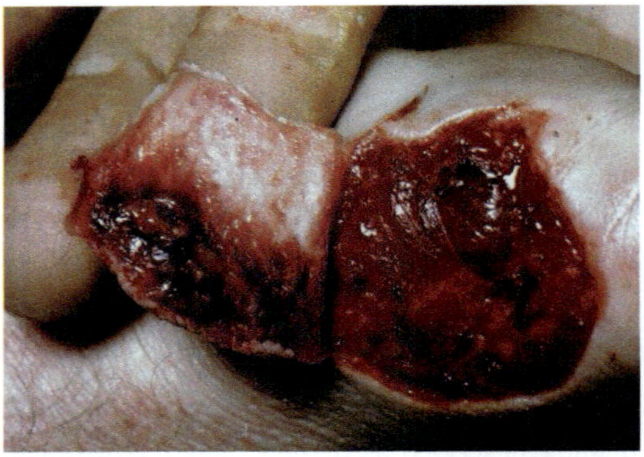

Fig. 10.21 On the same day, half the flap is shown trimmed of fat prior to removal of the remainder. The 'graft' still attached, was then replaced and held in place by tapes

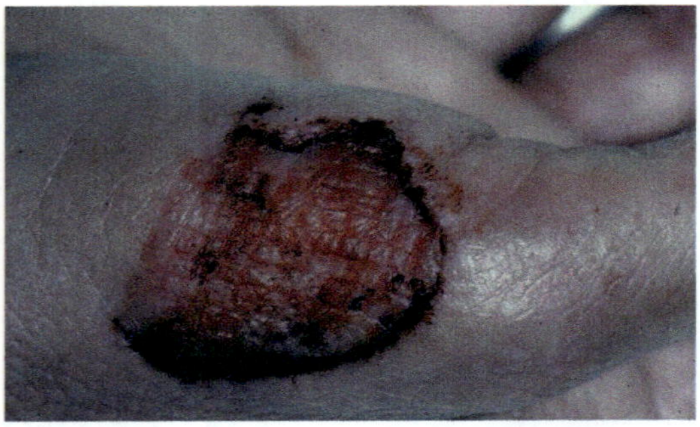

Fig. 10.22 Result at 5 days shows that the graft has taken well and requires only a protective cover. It will match and wear well but will lack sensation

If the bed is in a good state initially, the skin is best replaced immediately. Separated skin will however remain alive for at least 10 days if it is kept moist in a saline swab and stored in an ordinary 4° C refrigerator. It can be reapplied as soon as a previously non-ideal vascular bed improves sufficiently with time and dressings [including negative wound pressure devices] to sustain the graft.

There is no limit to the area of skin that can be successfully replaced as a graft. It will all take if carefully reapplied to a healthy bed without bleeding, haematoma, or fat intervening. There is however a limit to the volume of tissue any bed can sustain as graft. It is therefore advantageous to remove all fat and stretch the skin back out to size, thereby both thinning it and also maximising the area of contact with the bed circulation. These technical responses are in total contrast to those designed to assist flap tissue which is suffering from venous insufficiency.

Detailed Skin Grafting Techniques

Keep all separated tissue moistened in a normal saline swab. Keep attached tissue sponged or repeatedly irrigated with saline. Always remove fat from skin being replaced as a graft. Curved iris scissors are the best for removing fat, with the skin stretched back over a finger. In the elderly, soft fat can sometimes be very effectively rolled off using a gauze swab. Very thin dislodgements sometimes don't need anything other than stroking the piece out to size again and holding it there accurately with tapes or tulle gras, after making a number of fenestrations to permit serous drainage. These can either be cut with a scalpel blade onto a spatula or snipped or poked through with the graft lifted. These holes allow any blood or serum to escape subsequently into dressings. If 'buttonholes' are made inadvertently during the trimming of fat, it doesn't matter, because these can be regarded as extra fenestrations for drainage. The scars related to these small slit-like openings are eventually invisible or very minor and certainly preferable to graft loss from haematomas. Tulle gras in sheets or strips as well as tapes can be used to tether grafts to intact skin. Tapes need to be applied to clean dry skin before using any tulle gras layers. Suturing thin skin back can be difficult and cause bleeding. Accurate absorbent gauze layers are applied next and crepe bandages with some form of immobilisation to the complete the procedure. In the elderly, bandages alone or bandages with a sling are probably safer than using casts, which can themselves sometimes cause damage or precipitate falls. In lower limb injuries, the two-bandage technique is essential [See Appendix].

Even when the skin remains attached, the clinical decision as to whether it should be treated as a graft or a flap is not difficult to make. If the tissue does not have a demonstrable circulation, it will die unless it can be given an alternative chance as a graft. Neither a 'wait-and-see' policy nor a 'hope-for-the-best' attitude at this point can possibly help at all. Treating tissue as a graft is an all-or-nothing commitment. Tentatively snipping some fat off a sick flap worsens the circulatory predicament by reducing the residual vascular network, while continuing to deny the skin the best possible access to graft circulation from the bed, because of any fat that remains. Such flawed thinking and technique set an especially poor example to all observers, who will assume wrongly that it is helpful, the best thing to do, and 'at least everything was tried'. Both are flawed assumptions!

Turning a Flap into a Graft

Whenever a flap looks either ischaemic or severely congested, turning the potentially dead skin into a graft must always be the next consideration. Why just wait for it to die?

MFK has recently had this experience with a H-plasty forehead flap in a 64-year-old smoker with a recurrent mid-forehead BCC. The left arm of the H-plasty [double advancement flap with Burow's triangles] looked decidedly ischaemic on day 1 when patient's dressings were changed. He decided to try topical daily Rectogesic ointment used for anal fissures and containing small amounts of glycerol trinitrate. The clinical outcome is illustrated below (Fig. 10.23a–h):

The correctness of the decision will soon be confirmed by the absence of dermal bleeding encountered as thinning begins. Commencing at the tip, the aspect most remote from the attached pedicle or the most congested section, the subcutaneous fat is removed with curved iris scissors, continuing towards the attachment until tiny dermal bleeders are encountered. The remaining flap then requires flap management, with only the thinned portion requiring fenestrations and stretching out to size as a graft. If tension from suturing the 'graft' portion out to size pulls on the flap part unduly, it can be physically divided off from the flap and sutured to the bed instead (Figs. 10.24: Chapple's models of flap

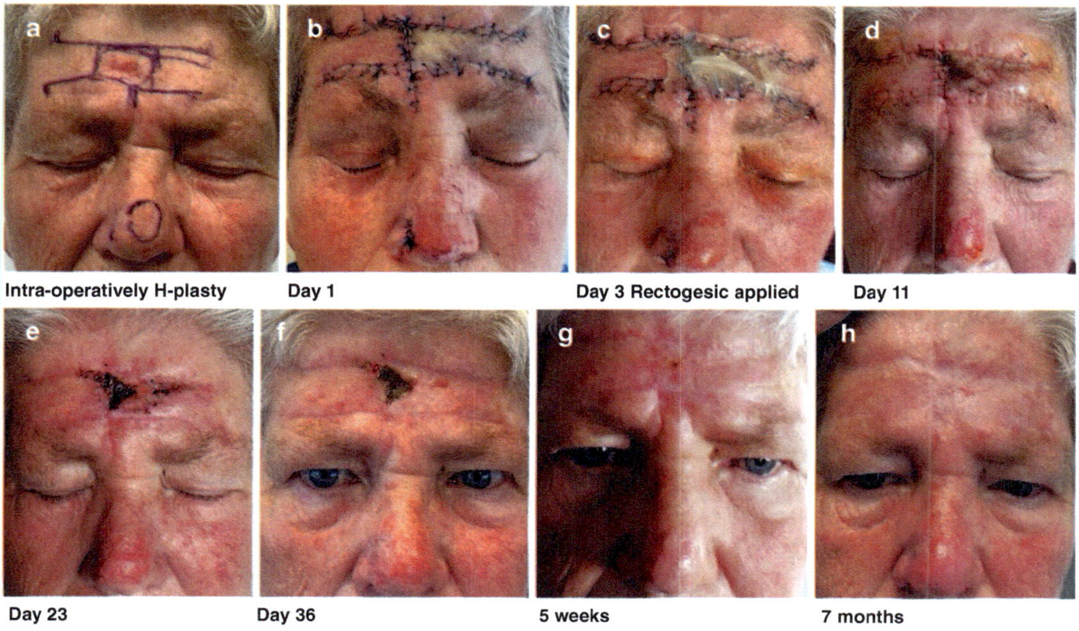

Fig. 10.23 (**a**–**h**) Ischaemic left arm of forehead H-plasty double advancement flap repair for wide excision recurrent infiltrating BCC [a decade since original excision]. (**a**) Pre-surgery appearance. (**b**) Day 1 view of ischaemic left H-plasty flap. (**c**) Day 3 when it was decided to try topical Rectogesic ointment to save the ischaemic flap. (**d**) After 8 days of Rectogesic. (**e**) Appearance at day 23 with small area of residual flap necrosis. (**f**) At 36 days, the area is almost fully healed. (**g**) Healed at 5 weeks post-surgery. (**h**) Result at 7 months

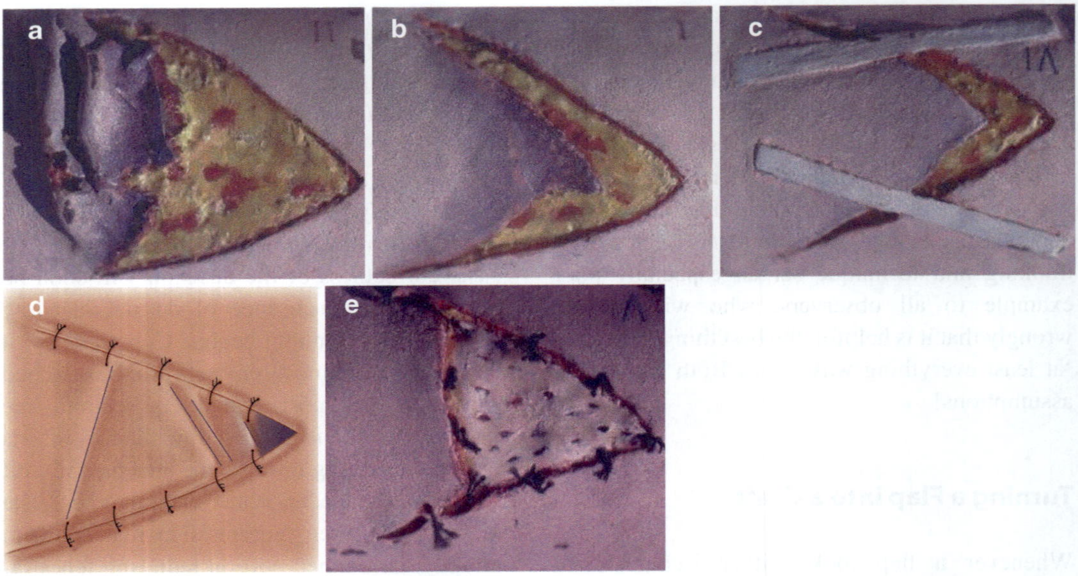

Figs. 10.24 (a–e) **Dr Joan Chapple's flap models for clinical teaching**. (**a**) This model shows a rumpled skin flap with venous problems at the tip, best salvaged by thinning all the fat from this congested portion and treating it as a graft. (**b**) The second model shows severely traumatised distally based flap, which will certainly die unless it is treated as a graft. (**c**) The third model shows a proximally based flap which is surviving as it lies, but will not stand any further replacement. Note the holding tapes. (**d**) The fourth model shows a traumatic flap, that has been sutured back with tension bands interrupting the circulation. (**e**) The fifth and final model shows the distal half of the fourth model trimmed of all fat, fenestrations made and replaced as a graft

salvage). The two different parts do not have a circulatory connection and the dressing will often be a lot simpler. The grafted area, with its underlying normal circulation, can cope with a little more dressing pressure than the flap portion, reducing the possibility of collections of blood or serum beneath the graft. The sutures can be cut long and used to tie over and stabilise the graft dressing. Immobilisation is usually necessary. It is useful to give grafted patients 3–5 days of antibiotics to prevent infection, especially by haemolytic organisms [like streptococci], which interfere with the initial fibrinous attachment of graft to the vascular bed.

Skin Losses

Whenever skin is missing, the first thing to do is to try and locate it. Even after considerable delay, it is usually possible, after trimming fat off, to produce a perfectly moist skin graft from a salvaged piece of tissue. If the original skin is not forthcoming, the next option must be that of simply dressing the wound until it heals. This is for small defects. For larger defects, a new split skin graft can be taken from a suitable donor site on the patient. Although this is easy with practice and whilst using a sterile grafting knife, it may be best to refer the patient to a plastic surgeon. Although such grafting can be done immediately, a few days delay is also acceptable. Always stop the bleeding and institute wound dressing with tulle and gauze, whilst organising referral for grafting.

Losses from Fingertips

Sometimes substantial pieces of finger get sliced off, or nearly so, and in many cases, this specialised skin may be invaluable, replaced as a graft. Arising from the convex surfaces like the pulp of a finger, the defatted piece may become both hollow and too large to reapply accurately (Fig. 10.25).

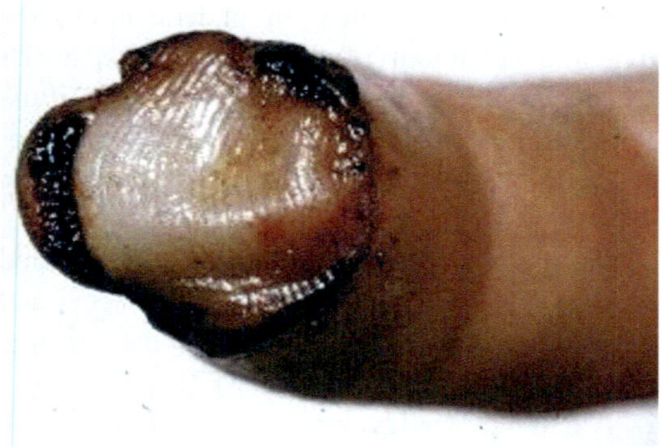

Fig. 10.25 This reapplied fingertip skin had fat trimmed out, but the concave piece then didn't fit or survive. Cutting a central flat new graft from such a piece is often better

It may be better to cut a new 'pinch' graft from the centre of the piece. This will be thickest in the centre and is also smaller than the original, so that it will sit well on the flat bed without overlap, with any bleeding escaping easily between fixation points. The small circumferential gap will heal quickly with a good junctional scar. Palm and pulp skin is specialised and should never be discarded lightly. If the specialised skin is unavailable, spontaneous healing of a fingertip is usually preferable to using a split skin graft from another part of the body. See Chap. 12.

Graft Re-Dressings

Dressings for grafts are not usually changed for 5–7 days. A successful graft has at this stage a uniformly dusky surface and sluggish return of circulation can be demonstrated in it following localised pressure. Haematomas are localised collections and should be released (Figs. 10.26, 10.27, and 10.28).

Serum collections should also be evacuated before grafts epithelialise on their under surface. If this happens, they will never stick down. Overlapping grafts may 'take' for an additional millimetre or so. This excess needs to be actively trimmed off at the first opportunity, so as to minimise junctional ridges. This procedure is completely painless but may cause a little temporary

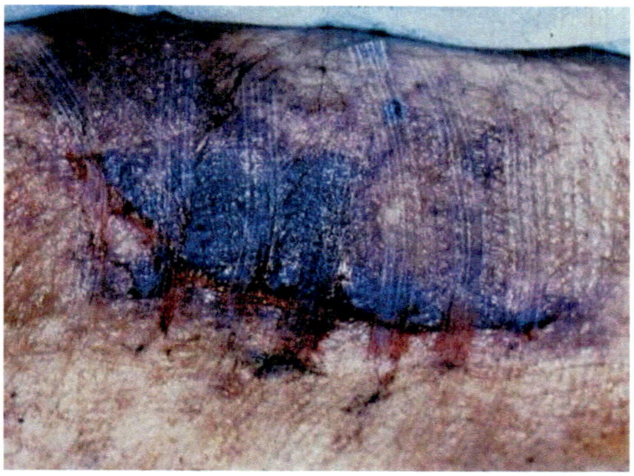

Fig. 10.26 Leg flap showing venous stasis and haematoma. 5 days post-injury. Flap death is likely

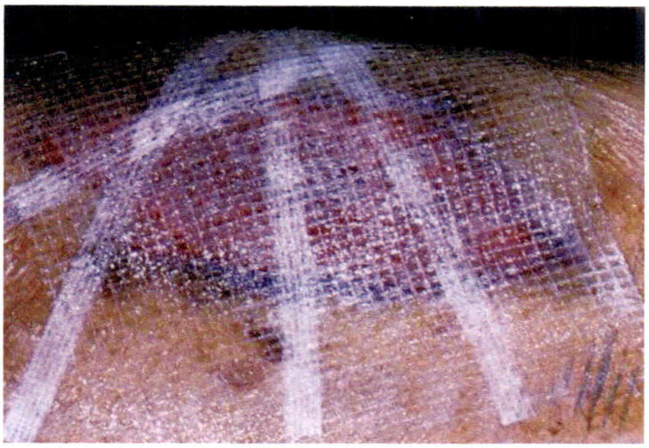

Fig. 10.27 Same day as 10.26, flap trimmed of all fat, haematoma removed and skin reapplied as a graft, held with tapes

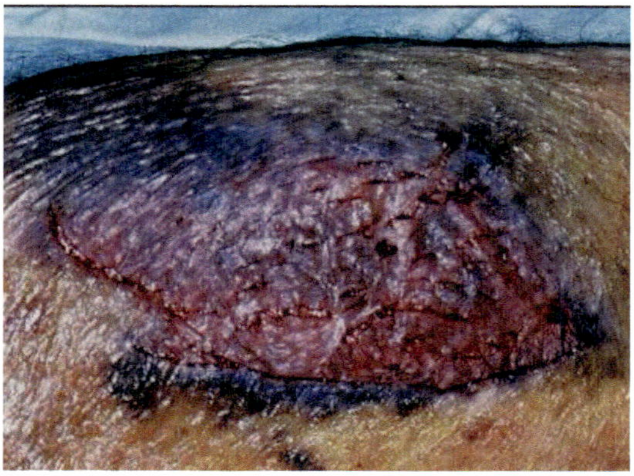

Fig. 10.28 One week later, the graft has taken successfully with minor bruising of surrounding skin. Note the fenestrations

bleeding. Within a week or 10 days, a successful graft looks pinker, shows a brisk capillary return when pressed on, and can be left out of dressings except for protection. The grafted skin may need lubricating with some moisturiser or oil if it is dry or scaly. Grafts on the leg need supportive bandages for several weeks to prevent the development of spontaneous blood blisters. Grafts shrink for several months before reaching a final smooth state. They never regain surface sensation. Contour defects, where fat has been trimmed off initially, continue to fill out somewhat over many months and years.

Although this graft/flap scenario may seem complicated, it is by no means an uncommon clinical situation to be faced with. Working through the detail of physiological requirements in complex wounds, patiently and logically, usually makes it possible to regularly achieve favourable outcomes, notably in elderly patients with leg injuries. Applying an additional firm bandage whenever patients get up also makes it possible for them to be managed successfully as outpatients. They must still rest their legs up within non-tight bandages for most of the first few days. [See Appendix].

Commentary by Dr Michael F. Klaassen FRACS–Co-editor with Dr Peter Charlesworth FRACS

In this well-illustrated chapter by Dr Joan Chapple, the lifeblood and core methods of every plastic surgeon's skill-set are demonstrated. Although her focus is mainly the traumatic flap scenario which is common in fingertip injuries and degloving leg injuries in the elderly, the essential comparison between flaps and grafts is well defined. As Shakespeare's Hamlet would ask 'To be, or not to be?' The question is reformatted in 'To flap or to graft? That is the question! The idea of whether it is better to live or to die. Elective flaps with their intrinsic blood supply and variations adopted with the aid of delay, expansion, or prefabrication are outside the scope of this book but can be found well illustrated in the references [1].

Experience is critical in understanding the dynamic behaviour of flaps and grafts, as Dr Chapple implies. Her models, which are illustrated and were prepared from inanimate material, are suitably re-simulated in the modern surgical skills laboratory using porcine skin.

For the novice trying to get their head around the various descriptions of flaps [both local and distant], the editors recommend the Atomic Classification of David Tolhurst [2].

A flap may well be turned into a graft as a salvage procedure by removing all the fat and immobilising the defatted skin as a graft. I have found it easier to abandon the damaged flap, particularly if there is a degree of degloving or avulsion in the mechanism of injury and simply proceed after flap debridement to repair with a fresh thin split skin graft. Traumatised flaps are definitely better immobilised/secured in place with tapes rather than sutures, as espoused by Dr Chapple.

Grafts may sometimes be better than local flaps for the aesthetic outcome of head and neck defects after skin cancer excision, and this is particularly the case for the elderly using full thickness skin grafts. I have been impressed over the last 35 years of practice how well even split skin grafts can look aesthetically in the long-term.

Finally, the consideration of pharmacokinetics in the salvage of sick or dying flaps. This is with the modern use of GTN patches or the topical application of the glycerol trinitrate-containing Rectogesic™, anal fissure cream used so successfully in the forehead flap illustrated in Fig. 10.23a–g.

Inevitably flaps or grafts may die, that is then the second question [What to do now?] and the important principle of Sir Harold Gillies [1882–1960]: Have a Lifeboat!

References

1. Klaassen MF, Brown E, Behan F. Simply local flaps. Cham: Springer; 2018.
2. Tolhurst DE. Fasciocutaneous flaps [thesis for PhD], Drukkeru Pasmans B V. 's-Gravenhage. 1988.

11 Dressings and Rehabilitation

Summary
The main aim of dressings in acute wounds is to absorb seepage and support the injured tissues. Bleeding must be stopped as an integral part of treatment, in order that bandaging tension can be reduced, so as to accommodate any degree of reactive swelling without restricting the circulation. Later dressings are designed to prevent the desiccation of exposed living cells until healing is re-established, minimise exposure to bacterial infection, absorb discharge, and assist with the softening and separation of slough.

The best rehabilitation of all is seamless, with the injured person making a rapid and comfortable recovery from injury to full function. Undue or persistent pain is particularly counterproductive. Problematic rehabilitation can be related not only to situations where there has been serious structural damage but also to circulatory complications and scarring arising out of inappropriate treatment. The protection of joint function by explicit posturing and splintage during the acute phase can also be crucial to a full recovery. The patient's understanding and involvement always plays an important part in the recovery of function.

Dressings

Dressings merely accompany healing, they do not do it. Their first role is to absorb blood and serum from open wounds and prevent sticking to clothing and bedding. Dressings support and protect wounds, plus their general constraint can be used to encourage closure. They splint injured tissues. Other important roles for dressings are to maintain a moist, non-toxic environment for exposed tissues and prevent access of airborne bacteria until healing re-establishes the protection of intact skin. They facilitate the separation of dead tissue by helping to soften it with creams or gel and absorb discharge. They can be used to administer topical antibiotics. Designing dressing regimes involves assisting with whatever the wound is up to at each stage and also accommodating the patient's needs.

Wound Dressings and the Circulation

Acute wound dressings help to stabilise the circulation and encourage clotting to occur. While temporary pressure may be used to achieve haemostasis, dressing tension above venous pressure has no place in the eventual bandaging. Continued elevation and splintage are used to rest the wound and maintain haemostasis, with specific posturing to assist drainage from any congested tissues. After all injuries to the lower limb, **a two-**

P. Charlesworth, M. F. Klaassen, *Chapple's Principles of Wound Care and Healing*,
https://doi.org/10.1007/978-3-031-53104-0_11

bandage regime needs to be made an integral part of the management, applying the second bandage before the patient gets out of bed. This is detailed in the Appendix and provision of an instruction sheet to the patient is recommended. A potentially perfect result can be ruined by not adhering to this aspect of dressing management. The patient who doesn't use the additional bandage may disrupt their wound with bleeding and/or haematoma, when their leg is dependent regardless of whether or not they are weightbearing. A tight permanent bandage that prevents bleeding and haematoma not only causes undue pain but may also restrict the circulation enough to debilitate or kill tissue. In the lower leg, this less visible complication can be as adverse for graft survival as it is for tissue with a sluggish circulation. A localised wound dressing beneath a firm bandage is also one of the most effective ways of administering detrimental focal pressure and adding insult to the injury (Figs. 11.1 and 11.2).

Tulle-Gras Dressings

It is desirable that the inner layer of a dressing does not stick to wounds or allow them to dry out. The most usual and useful material for this purpose is tulle-gras [Vaseline gauze, Jelonet™, Bactigras™, Adaptic™ or Atrauman™]. Tulle is best if it is soft and greasy. This is best achieved

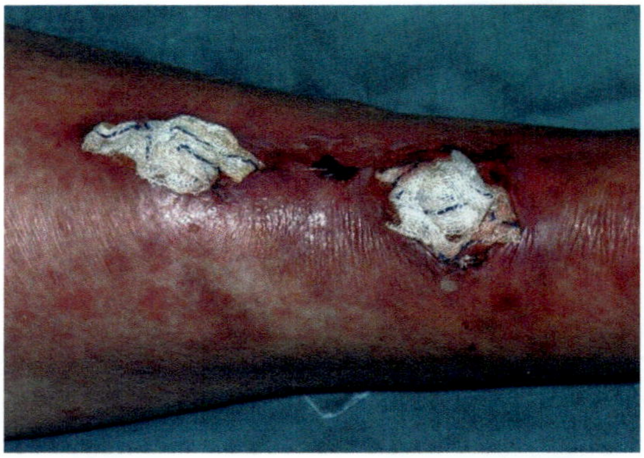

Fig. 11.1 Surface packing in place 3 days after a scraping injury to the shin. The leg was also firmly bandaged to prevent bleeding

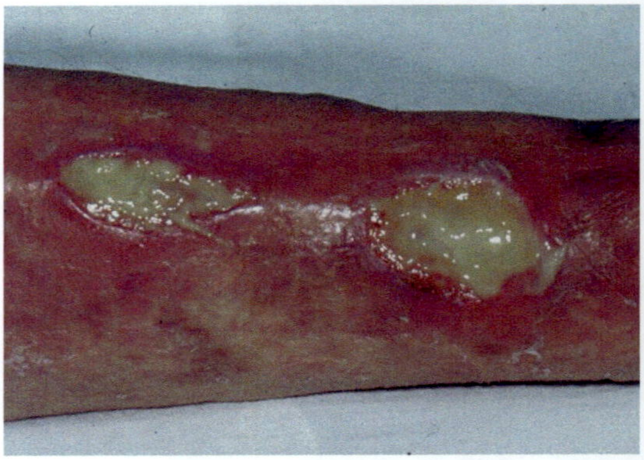

Fig. 11.2 The destructive effects of the pressure on the base of these areas is evident 3 weeks later. These areas took 3 months to heal

by storing multiple-pack boxes upside down. It is important to open the containers as briefly as possible, keep them as sterile as possible and to always handle tulle with sterile instruments before starting the procedure. It is poor technique to leave the box uncovered or ever place it inside the lid. Individually packaged tulle does not usually have sufficient grease to use in tulle moulding nor keep wounds adequately moist. It is also sometimes springy. When tulle is used to achieve general support and encourage closure, it needs to be well-anchored onto surrounding skin. When there is skin loss, the tulle layers should be larger than the raw surface in order that edge fibres cannot become incorporated in the wound. Overlapping tulle onto intact skin also keeps dressings and local applications accurately located to the raw surface.

Tulle, contrary to a widely held myth, cannot make intact skin unhealthy. The exception is true allergy, which is almost unknown. Joan Chapple frequently applied greasy and oily preparations to dry or scaly skin to lubricate and improve it. Tulle makes skin greasy, that's all it does, and what makes skin look white and moth-eaten [macerated] is exudate, blood, saline, bathwater, showers, swimming pools or rain—in other words wetness. The dead layers of skin simply become hydrated as they do when you've been in the bath too long. Palm and sole skin looks particularly bad when wet because it has such a thick keratin layer (Figs. 11.3, 11.4, and 11.5).

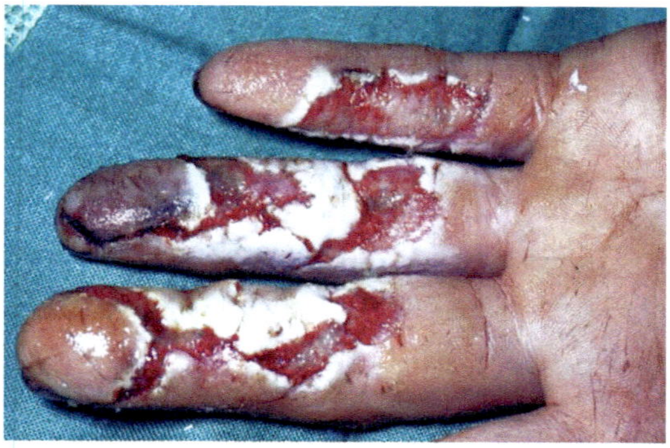

Fig. 11.3 5-day appearance of crushed fingers. The flaps have been held with tulle strips with the fingers rested on a splint and are largely healthy. The white skin is just wet

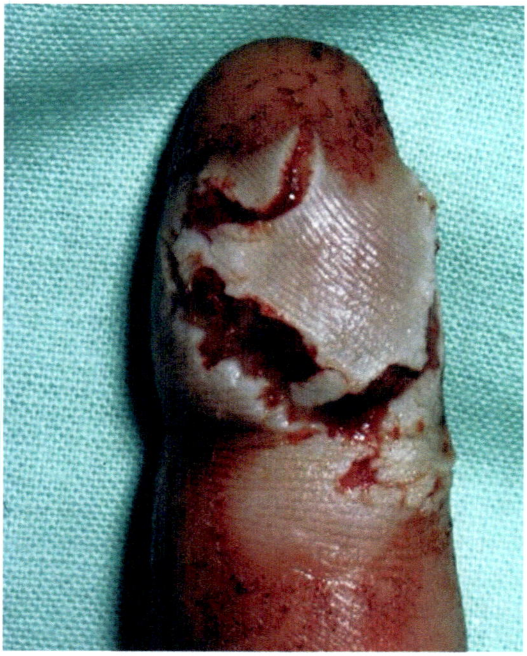

Fig. 11.4 Crushed fingertip treated without sutures showing 5-day result with wet [white] but not unhealthy skin flaps. Healing progressed well

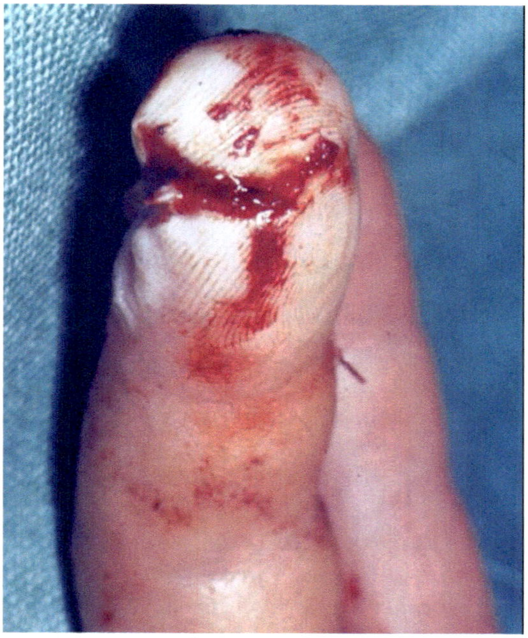

Fig. 11.5 White wet skin adjacent to crush lacerations at 5 days. The unsutured fingertip healed uneventfully

Wet skin however is not necessarily unhealthy either. It dries in the air within minutes and its layers remain cohesive as long as there has not been significant injury or infection, in which case it peels in a partial thickness manner leaving the living layers behind. Skin suffers and dies only from circulatory insufficiency, not wetness. Persistent wetness over weeks may allow yeasts to flourish, and such infection may then break the skin secondarily. If the fluid has enzymes in it, like saliva or bile, around sinuses or ostomies, the skin can get genuinely broken down, allowing infection in. Protecting it in these circumstances with adhesive film or barrier creams is helpful.

The use of tulle on sutured or closed wounds prevents dressings sticking to either sutures or the wound clot. Post-operative oozing comes through the tulle layer into the absorbent gauze material, leaving clean greased skin and discrete greased sutures when dressings are removed (Fig. 11.6).

A healthy sutured wound can usually be left without dressings after 4–5 days, showered on, greased again, and thereafter only covered for protection. Taped wounds can also be showered on, but may need retaping afterwards if the tapes are dislodged.

Editor's Comment [MFK] *I find modern tulle-gras [Jelonet ™ and others] tend to dry out and in reality, the modern tulle is not as good in terms of greasiness as Joan Chapple's old tulle-gras.*

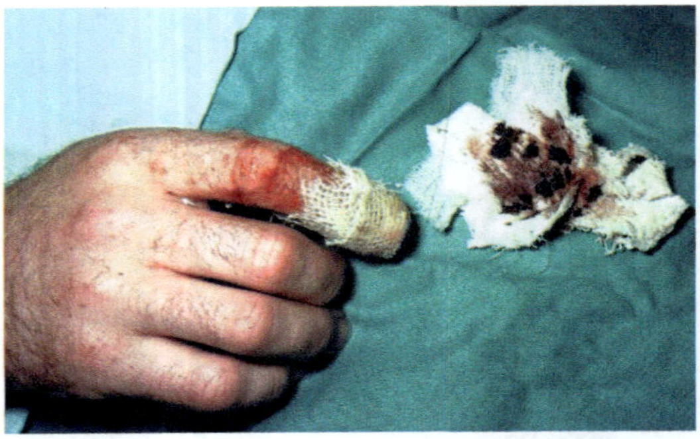

Fig. 11.6 Tulle, gauze, and crepe bandages have encouraged all oozing out into the gauze layers in this fingertip wound. The dressing was easy to remove

Instead, my preference for hand and finger dressings is wet saline-soaked gauze in strips longitudinally as a mould. These are removed easily by re-wetting them with saline at either day 1 [my preference] or whenever the first dressing change is planned for [4–5 days]. Bill Norris FRCS taught me this trick for hand dressings, when I was his registrar at East Grinstead, England, in the early 1990s. It works brilliantly, in my 35-year experience. I also allow my patients to get their wounds wet in the shower after 24 h, when the wound has sealed. So many years of surgical experience have convinced me that most patients require a dressing change of some sort at 24 h, to remove soiled, bloodied dressings and allow a new clean dressing option to be considered.

The use of antibiotic-impregnated tulle should be restricted to wounds with non-invasive infections because it cannot address invasive sepsis. Tulle-gras can be used to administer topical antibiotic creams or ointments, locating these by deliberately overlapping tulle onto the adjacent skin peripherally. Antibiotic powder is not a good way to deliver topical antibiotics as it is desiccating and the concentration as it dissolves cannot be controlled (Fig. 11.7).

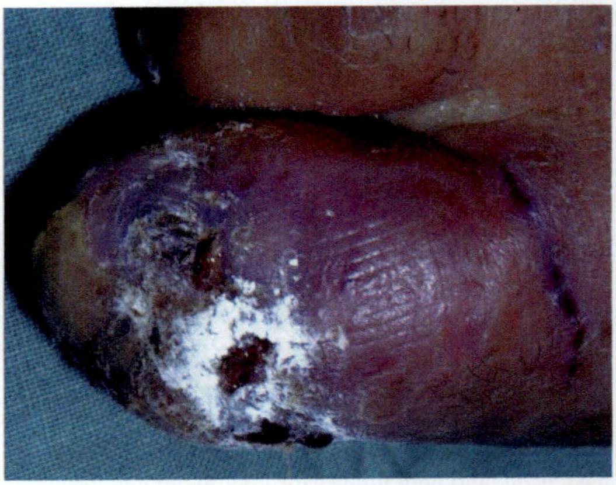

Fig. 11.7 This granulomatous wound after an ingrown toenail operation is being treated with antibiotic powder. This is a desiccating and inappropriate treatment

Tulle-Gras Moulding

When tissue is so badly traumatised that suturing is clearly inappropriate, it can be safely and accurately repositioned by using tulle-gras as a form of closure. Although the tulle ends up also dressing the raw surface, its very specific closure role is achieved by stroking the tulle broadly onto intact skin on one aspect of the wound, replacing tissue accurately with fingers or forceps, or both, and stroking the tulle out onto intact skin on the other side of the wound. If the injury is a large wound or a flap, the tulle can be used in sheets. Several sheets are usually needed but each is best applied separately as this is a closure technique, not an exercise in just slapping a wad of tulle-gras onto an open wound! Tulle does not make skin unhealthy [a widely held misconception in Joan Chapple's time?] and the more it overlaps the more support it gives. For digits, it is important to cut some tulle into strips no wider than the width of the digit so that these don't create dog's ears when applied over the end (Figs. 11.8 and 11.9).

Tulle strips are best applied in an oblique or spiral manner to fingers so as to avoid circumferential constraint. If there is skin loss, it is helpful to avoid pressing tulle-gras firmly onto this, arranging instead that it tent over the raw surface, the hollow being usefully allowed to fill with fibrin, clot, tulle-gras grease, or aqueous cream. This will make the first dressing change much easier. In digital moulding, there may eventually be 5–6 layers of tulle creating a greasy tube

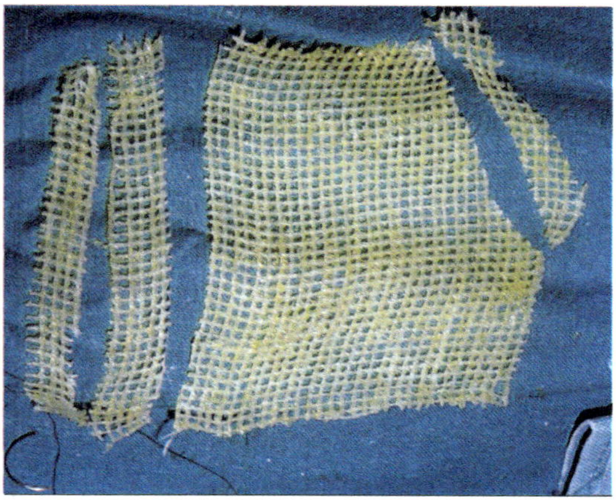

Fig. 11.8 To make useful strips, tulle must be cut parallel to the fibres. Obliquely cut strips just disintegrate

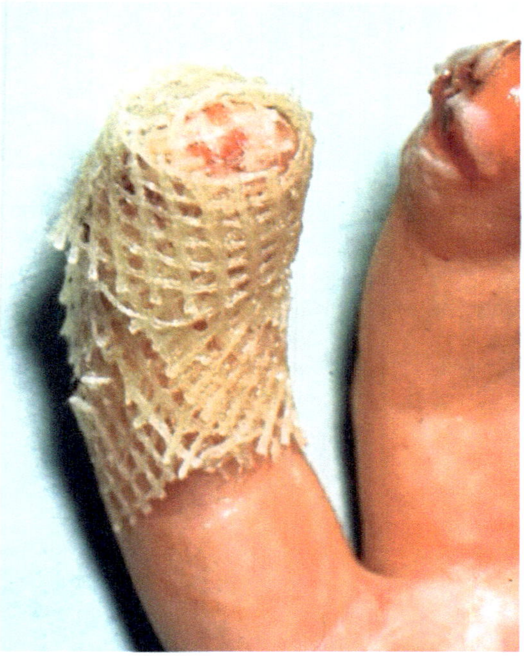

Fig. 11.9 Crushed fingertip after the application of tulle strips. The finger now simply needs protecting

within which a damaged digit can be surprisingly, accurately coaxed back to health.

A tulle mould should always try to start from the more mobile side and be attempting to replace tissue. Posturing joints can often assist replacement and should be done before any attempt at closure. At the end of the procedure, this posture must be maintained by splintage. It is particularly important that the tulle used for such moulding be soft and very greasy. The multiple-use tulle container can be stored upside down to achieve this and kept particularly sterile by only ever opening it briefly. Most individually packaged tulle tends to be too dry and springy after removing paper from both sides to mould onto skin properly. In the first 2 days, the tulle slides as tissue swells, maintaining the accurate disposition. Further closure often occurs during this time. Such a wound does however remain vulnerable to disruption by movement. Bleeding can also be readily started again. For both these reasons, complex wounds managed with tulle-gras usually require immobilisation. All patients with leg injuries should either have their leg elevated for the first 48 h in bed or be managed with the two-bandage regime [See Appendix].

Gels and Slough Digesters

Gels are non-toxic and can help to hydrate slough, but they are expensive and do no more for raw surfaces than tulle can. Aqueous cream on tulle is effective in softening dead tissue, and intermittent sharp dissection does wonders in helping to remove it. Enzyme-containing preparations do not distinguish clearly enough between slough and adjacent debilitated tissue, so they are liable to extend and deepen chronic ulcers. They usually cause painful wounds and certainly inhibit epithelialisation (Fig. 11.10).

Gauze and Tubegauze

Plain cotton gauze swabs applied singly or cut into suitable pieces make the best absorbent material (Fig. 11.11).

Seepage finds its way out into accurately applied gauze layers (see Fig. 11.6).

Poorly applied gauze can administer uneven pressure (Fig. 11.12).

Gauze needs holding in place as crepe bandages are applied, remembering that even the bandage turns are best applied in the direction

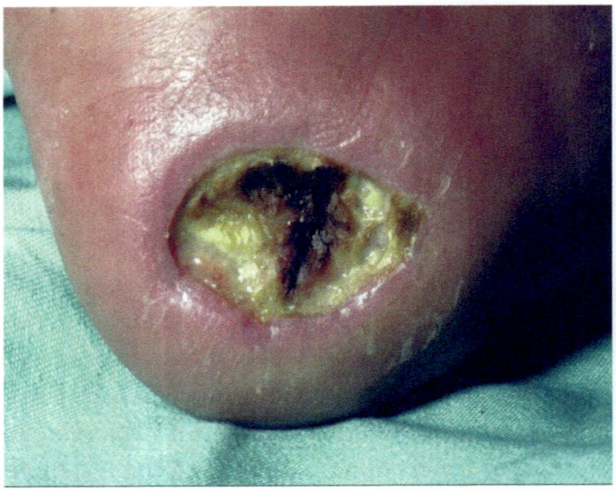

Fig. 11.10 Deep necrotic heel ulcer has been packed with enzyme-soaked ELASE™ ribbon gauze for more than 3 months. The prospects for healing are extremely poor

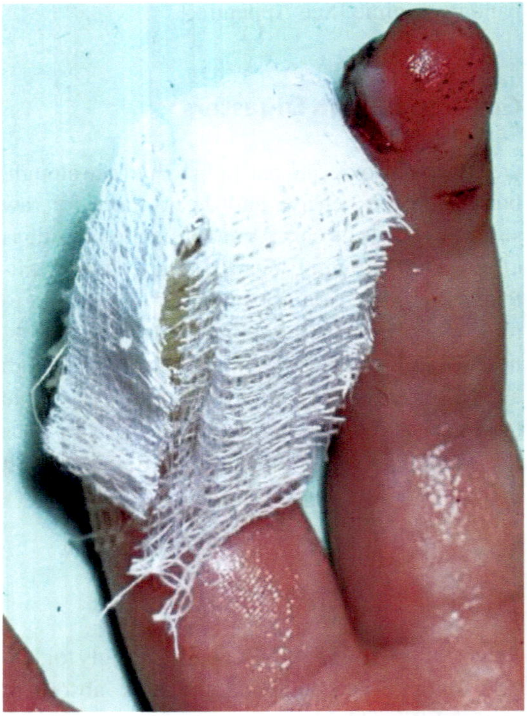

Fig. 11.11 Gauze strips are applied carefully over the tulle-gras

encouraging replacement rather than the opposite. Tube-gauze is not accurate enough as an acute dressing (Fig. 11.13).

Burns and wounds which have had abscesses or haematomas drained need greater bulk of

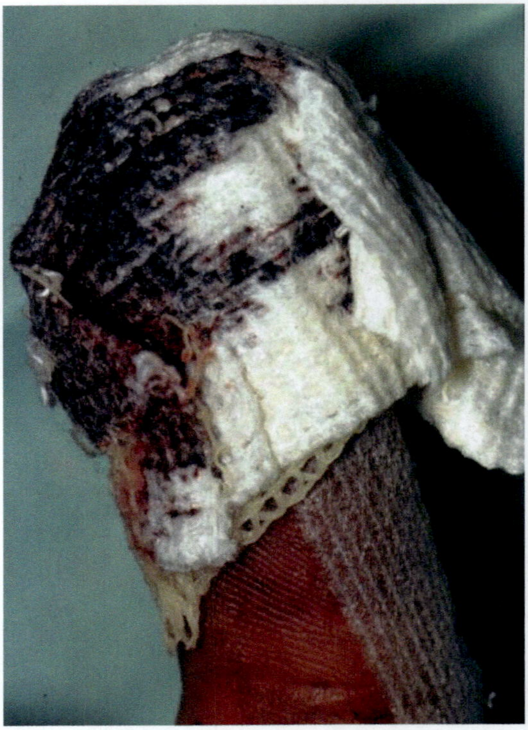

Fig. 11.12 Inaccurately applied gauze allows tissue inaccuracies and can also apply uneven pressure

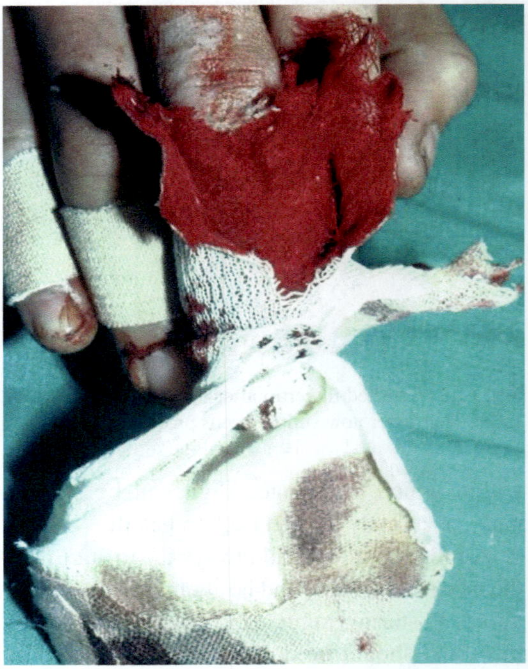

Fig. 11.13 Tube-gauze is not accurate enough for acute injuries. It is however fine for most later dressing regimes

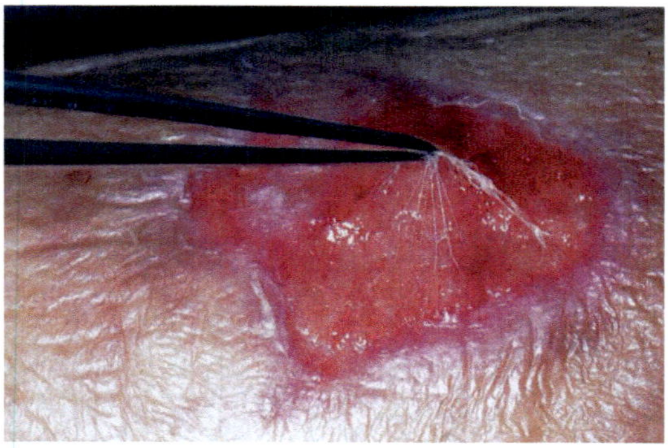

Fig. 11.14 This raw surface is not healing because of incorporated cotton wool fibres, which must be removed

absorbent material for the first few dressings. Cotton wool or lint is liable to stick, leaving fibres behind which can become incorporated in granulation tissue and interfere with healing (Fig. 11.14).

Saline Gauze Dressings

Damp saline gauze is a physiological dressing, but it must be either re-moistened regularly with saline or covered with tulle or GladWrap™ in order to keep it moist. Adherent gauze dressings need soaking with saline prior to removal. All procedures that produce bleeding are clearly interfering with healing. Intensive saline dressings are best restricted to a short period to remove the last shreds of adherent slough or to remove tulle- gras in the last dressing before skin grafting. Unfortunately, intensive saline regimes tend to be wheeled out when progress is slow, assuaging guilt or impatience or both, by giving the impression that all stops are being pulled out. All that is actually being achieved is extravagant nursing workload, with undue disturbance to both the wound and the patient. This has no advantage over a standard tulle/gauze dressings changed on alternate days.

Other Dressings

Dr. Joan Chapple strongly believed that **expensive,** individually packaged dressings of all kinds are actively marketed these days by medical companies who like to imply that these are essential if you really want to give your patient the most modern treatment.

Dressings made up of lint and cellophane are more of a nuisance than a help. They absorb only through tiny holes in the cellophane and wrinkle instead of moulding around contours. Seaweed/alginate dressings are fashionable and expensive, but when hydrated with saline are probably quite physiological. However, they start to dry off unless hydrated with saline and leave a good deal of debris around the wound. They are not actually better than tulle-gras at anything. *Editor MFK would challenge this statement based on his modern-day wound care experience.*

Other dressings have been devised for infected wounds. Topical antibiotics have a tendency to cause localised dermatitis, so they should only be used when pathogens have been confirmed as the cause of non-healing and there is no invasive sepsis. It is important not to use toxic topical chemicals on open wounds, e.g. Mercurochrome or Hydrogen Peroxide. *Editor MFK: I have used diluted Hydrogen Peroxide for years in the management of acute hand and limb injuries. In the right clinical scenario, its wound cleansing characteristics are second to none in my view!*

The most accurate and the least bulky dressings are usually the most comfortable. *Sometimes practicality overrides comfort.* After the first two or three changes, most patients can do their own dressings if some supervision can be arranged. In this era of user-pays, dressings can be enormously expensive. Patients can make saline for washing wounds by adding salt to boiled water. They can keep their own tulle-gras in the fridge and make perfectly satisfactory absorbent dressings out of old clean cotton material that has been washed, hung in the sun to dry, ironed and kept somewhere clean. There will be no problems as long as patients return if they are unwell, have any increased wound pain or notice that healing *has stalled.* People can better coordinate their own dressings with their daily lives, in particular with having a proper shower to suit themselves. No wound ever suffers from being washed in the shower. With the emergence of an increasing variety of antibiotic-resistant infections, it is becoming desirable to keep patients away from unnecessary contact with hospitals and professional clinics. *Editor MFK: in times of need and crisis [war, natural disasters, cyclones, floods, earthquakes, tsunamis—these adaptability principles may be important until proper medical aid arrives?].*

Bandages

Crepe bandages are easy to apply and make a tidy job. They are however elastic, and each turn adds pressure to the underlying ones. Avoid using pressure to maintain eventual haemostasis or to try to prevent reactive swelling, as this also reduces the circulation. Finger bandages need to be narrower than the width of the digit (Fig. 11.15).

If the bandage is too wide, dog-ears otherwise get left by turns over the tip. If a bandage does need to be cut down, always cut a strip off the machined edge and then roll it up again before use. Bandages work best from a roll with the bandage coming off the underside of the roll, not from the top (Fig. 11.16).

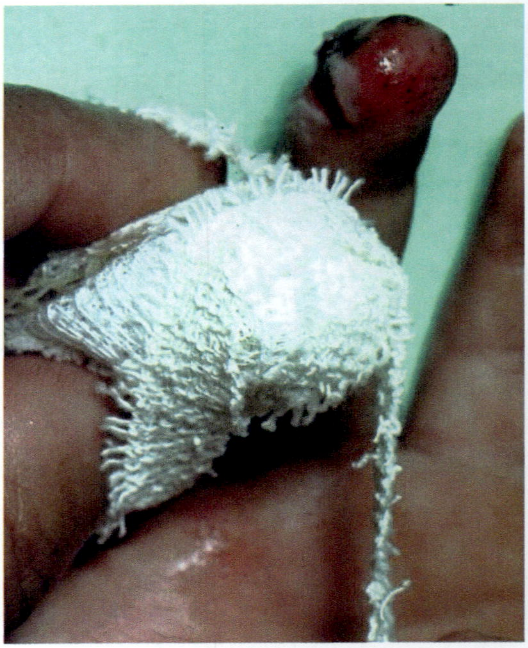

Fig. 11.15 An accurate, correctly sized [<width of digit] crepe bandage completes the finger dressing

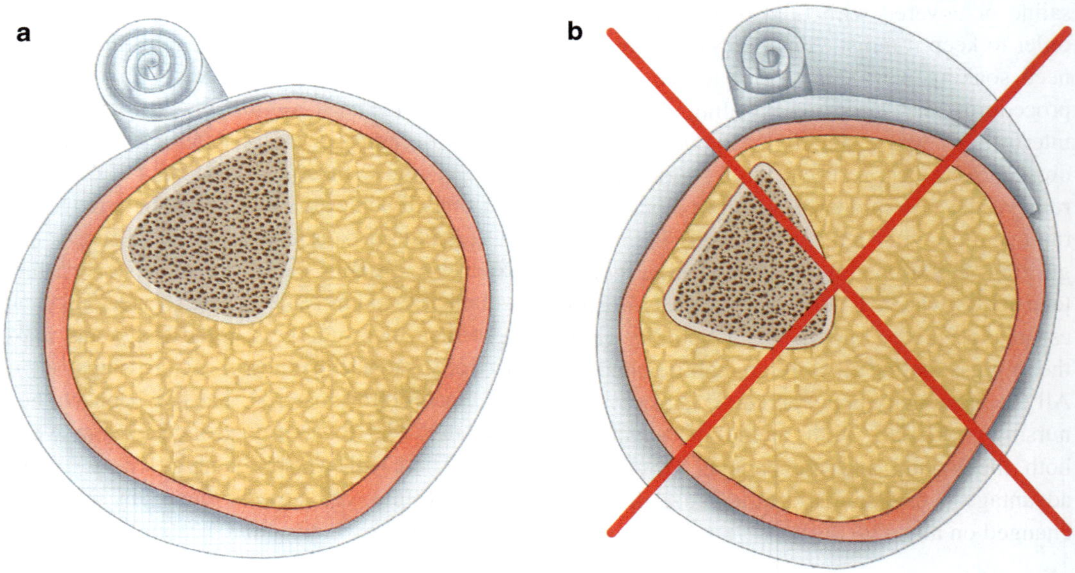

Fig. 11.16 A crepe bandage can only be accurately controlled if it unwinds from the underneath of the roll (**a** Correct, **b** Incorrect)

Sometimes a half-twist of a bandage will create a useful fixation point or suitably alter the direction of the bandage. A further half-twist should be made as soon as possible to reinstate it coming from the bottom of the roll.

Practice bandaging—The end of a bandage can be tucked in, pinned, or fixed with tape. Any circumferential non-elastic tape or splint applied over bandages will immediately convert the mechanism to an inextensible one, able to create relentless pressure as the tissues swell (Figs. 11.17 and 11.18).

Other elasticised bandages are available [Coban™ or Handygrip™] but as they are all capable of applying compounding pressures, these need to be used with considerable caution until their individual properties are thoroughly assessed. Bandaging can be as important as any aspect of the treatment. Elasticised tubular net is often very useful for holding dressings in place.

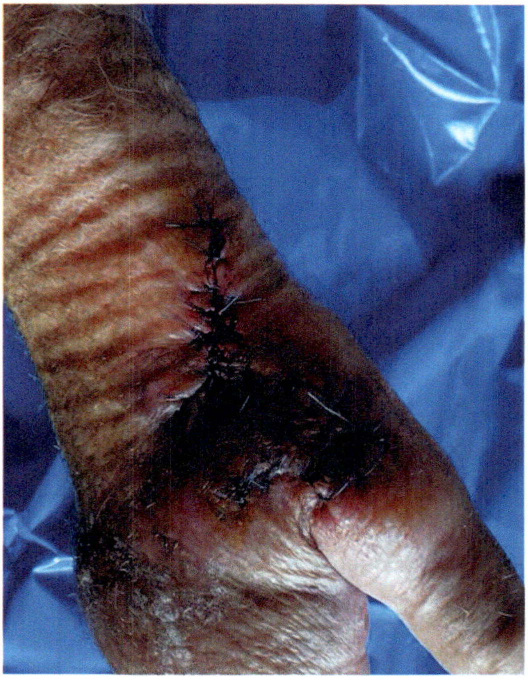

Fig. 11.18 MFK case—Elderly gentleman 1 week post excision SCC base of right thumb and repair with local flap + FTSG. Tight bandage aggravated by patient not elevating his healing hand

Tapes and Sticking Plaster

Sterile skin tapes [Steri-Strip™] can be used instead of sutures, but are capable of restricting the circulation if used unwisely, e.g. across new flaps or applied circumferentially in digits (Fig. 11.19).

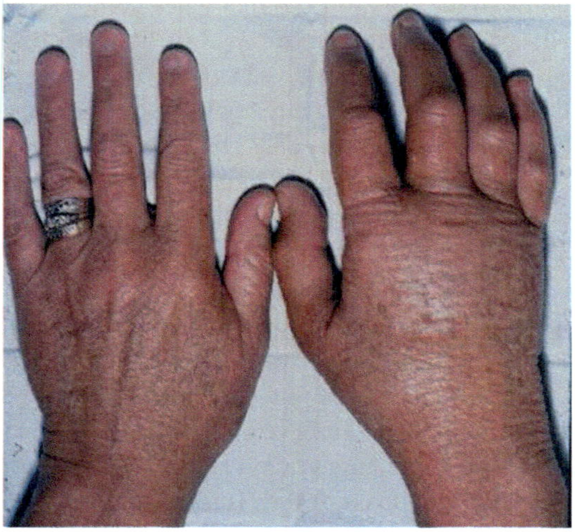

Fig. 11.17 Persistent swelling of right hand 3 weeks after carpal tunnel decompression caused by tight initial bandaging. This patient never regained full flexion or full use of her hand

They can also be used to enhance the security of a tulle closure, but need to be applied before the tulle to dry prepared skin, if they are used in this context. They can be used in addition to support a sutured wound, reducing tension generally and reducing the number of sutures needed. They should always be used when sutures are removed early (Figs. 11.20 and 11.21).

Tapes help to support wounds for a week or so after ordinary suture removal. It is always useful to cut the corners off tapes and sticking plasters to prevent them lifting by the corners. Most producers of Band-Aid™ equivalents finally seem to have cottoned onto this and are now rounding the corners of their products. Sticking plasters can be tailored for use on digits (Fig. 11.22).

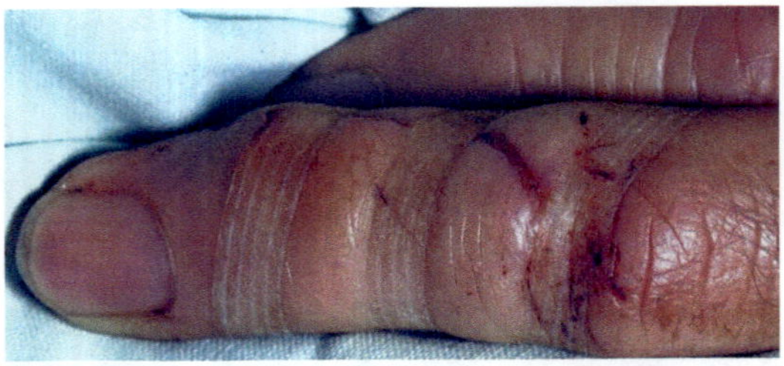

Fig. 11.19 Inextensible circumferential tapes [Steri-Strips™] have trapped the reactionary swelling and the finger has been very painful for 3 days. Tulle-gras or a non-circumferential tape closure would have been safer

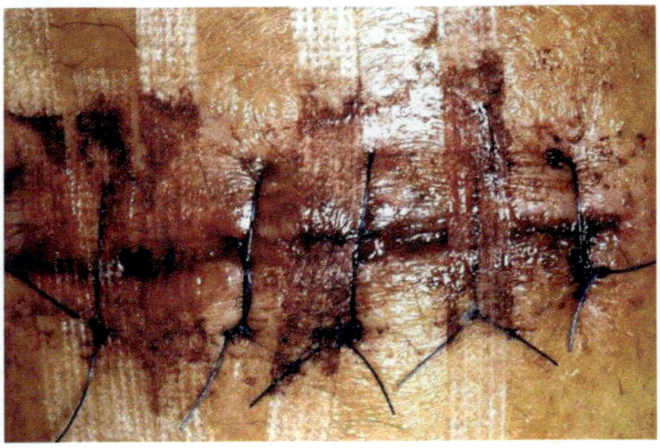

Fig. 11.20 A combination of sutures and tapes are providing fairly safe closure at 3 days. Note slight oedema of the edges

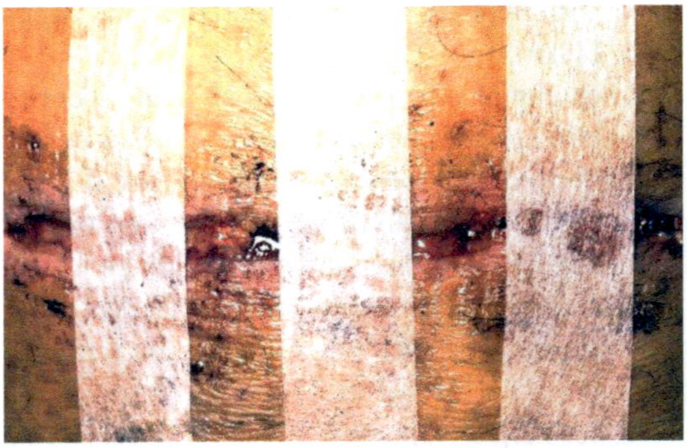

Fig. 11.21 Sutures were replaced by tapes with a much quieter wound at day 6

Modern non-elastic medical tapes such as Micropore™ are much less allergenic than those with Zinc Oxide adhesives. Longer strips to reduce tension in the vicinity of a wound can be made with 1 cm wide medical tape off a roll. These may need to be 30–40 cm long. To stop this sort of tape sticking to a flap or other com-

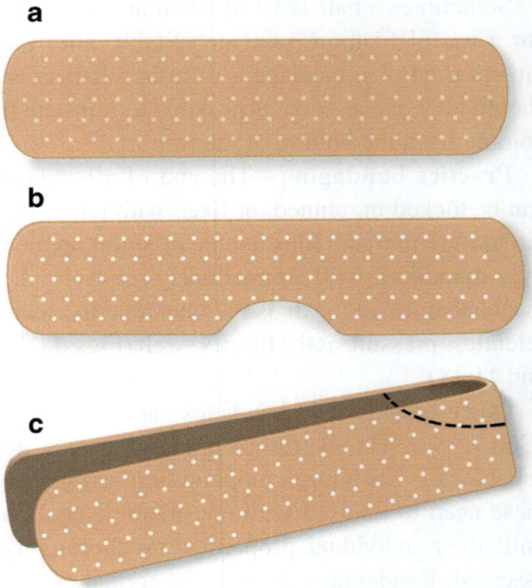

Fig. 11.22 The tailoring of sticking plasters: (**a**) Round the corners if this has not already been done in the manufacture. (**b**) Piece cut out to apply around the base of a finger dressing. (**c**) Cutting out this piece is best done by folding the strip back on itself

plex injury it may be passing over, a section can be rendered non-adherent by sticking tape to the underside. Sometimes it may be necessary to build up the 'take-off' so that tapes do not actually press onto the prominence of wounded tissue. Additional security can be conferred on a tape closure by eventually applying another tape transversely across the ends (Fig. 11.23).

Posturing of adjacent joints may be helpful and immobilisation usually needs to be added to all these other manoeuvres.

Inelastic tapes of any kind can provide a wonderfully effective closure and stabilisation when applied across painful skin cracks such as develop beside a thumbnail or in the thick keratotic ridge of heel skin. Pain is relieved instantly and healing follows within hours or days, especially for people who develop cracks whilst out tramping. The brittle skin ridges can be dealt with later.

Elastoplast and Elastic Dressings

Elastoplast™ sticks much better to itself than to skin and keeps a crepe bandage in good condition, particularly if the end sticks to itself somewhere. It should never be stretched on, especially around fingers. Never apply any kind of tape by pulling it from a roll onto either the patient or dressings. The tension transferred will depend on the stickiness of the product and such variables as the temperature/heat of the day. Elastic sticking plaster can apply enormous pressure, and circumferential tapes are capable of restricting circulation as tension builds up in the wound area (Fig. 11.24).

Elastoplast™ can be very useful for small wound dressings and also around the base of a crepe or Tubegauze [Tubular-Gauze™] finger dressing, where it needs a crescent cut out to allow finger movements, but should not be stretched on and must be long enough to stick to itself (Fig. 11.25).

3M Microfoam™ is less allergenic than Elastoplast™ and stretches in all directions. It is an exceedingly useful material for awkward wounds, but caution is needed when it is used as a bandage. Adherent plastic dressings can be useful for grazes and donor surfaces, especially to apply and contain a small amount of cream. They are not a true substitute for skin and mainly useful for partial-thickness losses.

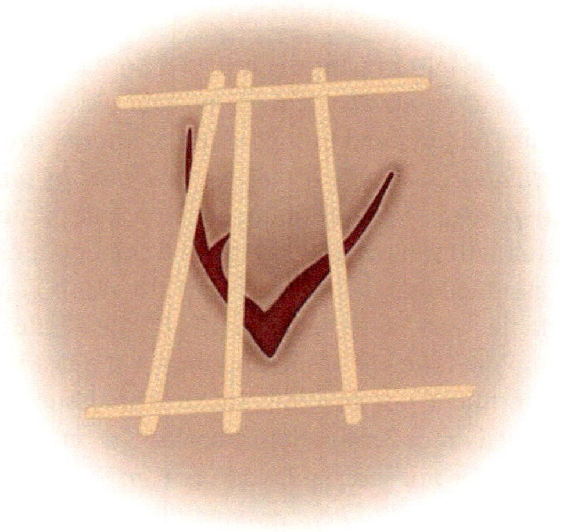

Fig. 11.23 This slightly ragged flap is showing some venous congestion, which makes it unsafe to replace more fully or to suture. The main tapes are longitudinal and have been further secured with a transverse tape across their ends

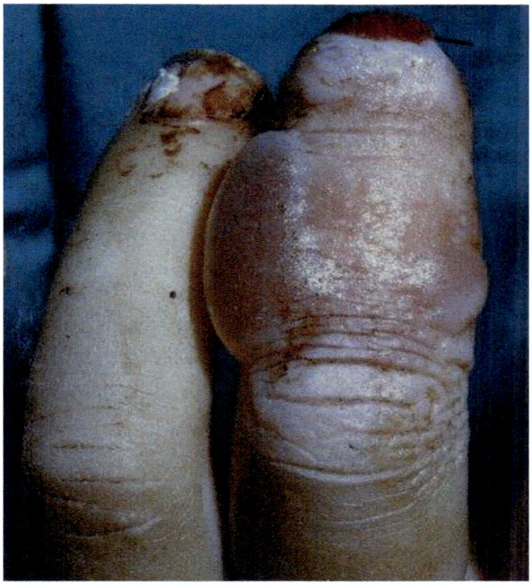

Fig. 11.24 Blistering caused by a tight Elastoplast™ around the base of a bandage

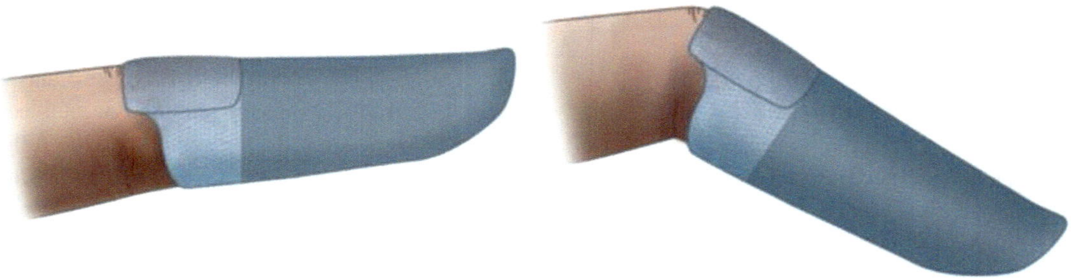

Fig. 11.25 Tidy Tubular-Gauze™ finger dressing. The circumferential Elastoplast™ should not be stretched on, be cut away to allow full PIPJ flexion and be long enough to stick to itself

MFK favours Fixomull Stretch™ or Hypafix™ as a flexible breathable initial dressings for fingers, hands, and other mobile areas where surgery has been required. He does also like three-inch Elastoplast™ for securing the outer dressings of skin graft donor sites on thighs.

Immobilisation

External splintage is as important in the management of circulatory instability as it is for fractures and dislocations, especially where wounds are being managed without formal suturing. Splints can be made with moulded thermo-plastic, metal, Plaster of Paris [Gypsona™] or fibreglass; all preferably used as slabs. When these are not available, makeshift splints can be devised. Plaster-of-Paris is not only the cheapest technology for immobilisation, but is the least toxic to use. Both its production and disposal is significantly more acceptable environmentally than fibreglass, which may be justifiable where light, waterproof immobilisation is required for a long period.

Complete casts must always be fully split after acute trauma for circulatory safety. Fractures are nearly always associated with soft tissue injury in the vicinity, making it even more imperative that swelling is allowed for by using a slab or split cast. A 1 cm-wide strip can be cut out of a complete cast to allow for swelling, without having to apply any bandages or tape over the gap. Underlying bandages can be accessed easily and divided if necessary to relieve pain. The position of any fracture is unlikely to lapse if the split plaster is supported by re-bandaging as swelling subsides.

Removal of Dressings and Redressing

Wounds ideally need several days' rest to recover. It can be quite useful to gently change outer dressings or reduce them while they are still moist. Throbbing pain is often relieved by reduction of bandage tension. If this doesn't happen, it is worth looking at the wound more closely to see if there are tight sutures and/or a haematoma, both of which should be released. If the 'haemostasis-before-final-dressing' technique has been used, the dressings are unlikely to be involved in a heavily blood-soaked mess. Any wound, which instead of beginning to settle after the first 2 days gets steadily more painful, also needs to be examined closely as infection may be developing. *After 35-years-experience of managing surgical and traumatic wounds, MFK strongly believes that they all need a dressing change at 24 h and if necessary, this may need to be performed as an EUA. The principle is to remove any blood-stained dressings which are a risk to normal, rapid wound healing. He also believes that the primary surgeon should do this dressing change.*

Removing dressings is less of an ordeal if it is done rather slowly and if possible, with the patient helping and co-operating. *Children are a particular challenge if they are attended by anxious parents.* Verbal communication and participation will remove a good deal of anxiety. It can be assumed that the wound is healthy if it is comfortable and does not smell of dead flesh. Complete removal of the dressing or the last layers of tulle is not then imperative. The tissues are obviously recovering. Saline soaking is only ever helpful for non-greasy layers. *For greasy layers, use Paraffin oil to help remove the tulle if it has dried.* In the digits, removal of dressings is often best done by splitting the outer layers longitudinally with sharp, blunt-ended dressing scissors, opening them like an oyster shell rather than unwinding every layer, leaving clean tulle-gras layers to be similarly cut and eased off towards the wound.

If dressing removal does become an ordeal, giving the patient and yourself a welcome rest now and then is a good tactic. The best plane to work in to remove dressings is the one between the gauze and the tulle [or sometimes the tulle/skin junction], rather than painfully removing layer after layer of stuck material. It is best to gently lift the tulle off rather than tugging at it. Always lift dressing material off from each side towards the wound in order to minimise distortion of the most sensitive tissue. Patience is a sublime virtue in dressing removal. *MFK's view is that the primary surgeon is the best professional to change the first dressing and subsequent one because they know exactly what is beneath the layers of dressings and ideally, they will have applied the original dressing. This is a fundamental skill taught to junior plastic surgical trainees by experienced plastic surgical nurses. His experience is that community nurses are also very skilled at dressing changes and he involves them, if the clinical circumstances of the patient demand this. Open communication using digital photographs and emails facilitates a co-ordinated team approach to the patients' dressing management until final healing is achieved.*

In rare situations, where the dressing removal is a real challenge, the use of local anaesthetic is recommended by Joan Chapple.

Tulle-gras mouldings can be repeated but it is usually more appropriate to be coaxing wounds to close with tapes after the first few days. For taping, the skin needs to be cleaned of grease with solutions such as ether or painted with Tincture of Benzoin, which after drying the tapes will stick to more effectively. Tapes also function well as a local splint so other splintages may be discontinued as long as there is no underlying bone or joint injury. Residual raw surfaces need re-dressing with tulle-gras over the tapes, then gauze outer dressings until wounds heal.

The main purpose of a continuing dressing regime is to prevent the drying of residual raw surfaces (Fig. 11.26).

Several layers of tulle are needed if the wound is going to be left for a few days between dressings. It is a bad technique to leave raw surfaces to dry if the dressing procedure is ever interrupted or while waiting for someone else to inspect the wound. Always leave raw surfaces under a saline-soaked swab or at least return the tulle temporarily to prevent drying. *Warm, moist wound conditions are the best for granulations and epithelialisation. In contrast, desiccating conditions are the worst.* Following complete healing, there is sometimes a place for supportive or protective dressings. *MFK believes in taping scars with flesh-coloured Micropore™ for up to 3 months until the scar has regained significant tensile strength. This will provide the patient with the highest chance of an excellent long-term scar from an aesthetic perspective.*

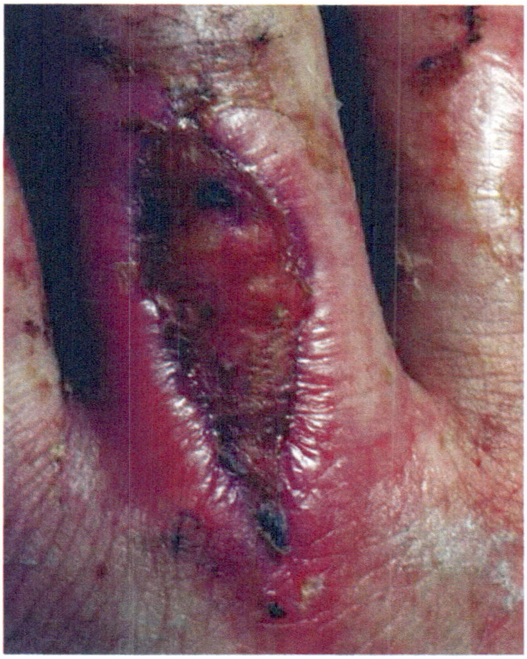

Fig. 11.26 This unhealthy wound now has a dry surface, which cannot support healing until it granulates again

Chronic Wounds: Diagnosis and Dressings

Dead tissue and infection in a wound are the most common causes for delayed healing. A dressing regime to hydrate slough and help it to separate can be assisted greatly by intermittent sharp dissection with fine curved iris scissors or a #15 scalpel blade. Enzyme digestion of slough is dangerous as it does not distinguish clearly enough between dead and debilitated tissue. As soon as dead tissue has separated, the wound can set about producing granulations and it is much less likely from this point to get infected. Epithelium from the edges or from islands should begin to spread rapidly across a healthy granulation tissue (Fig. 11.27).

If it is not doing this, the wound is still unhealthy no matter how clean it looks. The

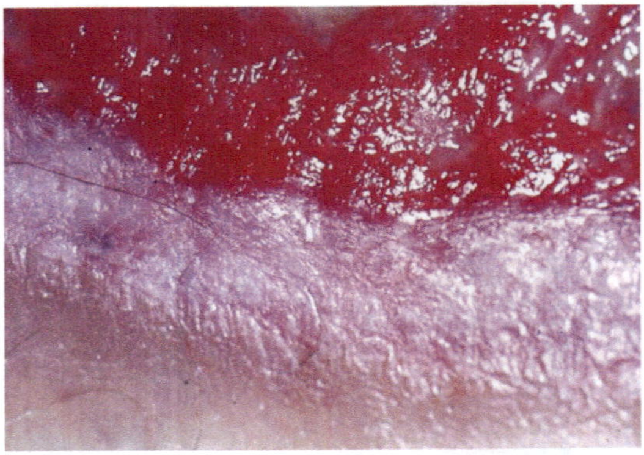

Fig. 11.27 Healthy raw surface showing a rapidly advancing epithelial edge

source of the delay at this stage can be due to one of several factors. These need to be systematically excluded rather than simply going on and on changing dressings.

Causes of Delayed Healing

1. Healing can be reduced or stopped by **pathogenic bacteria.** A swab must always be taken from unhealthy wounds to see if these are present. If there is no invasive sepsis, the appropriate response is to use topical antibiotic cream or lotion administered on a dressing and changed daily. Invasive infection requires systemic antibiotics, making topical antibiotics superfluous. Infection can destroy skin and produce abscesses, both of which delay healing.
2. The surface may be damaged by **drying.** Epithelial cells cannot migrate on a desiccated wound surface.
3. There may be **foreign material/foreign bodies** in the wound, including sutures, dead tissue, dirt from the original injury, or strands of dressing material including tulle-gras and cotton wool. Such a wound is in 'foreign-body-rejection' mode and cannot heal until the situation is remedied. The persistence of a discharging sinus or non-healing granuloma can be related to dirt, dead bone, or fibrous tissue, as well as non-absorbable suture material. Active excision of dead tissue and removal of haematomas is always helpful.
4. The wound may be being **chemically discouraged** from healing, e.g. by having toxic solutions applied to it, usually in an attempt to prevent or treat infection. *MFK has inherited patients being treated with a variety of unorthodox, alternative medicine poultices, black salve, and even one patient who was dressing his chronic leg ulcer with a solution of his own urine! Healing was compromised by these approaches.*
5. **Interference** with a wound by the patient, also known as factitious wounding. Very rarely a patient may be wilfully discouraging healing by mechanical or chemical means and even by introducing foreign material. *John Bennett FRCS, one of MFK's mentors at East Grinstead in England, used to see at least one patient with a factitious chronic wound* per annum *in his practice.* A dressing must be cleverly engineered to prevent direct access to the wound. Healing will proceed apace when harmful influences are stopped. Some part of the psyche of most of these patients usually wants to be healed again, so it is best to raise the possibility of wound harm as a somewhat abstract concept with the patient, allowing the patient to come out of the situation with some honour. Encouragement rather than blame or anger will be most likely to achieve a successful outcome. *In the most challenging cases, often involving younger patients with dysfunctional family dynamics, psychological services may need to be involved. MFK has found that after all other possibilities for the delayed healing have been excluded, direct challenge is the only way forward and the patients/families will either accept psychological counselling or discharge themselves.*

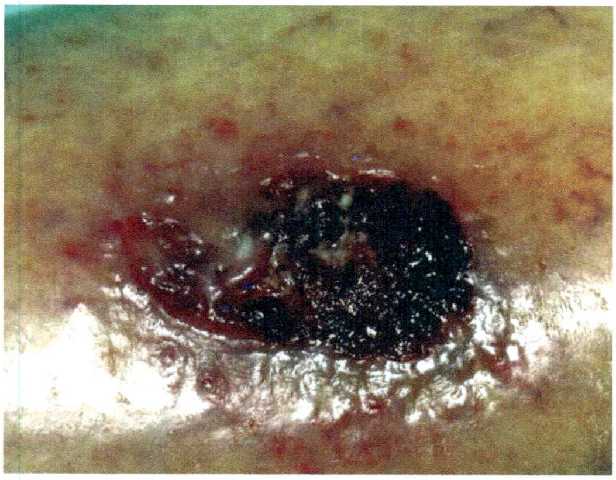

Fig. 11.28 A chronic leg ulcer of 3 years' duration which was diagnosed as a basal cell carcinoma [BCC] by a small biopsy, after excluding other causes of non-healing. It was treated successfully by wide excision and a graft

Rarely they may invoke a medico-legal challenge, so documentation, photographic evidence, and a chronological record are essential.

6. A granulating unhealed wound may occasionally be the **surface of a low-grade neoplasm.** An incisional biopsy may be indicated once other causes have been eliminated. An ulcerated or rapidly growing tumour obviously does not come into this category and requires at the very least an excision biopsy (Fig. 11.28).

Really Chronic Ulcers

Most chronic ulcers have a serious underlying circulatory problem for which there is no specific treatment. The locality may not even have enough circulation to reject slough, let alone produce granulations. Infective episodes are often a recurring problem. Desiccation has a particularly detrimental effect on such poor-quality tissue. The patient should be assisted to design and manage a dressing regime to fit their lifestyle and be reminded to report promptly any new exacerbations of infection. The throbbing pain of invasive sepsis may or may not be associated with inflammation but usually responds well to the appropriate antibiotics. Non-infective pain occurs sometimes and is well worth treating with medication if sleep or quality-of-life are affected. It may also be worthwhile trying other dressing materials and regimes for chronic ulcers that remain painful despite infection being controlled. Patients may want to try various remedies of their own including Manuka Honey and its antibacterial qualities or medicinal marijuana.

The 'Gate' Dressing

If a dressing regime is likely to be prolonged, it can be useful to design a mechanism to hold the dressing in place so that sticking plaster and tapes are not having to be frequently pulled off the skin. One of the most useful of these is the 'gate' dressing. It is a very old technique dating from the pre-antibiotic era [pre-1940] when discharging wounds sometimes required dressings for months or years. It requires the careful preparation of at least two pieces of wide sticking plaster, which have rounded corners and about a third of their length folded back over a swab stick. Several small holes are cut beside the stick, and after preparation of the skin with Tincture of Benzoin, one of these plasters is applied on each side of the wound with a space between them for the dressing to be laced in with ribbon-gauze. It is of course possible to use another two of these sticking plasters at right angles to the first pair. While this mechanism is usually incompatible with showering [except when it all needs replacing], it is a much better regime for the skin. It makes dressings much easier and often enables patients or their families to do the dressings (Fig. 11.29).

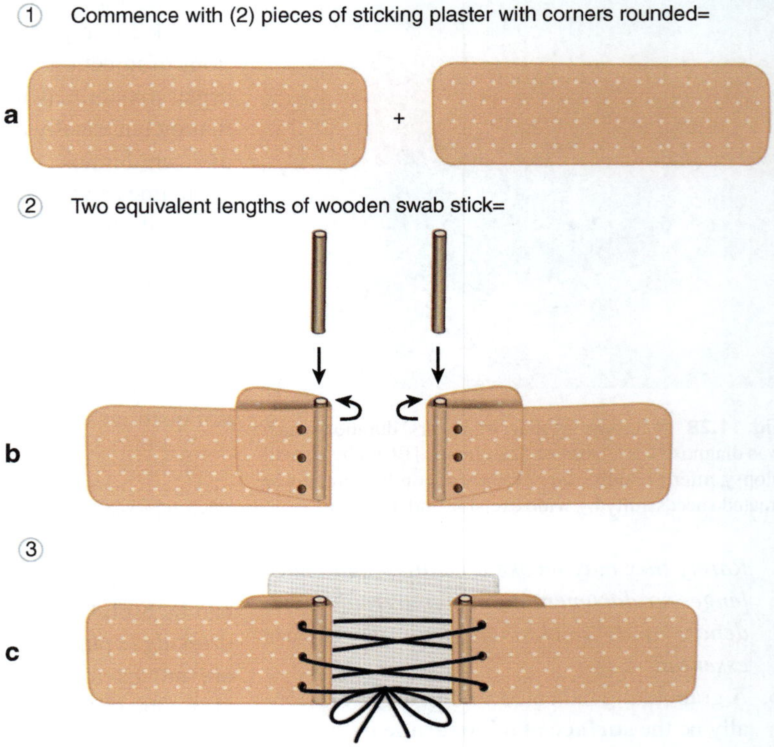

Fig. 11.29 The Gate Dressing. Each sticking plaster strip (**a**) has one end folded back over a swab stick (**b**). After holes are made for lacing, one strip is applied on each side and the dressing can be tied in place (**c**)

Rehabilitation

Communication

Rehabilitation is always about the whole person and begins at the first communication. Injured people usually remember quite clearly what is said to them initially. Reassurances that they will be able to cope with everything are what most people need to hear. It is always the unknown that is most scary. Patients also need to know that they will have the necessary assistance with pain management. A great deal of unnecessary anxiety is experienced if patients are fearful that they might somehow let themselves and everyone else down. They cope remarkably well if they are given enough information and encouragement, as well as being helped by the people who are important to them.

Patients rarely need a complicated medical dissertation about the differential diagnosis, an over-emphasised account of all the possible risks and complications, or a voyage into the worst-case scenario. A confident positive communication is important, e.g. *'It probably looks pretty terrible to you but there's no tissue lost and it all looks very much alive, so there shouldn't be any problems with healing. Luckily you haven't damaged anything really important'*. Or *'You'll be healed by this time next week and should be back to doing everything again in 3–4 weeks'*. Or *'We'll be able to put it all back together alright but it will take a while to heal because it's been pretty badly crushed. It's going to swell up for a few days but it won't ever get too sore. You'll be able to start walking about a bit in a week or so'*. Or *'You have damaged this or that which needs repairing, but it will take a while to find out how well it's all going to work. You may find that you do things a different way for a while, but you will certainly be able to eventually do everything you did before it all happened'.*

Reassure patients that improvement in their scars and function will continue after healing for many months or years. Ask them if they have any questions they want answered and make the answers as straightforward and honest as possible. Be both optimistic and realistic. Joan Chapple believed that it was a good thing to encourage patients to look at their own wounds, so they could begin to engage with the reality of the situation and fully understand their treatment. In this way, the patient can greatly assist in their own recovery and are involved in each new stage as a participant. This makes a great difference to their rehabilitation.

Pain

Next in the rehabilitation plan is pain management. Initially, intravenous analgesia injected slowly provides the most immediate relief of pain from acute wounds and ensures that the dosage is adequate. Responding properly to a patient's initial pain is the first opportunity to express practical caring, helping to establish a relationship that the patient will need to rely on and be supported by throughout their rehabilitation. Many people have previously experienced or witnessed intolerable pain situations and need reassuring. If tissue is treated appropriately, pain should never become intolerable. With uncomplicated wounds, oral analgesia is usually all that is needed after the initial IV injection, and this may be required for several days. Severe throbbing pain during the first 48 h indicates that all is not well and there must be clear instructions and a way for patients to return promptly for relief of dressing tension. If this does not relieve the pain, wound inspection is indicated. Snipping of sutures or even further decompression may be necessary. Pain ordinarily decreases steadily and quite rapidly after the first few days, unless infection supervenes.

Comfort in the first few days indicates a good level of perfusion, allows restful sleep, and sets the scene for uneventful recovery and rehabilitation. It is helpful initially to have the painful part protected and immobilised. Dressing bulk can be reduced as soon as possible and a little comfortable early movement plus light touch can be encouraged even in the dressings. This helps maintain neuromuscular patterns of function. It should be commendable rather than disconcerting if any patient returns with their outer dressings mildly dirty from useful activity! Splintage must be used if movement and use is to be absolutely prevented.

Excessive pain in the first few days is always related to tension and vascular insufficiency. If unrelieved, this sets a bad scenario in train. Nerves get thoroughly jangled up, the circulation remains destabilised and additional muscle tension exacerbates the pain. Patients become sleep deprived and anxious, with a low tolerance for everything, especially pain. They get worn out, frustrated, or depressed by constant pain and before long quite ordinary sensory stimuli begin to get misinterpreted as painful, greatly discouraging use. Many disabling complex regional pain syndromes begin in just this way. They are often associated with the physical changes that follow circulatory insufficiency. Necrosis and/or haematoma can become a basis for invasive infection, which causes renewed and additional pain, swelling, and diffuse scarring, all of which are likely to interfere further with and prolong rehabilitation. This is represented diagrammatically in a Pain/Disability chart (Fig. 11.30).

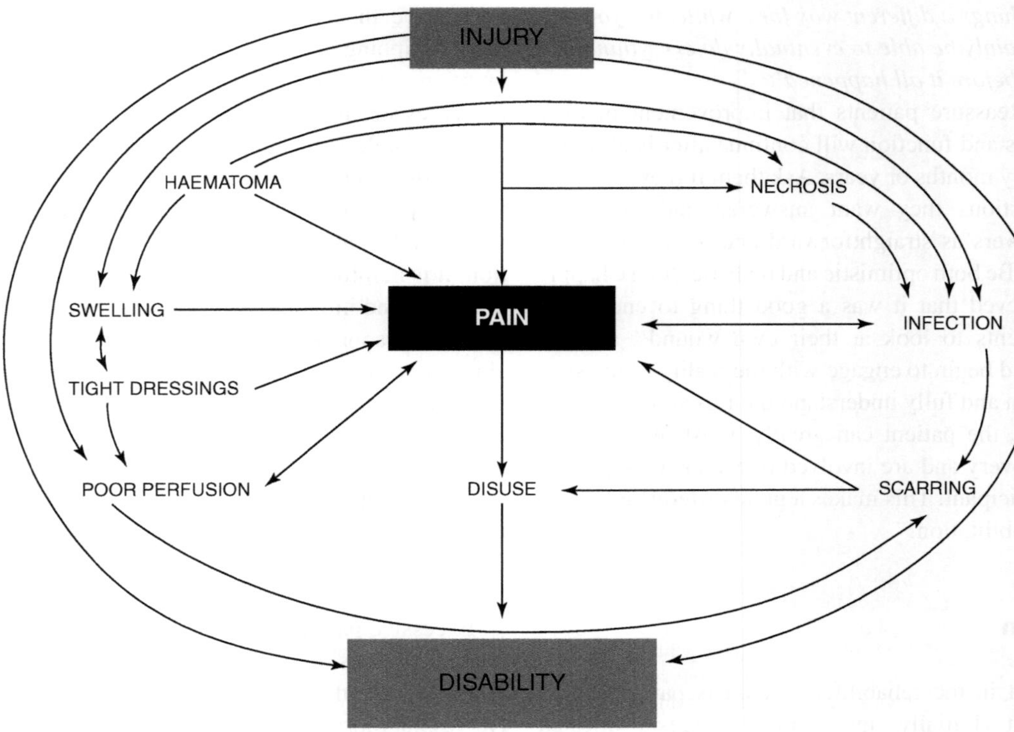

Fig. 11.30 Pain/Disability chart

Oedema

Since traumatic oedema is an indication of cellular injury, maximising the circulation is the best way to help. Pressure bandaging, in an attempt to either prevent or treat swelling, is therefore completely inappropriate. Encouraging direct seepage from a semi-closed wound by gravity reduces oedema and tension, which facilitates early mobilisation and encourages further seepage. Elevation should remain part of the regime until swelling resolves and sustained active movement, which disperses oedema, should be commenced as soon as this is comfortable. Passive movement while the part is still swollen merely rearranges oedema at the expense of the opposite movement. Forced or painful passive movement can actually reduce the range of movement by producing additional injury and new reactive oedema. Patients should be warned that for some time there will be an exaggerated tissue response to even further minor injury or excessive use. They need to be made aware of this before assuming that they can resume a demanding sports or work programme just because the skin is healed. Provided that patients are able to increase their activity gradually, within the constraints of pain and swelling, the return to some use and work is very beneficial. Woody oedema which persists after 3–4 weeks often has its origins in early circulatory deprivation, infection, or inappropriate therapy, rather than just severe trauma. By this time, diffuse fibrosis is also occurring and rehabilitation can be delayed or incomplete.

Splintage

It seems reasonable that the body's resources can be more adequately focused on the early recovery of the injured tissues, if both the person and the part are rested. The injured person intuitively seeks peace and quiet. Splintage assists the wound greatly.

Mechanical rest to the injured part has several benefits.

1. It helps stabilise the circulation, assists recovery from circulatory spasm, and helps to maintain haemostasis. Posturing adjacent joints to reduce wound tension in the first 48 h facilitates venous drainage of congested tissues.
2. Immobilisation assists the rapid establishment of additional capillary circulation.
3. Immobilisation minimises pain, anxiety, and associated muscle tension.
4. Protective splintage prevents any disturbance of the wound, particularly where alternatives to sutures have been used. It confers comfort and security, particularly during sleep.
5. Splintage provides mechanical stability while fracture and/or joint injuries heal.
6. Splintage in the position of function protects the joint function while injured or inflamed tissues are swollen and recovering.
7. Immobilisation of the injured part can often permit the early resumption of function in the rest of the body.

Posturing

The posture required to safeguard or improve a precarious circulation must initially take precedence over the best joint position, if these conflict. The posture must be restored to the optimal one for joint function as soon as the circulation is assured. The functional posture in which to immobilise a joint is that in which its major ligaments are kept stretched during the period of reactive swelling (Fig. 11.31).

When the main ligaments are slack as allowed by the rest position without splintage, they will shorten very rapidly. It can then be very difficult to regain a full range of movement. Wrist and ankle joints are at particular risk in the unsplinted rest position. The wrist should ordinarily be immobilised in 15–20° of extension. Functional posturing of the hand should ensure flexion at the finger MCPJs with the PIPJs in full extension. Immobilising the ankle at a right angle until patients are weight-bearing again is especially important in protecting ankle function.

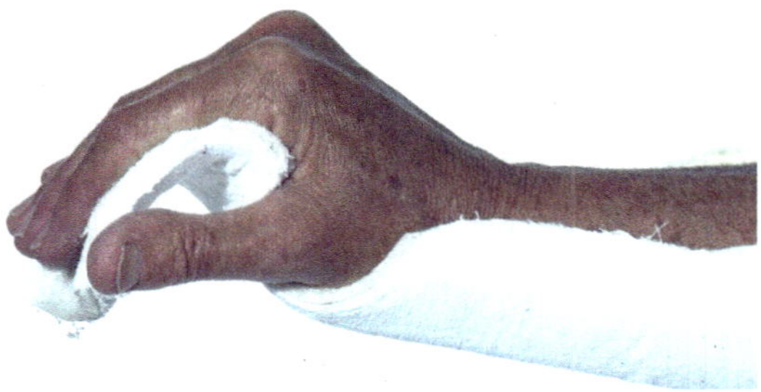

Fig. 11.31 Functional safe position for an injured hand or digits. This optimal position keeps all the major ligaments tensed and this prevents shortening which can restrict later function

Sensory Rehabilitation

Comfortable early touch is the best sensory rehabilitation of all, and pressure stimulation can commence through bandages. Specific sensory rehabilitation is not usually needed unless early pain levels have been excessive or there has been nerve damage resulting in altered or absent sensation. In these cases, gentle touching, patting, stroking, and repetitive percussion of the affected areas or scars assists the return of acceptable sensation. Patients can do this themselves. Sensory improvement will continue over many months as nerves recover, regrow, are released from scar and grow in from adjacent skin. Recovery is also assisted by re-education and adaptation. Sensory recovery after nerve injuries is always much more accurate and impressive in children. Permanently painful sensation or sensory loss, especially around the hand and face, can be particularly disabling. Patients with sensory deficits, paraesthesia, or pain have relatively greater disability than those with purely motor losses, although this is not nearly as obvious to other people.

Motor Rehabilitation

Regaining movement is encouraged by use but it is important that regular sustained active stretching movements aimed at extending any reduced range are also practiced. The maximum movement needs to be held for 30 s before changing to the opposite one, each session lasting no more that 5–10 min, several times a day. Hands may need to be temporarily taken out of their functional splints to do this work but must be returned to these after more severe injuries, for at least 10 days. Rapidly alternating or waggling movements do not achieve anything more than a sense of freedom. Passive joint movement is not needed unless nerves have been injured and should never be forceful or exceed the pain threshold. Occasionally people do too much additional exercise and can experience a loss of movement, rather than a gain. All of us normally alternate muscular use with inactivity and recovering tissue also needs to be rested. It is best to advise careful ordinary use with short periods of additional exercise several times a day, until full capacity has been regained.

Physiotherapy

Patients usually pass from the early painful phases of recovery into one of recovering both function and movement quite seamlessly, within 2 or 3 weeks. This is just when most physiotherapy is added. It is hardly surprising that in most cases, the rapid progress that follows tends to be attributed to the therapy, when it was going to happen anyway. The conditions that are resistant to physiotherapy generally arise out of something very different. Problems can be associated with severe initial damage but much too often there is also a significant contribution from early circulatory insufficiency. Recovery in these cases has frequently been unduly painful as well as slow. Persistent oedema may be present. Atrophy and stiffness are often long-term features and may persist despite prolonged physiotherapy.

In severe injuries, the excursion of injured joints may not be regained until the scar tissue softens. Ordinary use needs to be supplemented by sustained active exercises over several months to extend any reduced range. Active and passive movements always need to be kept within the limits of pain, because they can otherwise both produce oedema, which reduces the range of movement. While the hoped for range of movement might be regained earlier by more aggressive therapy, instability of joints can sometimes occur when scar tissue eventually matures and lengthens. Patients accepting of somewhat reduced but useful range of movement in the first few months and gradually increasing this may get the best final outcome.

The maintenance of a full range of movement of uninjured joints requires a concern by both patient and all professionals to retain this. Elderly people are most at risk. All patients with their arm in a sling for soft tissue injuries need the full range of shoulder and elbow movements demonstrated and then practised daily out of the sling. Patients with hand injuries need to do this, whether or not they have injuries further up the arm. It is particularly unfortunate to end up with a satisfactorily healed and useful hand, but a frozen shoulder! While patients usually enjoy regaining function, they don't always think of this maintenance aspect themselves.

Disability

Rehabilitation is the re-establishment of the confidence and ability to do everything that was done before the injury. Disability has complex causes, is always subjective, and not directly related to physical abnormality. Dr. Joan Chapple once asked an elderly woman with severe rheumatoid hand deformities, if there were any things she couldn't do (Fig. 11.32).

'What do you mean?' she replied indignantly. *'If I can't do it with one hand, I simply use both!'* The fact that her deformities had come on gradually, combined with the fact that she had no sensory loss or residual pain, meant that she could

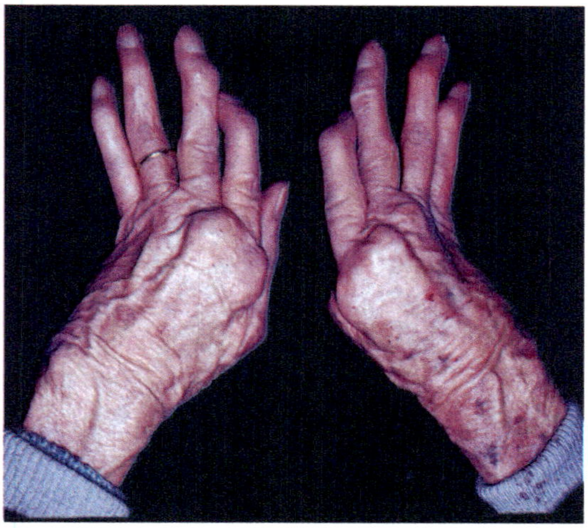

Fig. 11.32 Severe rheumatoid hand deformities in a 70-year-old who wound not acknowledge any disability whatsoever

manage everything on her own and did not see herself as in any way disabled.

Patients who don't make a full recovery may need encouragement or assistance to do things a different way or they may be helped by specific tools or prostheses. They may need help with the acceptance of reduced function. The long-term responsibility for rehabilitation is otherwise best transferred to the patient, to encourage them to get on with things they want to do in life without undue risk. There may be considerable further improvement or adaptation to be had with time, but at a certain point, it becomes unhealthy to continue to focus professional attention on the things the patient can't do.

Commentary by Rosanne Bovey RN, Dip App Sci (Nursing Management)

Wounds have been observed and treated with surprising sophistication since words were recorded.

Every culture across the millennia found ways to engage the principles we use today.

- Clean
- Manage exudate
- Hydrate
- Protect
- Support

Modern day dressings have evolved around the scientific study of wounds and the individual patient's ability to heal. Our now more broad understanding of healing in relation to blood supply, oxygenation, systemic disease, medications, temperature, glycaemic control and nutrition, underpin wound management and the dressings we use. Current best global practice around wound protection and support remains unchanged from Dr Chapple's shrewd observations. Moist wound healing is now the accepted best practice and, as she notes, desiccation leads to much poorer wound outcomes.

Her thoughts on chronic wounds reflect an abundance of experience and understanding of pathophysiology. Although bandaging in venous stasis ulcers remains current management, most would see her Double Bandage technique for injuries to the lower limb as not sustainable from the nurse or patient perspective.

Experienced clinicians know that most acute wounds will heal irrespective of what we put on them and Dr Chapple was cognisant of this. From a Plastic & Reconstructive perspective maximising function and aesthetics are primary goals. Her writings on tapes and sticking plaster show a profound understanding of physics which still applies to our more recent products. Although Dr Chapple states emphatically that 'no wound ever suffers from being washed in the shower', I think most would disagree when it comes to skin grafts!

20 years on, however, many would challenge the first line of this chapter that 'Dressings merely accompany healing, they do not do it' with the more recent developments of 'interactive' dressings that alter the wound environment and interact with the wound surface along with the advent of negative pressure and haemostatic products. Another modern challenge is the plethora of dressing options with 'Big Medical' seizing market opportunity and most brands producing a similar array of dressing types, currently upwards of 35. All now in single use, of course. Dr Chapple would no doubt be scathing of the industry that has done away with multi-use products but I doubt that many of our patients would find home-made dressing an acceptable standard these days.

Many recent scholarly textbooks explore in detail specific types of dressings and their applications. The landscape changes rapidly in this field with new players and new products regularly appearing.

This reader, as a surgical nurse with 40-years-experience, has learnt some new techniques from Dr Chapple's writings and had paused for thought about some current practices. As such, I have circled back to what would now be thought of as 'old' products such as Tulle-Gras. Some of the newer 'replacement' products are much less malleable.

It is obvious that Dr Chapple thought deeply and comprehensively about dressings and their use. She had an understanding of the patient experience and her techniques reflect this. Threads of social justice and empathy are evident, along with an astute understanding of wound healing and the products available at the time. Though quite adamant in manner, her comprehension of pathophysiology and physics underpins not only this chapter but the whole book and as such her legacy lives on.

Commentary by Adam White BSc Physiotherapy, NZRP, HTNZ

I agree with MFK about allowing patients to get their wounds wet in the shower after 24 h, with the proviso the patient has a town water supply, and not tank water as many of our rural patients have.

There is an excellent point about cutting tulle-gras into strips for digits to avoid 'dog ears' as then if splints are needed over dressings they can be smoother, smaller and more rounded so less likely to get knocked and caught up on clothes, etc.

I was taught by an old orthopaedic nurse in the 1980s about applying the bandage from the underside of the roll, great to see this in print! I find the use of Coban TM extremely useful to hold on dressings, as long as it is applied under no tension. It keeps dressings slim so splints, if needed, can be made smaller. As Coban sticks to itself splints can be held on using Coban over the dressing Coban. This is much better than using tape or Velcro to apply splints, as it gives even pressure to prevent a damming effect on swelling as is shown in Fig. 11.19. Then swelling is reduced earlier and splints can be remoulded, for example, to gain Proximal Interphalangeal Joint extension as soon as possible after central slip repairs.

I like to agree with the comments about using Hypafix as a flexible, breathable initial dressing for mobile areas. The Hypafix needs to be applied correctly though as it only has stretch in one direction so if applied the wrong way it can limit range of movement.

Excellent points about getting patients involved in dressings and removal. In my experience patients that don't like to look or touch their injured hands are more likely to develop pain and Complex Regional Pain Syndrome (CRPS) problems and are less engaged in their own rehabilitation. In our Waikato plastic surgery clinics we have to resort to using nitrous oxide for the patient at times to be able to move old, stuck dressings!

We also use taping for scar management. However if scars are becoming hypertrophic, or adherent, products like Cicacare™, Silipos™, or silicone creams can be helpful. These products help to flatten, soften and reduce scar redness.

In the case of some patients with Factitious wounding, we have at times resulted to plaster casting over wounds to prevent patients tampering with them!

Rehabilitation

In my experience, patients only remember very simple basic things from their first communications with doctors. I agree that reassurance, simple explanations, and honesty reduce anxiety and improve compliance with future rehabilitation. Unfortunately, nowadays patients legally have to be informed of complications possible before any interventions often increasing fear and anxiety unnecessarily.

Given the amount of structures in such a small space in the hand and to maintain normal movement patterns, it is vital to be able to let the patient move as many joints/digits as possible in hand injuries.

To reduce the likelihood of CRPS and poor outcomes, it is very important to take patients reporting excessive pain seriously initially and changing dressings, casts, and splints immediately even if this needs doing multiple times, along with good pain relief and education regarding the importance of hand elevation.

Splintage

Another use of splintage is to reduce and prevent further inflammation, and hence pain and scarring.

Posturing

The ideal position of immobilising the hand depends on the injury and subsequent surgery. The described position of wrist extension, MCPJ flexion and PIPJ full extension, i.e. the 'Cobra position' is not really a 'functional' position, but prevents joint stiffness later on. What we call the 'functional' position would be used for the elderly, rheumatoid, or patients with severe Osteo arthritis which would be wrist extension 20–25°, mid-range MCPJ flexion, and PIPJs in approximately 30° of flexion. This position allows better function and use of the thumb with the fingers if stiffness becomes present. Of course in order to protect flexor or extensor tendon repairs and volar plate injuries, the joints are positioned differently.

Motor Rehabilitation

It is important in performing exercises, passive and active, not to increase inflammation as this leads to more stiffness later on.

Physiotherapy

As stated certainly in some cases, patients can recover seamlessly their function and ROM after a few weeks. However, we should not take away from the importance of physiotherapy/hand therapy. Nowadays, most hand injuries patients are seen by therapists often within a few days of injury or surgery to gain ROM, prevent and reduce oedema/atrophy and stiffness before it occurs. Early hand therapy input does much to reduce anxiety, promote normal movement patterns and use that will often disappear quickly with immobilisation resulting in tight intrinsic muscles and stiff joints. In complex hand injuries, early intervention including splintage to protect repaired structures and allow useful movement is vital. Much research in the last 30 years shows the benefits of early protected movement in preventing adherence and allowing safe motion to improve tendon repair strength. Often patients need to be taught specific exercises to perform with specific hand postures to protect repaired structures and prevent tendon ruptures and adherence, e.g. controlled active protocols like the modified Belfast, Manchester, Short Arc Motion Volar Plate, and use of relative Motion splints. Current practice of early movement is unlikely to cause instability of joints later as joint structures can be protected as needed, e.g. with buddy taping for ligament injuries or splintage of potentially unstable joints or those in danger of developing instability. The author seems to contradict herself by implying that patients may not need physiotherapy by saying they can recover 'both function and movement quite seamlessly within 2–3 weeks' and then stating the importance of early ROM and maintenance exercises which physiotherapy provides.

Disability

It is part of rehabilitation to provide tools to enhance activities of daily living for patients as needed at the end of and along their rehabilitation journey.

Hand Injuries

12

Summary
While all aspects of healing and wound care are the same in the hand as elsewhere on the body, the effects of complications can be disproportionately serious in terms of function and independence. There are many specialised structures in confined spaces. The hand is also richly supplied with nerves, and tension is reflected very early and accurately by pain. Techniques must safeguard the circulation, minimise pain, and facilitate an uncomplicated recovery. Complications often compound their effects. Optimal acute treatment is therefore extremely important. The protection of joint function by specific splintage is also critical to the recovery of full function.

Editors' Note *Hand surgery requires all the surgical skills that underpin good plastic surgery: knowledge of applied anatomy, gentle tissue handling, precise surgical repair, and successful functional outcomes. The long hours that plastic surgical trainees spend during the night repairing acute hand injuries are fundamental to their surgical development and are never wasted. General surgeons and orthopaedic surgeons who spend some time during their training in a plastic surgical unit similarly benefit very significantly from this exposure to acute hand problems. The concepts of plastic surgical reconstruction are universal across surgical craft groups.*

Hand wounds are common and behave no differently from wounds elsewhere. There are however many important structures in a relatively confined space. Whenever there is a motor or sensory deficit, it is always a good idea to refresh the memory by referring to anatomy books. *[Today there are also excellent Video Atlases such as Acland's Video Atlas of Human Anatomy/Volume 1: The Upper Extremity [1].* The richly innervated and specialised tissue on the front of the thumb and finger pulps confers the capacity to almost 'see' in terms of assessing size, shape, texture, and instant recognition of things. Hand injuries are not surprisingly relatively painful. All hand injuries are potentially serious, and there are usually hand specialists and hand units available for advice and referral in more complex wounds.

Hands confer independence and much of the ability to work. Their comfort and confident use is something that most people take for granted, until their hands are injured or stricken with disease. There is a high level of insecurity and emotion associated with hand injuries and their treatment/rehabilitation needs to take this into account.

The mobility between layers and structures is always essential to full function and comfort. This mobility function is at its most sophisticated in the hand. Flexion not only involves shortening and compression of all the tissues on the flexor

P. Charlesworth, M. F. Klaassen, *Chapple's Principles of Wound Care and Healing*,
https://doi.org/10.1007/978-3-031-53104-0_12

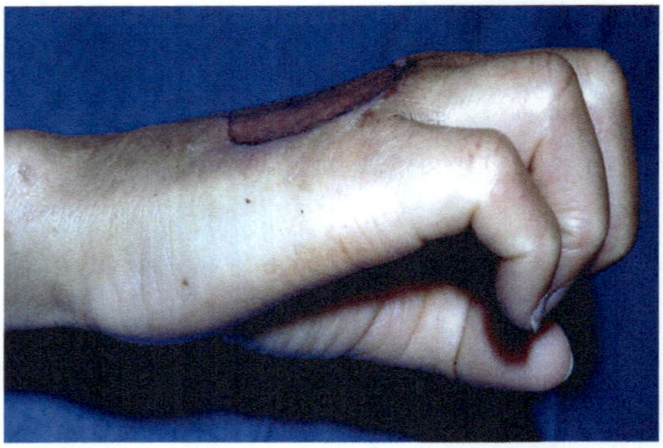

Fig. 12.1 These MC/P joints have stiffened in extension after splinting was omitted during the acute initial stages of a degloving dorsal injury. Patient is trying desperately to grip

aspect but also the coordinated relaxation and stretching of all those on the opposite aspect. The movement of capsules, ligaments, and tendons around joints is also critical (Fig. 12.1).

Figure 12.1 is the case of a young woman who caught the back of her left hand against a belt sander sustaining an area of friction burn and closed degloving of the dorsal skin. The skin initially looked white but was not torn and her hand was simply dressed by the local doctor. Both hand and fingers were swollen for several days and she kept her hand elevated. The damaged skin turned dark in colour and discharge appeared at the edges requiring regular dressings. Her fingers were less swollen but still very stiff and at a month post-injury she was referred to the hand clinic. She was admitted for initial debridement of the dead skin and a sizeable split skin graft 2 weeks later. The graft healed within days but her MCPJs had stiffened in extension and her IPJs in fixed flexion. Her wrist could also not be extended from a neutral position. Her hand function was severely impaired and despite prolonged physiotherapy and serial night splintage her hand movement improved only slowly. Her left hand was severely and permanently disabled and she was never able to play her guitar again.

Adherence between adjacent layers or structures can restrict the excursion of both. Diffuse scarring, such as that which follows infection or circulatory deprivation, has a particularly adverse effect on remobilisation. Tendon adherence to the tendon sheath after bacterial teno-synovitis can often inactivate tendon movement completely, despite full passive joint function because the joint itself is unaffected.

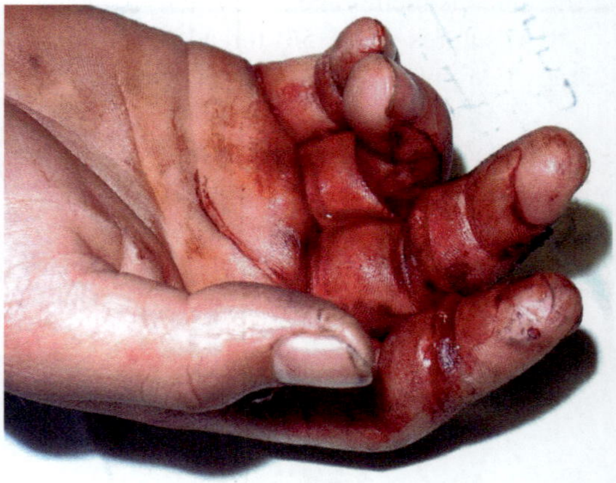

Fig. 12.2 Resting posture after injury, showing absent long flexor tendon function in both index and middle fingers after lacerations at PIP joint level. Sensation was unaffected

Hand skin is special. Dorsal skin is thin and mobile as compared with the fixed, thicker palmar skin on the front of the hand and digits, which is greatly specialised for wear and tear, grip, and touch. Another useful anatomical detail is that at the level of the joint creases in the digits, the skin is tethered directly to the flexor tendon sheath, without any intervening subcutaneous tissue. While this facilitates flexion it also means that the tendons are extremely superficial in these creases and can sometimes be severed without damage to either digital nerves or vessels (Fig. 12.2).

Examination and Assessment

Circulation

With two main arteries and lots of draining veins, circulation in the hand is not usually a problem. Each digit however is a relatively isolated unit and although each also has two digital arteries and several veins, the circulation can be readily affected. Circulatory restriction can be produced by circumferential tapes, Elastoplast and bandages, or by the bands developed by sutures (Figs. 12.3a, b, 12.4a–c and 12.5).

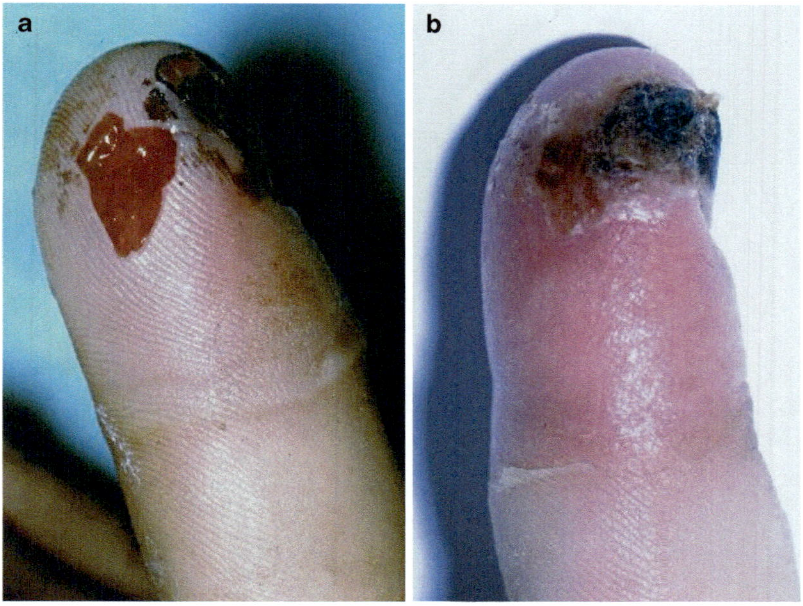

Fig. 12.3 (**a**, **b**) This shallow wound of a distal digit was bandaged very firmly for 3 days to stop the bleeding. The finger was very painful throughout. Three weeks later, the full extent of the bandage injury is evident. The loss of both bulk and sensation persisted

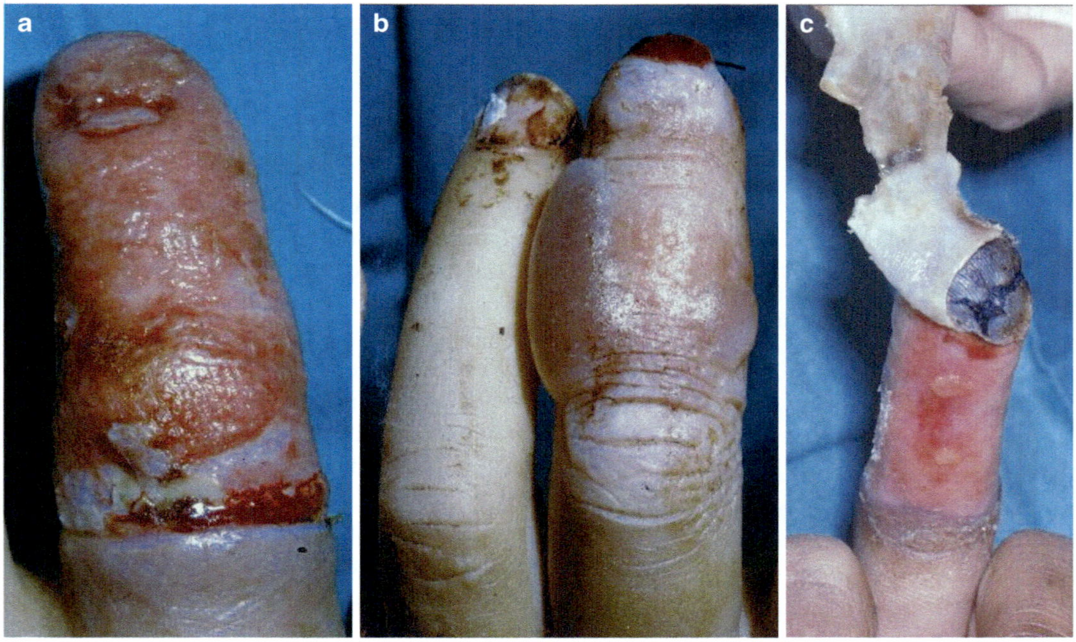

Fig. 12.4 (**a**–**c**) Clinical examples of the complications resulting from tight Elastoplast dressings causing nutritional injury to a finger in a crushed nail injury 10 days before. Blistering from a tight Elastoplast and finally gangrene of another crushed pulp after tight basal Elastoplast causing a more extensive injury

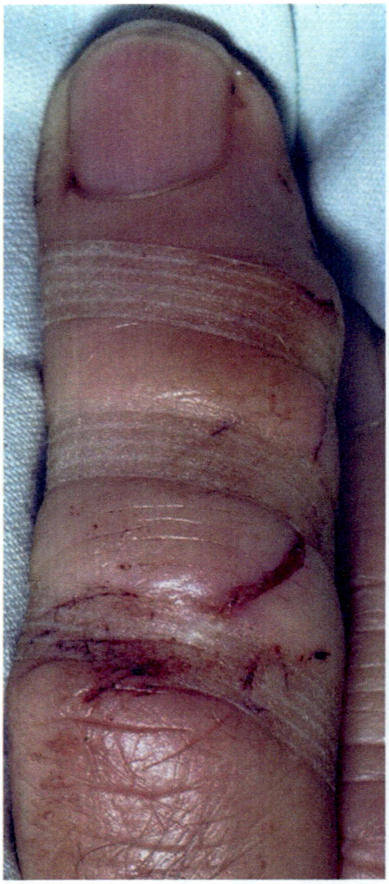

Fig. 12.5 Inextensible circumferential tapes have trapped the reactionary swelling and the finger has been very painful for 3 days. The shelving wound is closed, but a tulle or non-circumferential tape closure would have been safer

Although flaps in the hand need the same circulatory considerations as flaps anywhere else, the repercussions of necrosis may be much more serious (Figs. 12.6, 12.7a, b and 12.8a, b).

Movement

Each joint has a prime flexor and extensor, and these functions can and should be tested. In the fingers, the *Flexor Digitorum Superficialis [FDS]* flexes the proximal interphalangeal [PIP] joints and *Flexor Digitorum Profundus [FDP]* is the sole flexor of the distal joints. Both superficial and deep flexors contribute to the resting semi-flexed posture of the fingers at all three finger joints, and this will be altered if one or both are severed (Fig. 12.9). The thumb has only one long flexor.

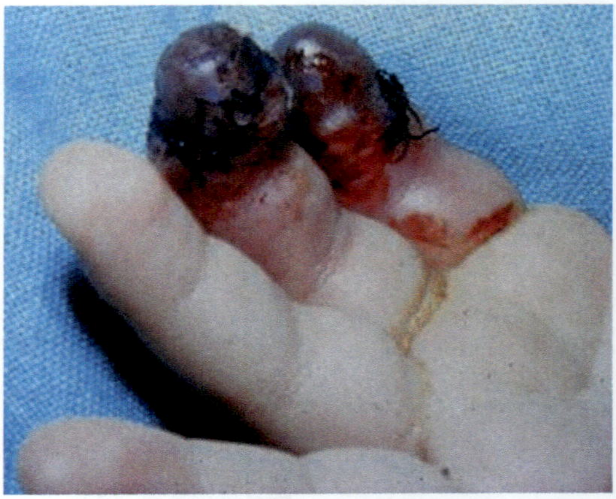

Fig. 12.6 Venous stasis in crushed fingertips has led to their death. This is being followed by invasive sepsis. Although the fingers have been accurately repaired, all the suturing has worsened their venous problems

Testing of Motor Function

In the palm, the *FDP* tendons lie deep to those of the *FDS*. Both enter the flexor sheath and *FDS* then divides with a slip passing around each side of *FDP* to insert along the sides of the middle phalanx. This means that a relatively superficial laceration in the proximal joint crease can sever the *FDP*, leaving the *FDS* functioning to flex the proximal joint and the nerves also intact. An important tendon injury can easily be missed.

The Profundus tendons are the sole flexors of the distal segments of the digits, so testing is straight forward. The *Superficialis* tendons can fortunately and elegantly be tested for by holding adjacent fingers out in full extension while asking for flexion in the finger under testing. The Flexor Profundus is thereby inactivated and a pure *Superficialis* movement [or its absence] is demonstrated. In the index and little fingers, this test may be less clear-cut than in other fingers and the performance should be compared with that of the

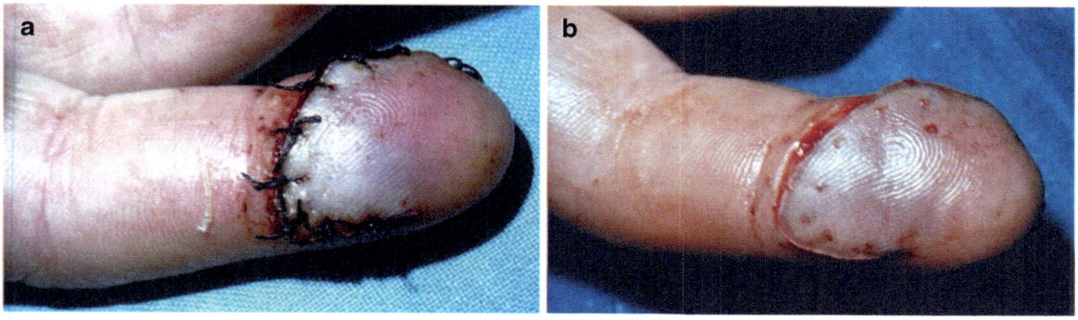

Fig. 12.7 (**a**) Impending necrosis of a pulp flap on the day of injury. The patient returned with severe pain later the same day. (**b**) Immediate relief of pain and recovery of circulation followed the removal of the sutures on the same day as previous figure. The finger proceeded to heal well in tulle dressings

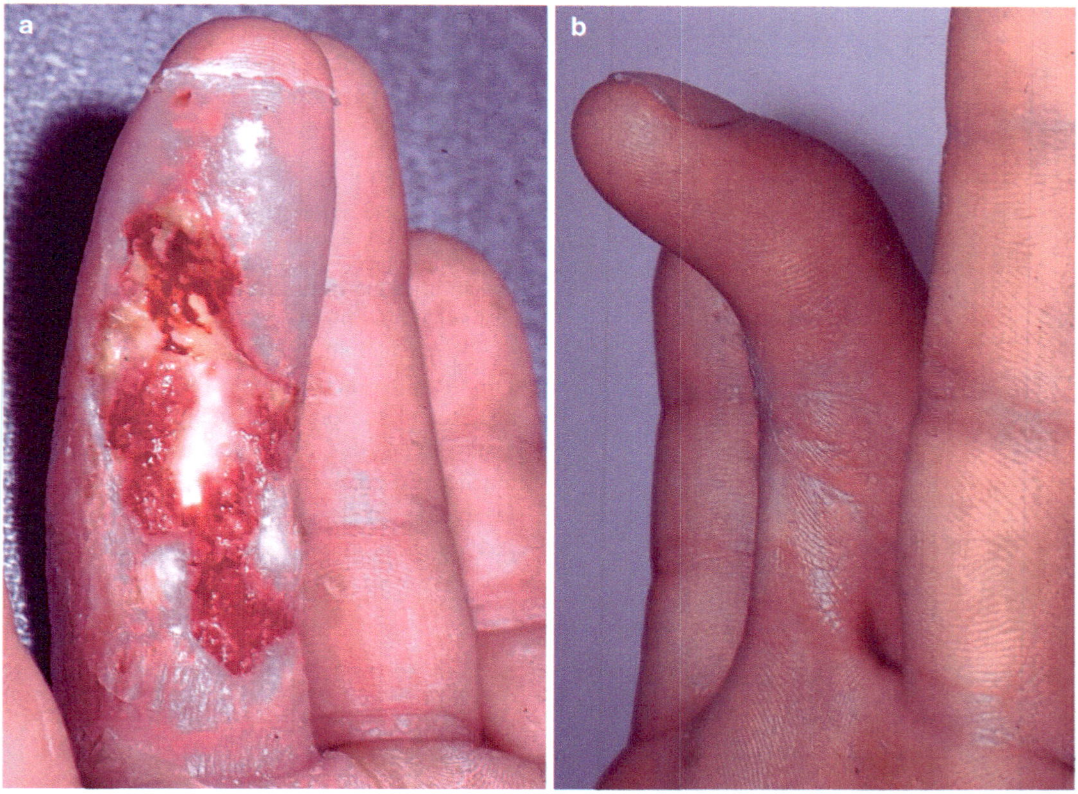

Fig. 12.8 (**a**) Deep destruction down to tendon followed the suturing of a burst finger. (**b**) Permanent and severe flexion contracture of the finger inevitably followed healing and was untreatable

patient's uninjured hand. If sensation is unaffected, patients may sometimes be unaware of an important tendon deficit.

The long extensors primarily extend the metacarpophalangeal [MCP] joints. The full extension of the interphalangeal joints is conferred by the intrinsic muscles, carried out by means of the complex extensor apparatus down the dorsum of the digits. The small muscles in the hand, supplied by branches of the median and ulnar nerves are very important in posturing, stabilisation, strength, and pinch grip (Fig. 12.10a–c).

Asking for metacarpo-phalangeal flexion with extension of the interphalangeal joints in both hands, after first demonstrating this to the patient, is the best test for intrinsic muscle function. This is sometimes called the 'intrinsic position'. When ulnar nerve function is lost, the index and middle fingers make some attempt to produce the intrinsic position, because they each have a median-supplied Lumbrical muscle, while the ring and little finger interphalangeal joints will curl up into a clawed position, with no flexion at all taking place at their MCPJs.

Figure 12.10a, b, and c illustrate the 25-year-old motor-mechanic who had healed well and recovered full strong flexion after a small penetrating hand wound in the central palm. A month later, however, he complained to Dr. Chapple that he *'couldn't use his hand properly'* ... *'I lose change through the gap and can't do my work properly'* he replied when asked what function he had lost. He also couldn't make a flat hand to get into his pockets or down in amongst engines, without knocking skin off his knuckles. He could not position his fingers ready to do anything. **This was a classic description of intrinsic muscle function loss, which Dr Chapple thought worthy of photographing.** He basically could not stabilise the middle and ring fingers strongly in MCPJ flexion and interphalangeal extension, which is the position from which one sets out to do most things. Fortunately, he recovered full function after another month of waiting for the nerve fibres to grow down again into the interosseous muscles.

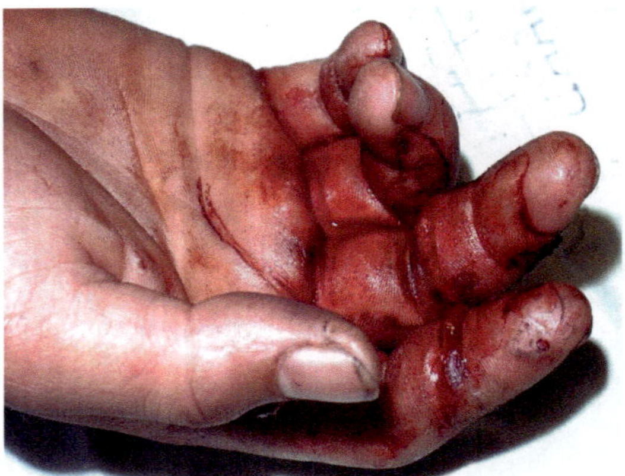

Fig. 12.9 Resting posture after injury, showing absent long flexor tendon function in both index and middle fingers after lacerations at PIP joint level. Sensation was unaffected

Sensation

Sensation in the front of the hand is mediated by the median and ulnar nerves, with the ring finger usually having half supplied by each. On the dorsum, the radial nerve supplies sensation down to the level of the proximal interphalangeal [PIP] joints. Beyond this, the median and ulnar innervation usually takes over. In the digits, there are sizeable digital nerves. The accurate repair of severed nerves is important and should be done by specialists with access to operating microscopes.

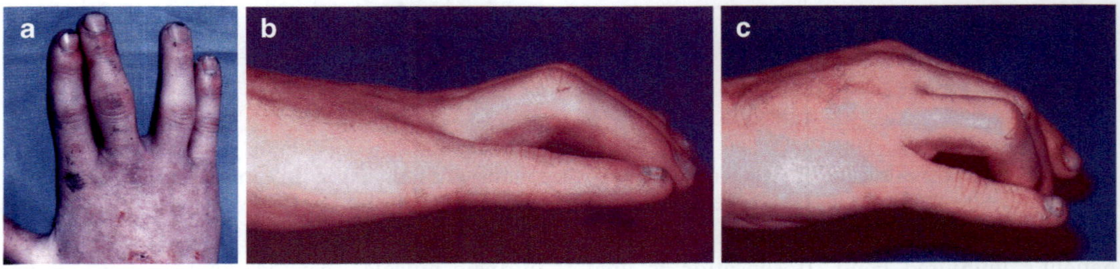

Fig. 12.10 (**a**) Right hand showing an inability to close fingers together, after interruption of the nerve to small muscles in the cleft. (**b**) Inability to make a flat hand with these two fingers in the same hand. (**c**) The same hand demonstrating the inability to posture the ring and middle fingers in MCPJ flexion. [see CASE STUDY BELOW]

Sensory Testing

Touch is easily tested with the end of an opened-out wire paper clip. Pricking with a needle is unnecessarily barbaric! Tests for proprioception and discrimination are not required in acute injury examination. With the patient's eyes covered *or closed,* the accuracy of light touch is investigated, starting in territory where sensation should be normal. In an irregular time sequence, stimuli are provided to the skin that may be affected in a persistent manner and with patience until a consistent response is elicited. Sensory loss with an anatomical explanation is usually clearly demonstrable. Sometimes after crush injuries, anatomically based paraesthetic sensation is present and is described as 'pins and needles' or a 'tingly feeling' when affected skin is touched.

Sensory loss that doesn't make anatomical sense can only have two explanations. It may be part of a previous injury or be hysterical aberration which is usually of a non-anatomical or 'glove & stocking' distribution in the limbs. Insensitively discrediting the latter is liable to produce other psychosomatic symptoms. ***Joan Chapple always found it more constructive to give the patient the benefit of the doubt and to explain that although sensation could sometimes be a 'bit funny for awhile' it should all feel pretty normal again before long. She expected it to have been recovered by the time she next saw her patients and mostly this proved to be true.***

Radiology

Where the mechanisms of injury, deformity, or pain with movement suggest a possible bone or joint injury, the hand should be X-Rayed (Fig. 12.11).

Bleeding should be stopped first. Unstable fractures of the hand should be referred to a Hand Specialist. Stable crush fractures of the distal phalanx should be moulded back into shape, supported by Tulle strips, treated with the

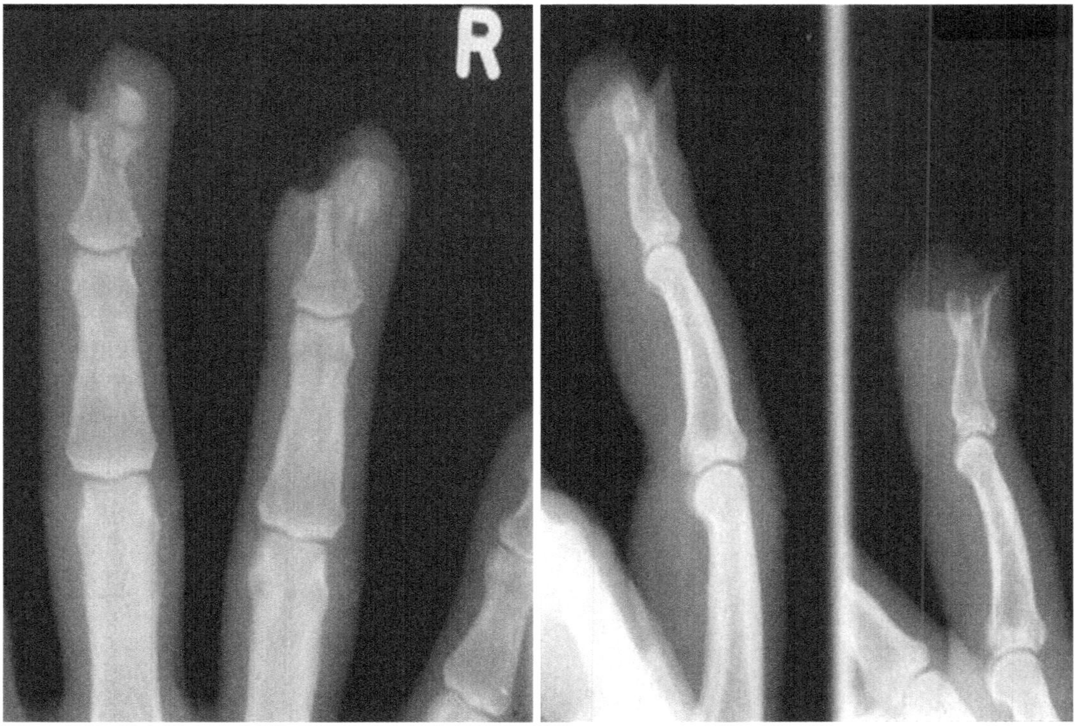

Fig. 12.11 X-ray of two fingers showing the phalangeal tufts resulting from fingertip motor-mower injury

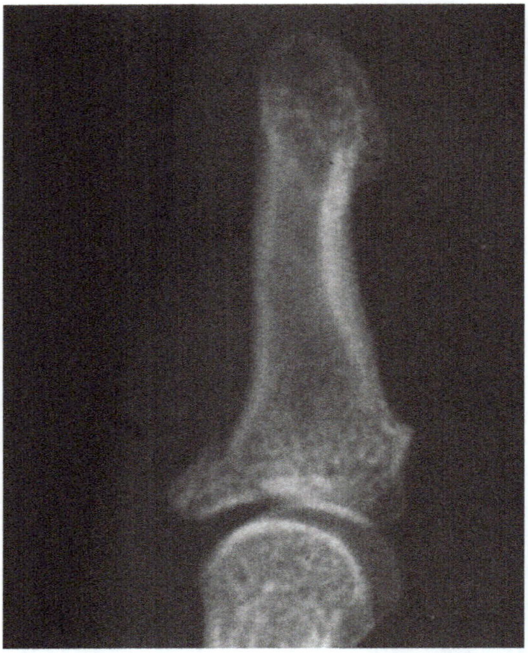

Fig. 12.12 A small fracture of the extensor insertion can give rise to a mallet deformity, which can be very successfully treated

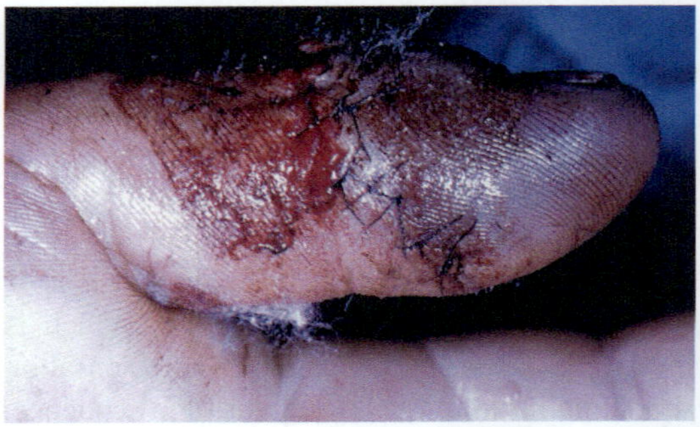

Fig. 12.13 Venous congestion of thumb-tip. Suturing has jeopardised the continuity circulation. This thumb tip did not survive

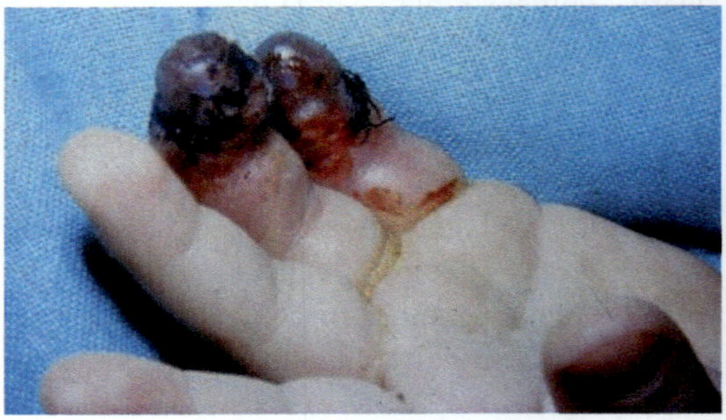

Fig. 12.14 Venous stasis in crushed fingertips has led to their death. This is being followed by invasive sepsis. Although the fingers have been accurately repaired, all suturing has worsened their venous problems

soft tissues, and rested on a splint. Patients presenting with a 'mallet' deformity or drooping of the distal segment of a digit should always be X-Rayed to exclude a readily treatable fracture (Fig. 12.12).

Finger-Pulp Anatomy

The distal pulp of the digits has its own particular structure and circulation. The finger pulp has highly specialised skin with a unique pattern of finger-print ridges with sweat glands opening onto them. The subcutaneous tissue is arranged into numerous richly innervated fibro-fatty compartments conferring special touch and pressure components to the sensory 'picture'. This tissue can develop a tension build-up very readily, especially when it is injured by crushing or concussed by power tools and/or motor-mower blades. Throbbing circulatory pain after pulp injuries is often marked and the imposition of further circulatory restriction by sutures is particularly dangerous (Figs. 12.13, 12.14, 12.15a, b).

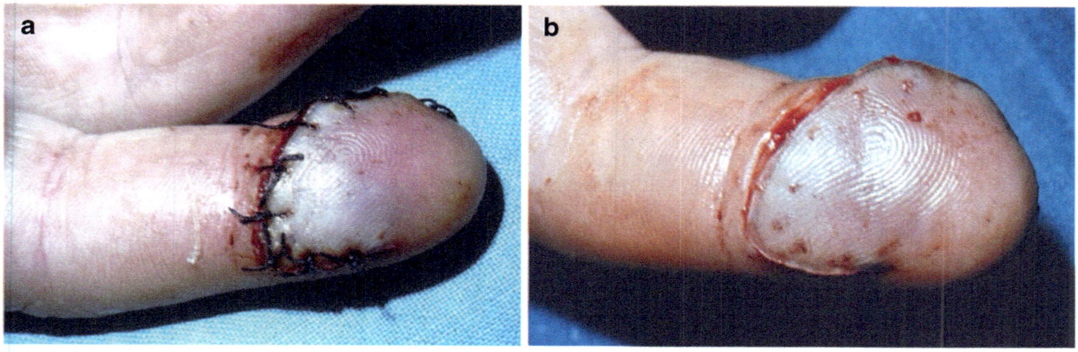

Fig. 12.15 (**a**, **b**) Impending necrosis of a pulp flap on the day of injury. The patient returned with severe pain later the same day. Immediate relief of pain and recovery of the circulation followed the removal of sutures. **b** is the same day as **a**. The finger proceeded to heal well with tulle dressings

General Principles of Treatment

All the principles of wound treatment already described apply to hand wounds. Always elevate the hand while working on it and avoid using a tourniquet. Posturing for circulatory purposes or to protect joint function should always be done before closure, so that inaccuracies and unexpected tissue tensions are not produced by later rearrangement.

Injuries to specialised structures like major vessels, flexor tendons, and nerves may require referral for microsurgical repair. Unstable fractures and complex joint injuries may also need specialist treatment. If possible, patients with these more complicated problems are best managed by the nearest Hand Clinic or Hand Surgeon.

Skin Grafting About the Hand

Skin that is devitalised or separated will take if it is replaced as a graft. On the dorsal aspects of the hand and fingers, the results of replacement are reasonable although loss of surface sensation will persist (Fig. 12.16a, b).

Where a small area of palmar skin has been lost, the best result is probably achieved by dressing the wound until it heals spontaneously, sometimes even if the 'bit' is available. Shrinkage will be incorporated into the healing process and the scar will eventually be stable, durable, and smooth, with the minimum area of sensory loss. With larger areas on the palmar aspects, the use of the original skin may be justified even though it maximises the area of sensory loss, because it is of much better quality than either a skin graft from elsewhere or an extensive scar. Although deep pressure sensation remains beneath grafts, this does not protect the surface from burns or sharp injuries. When the original skin is not available, it may be necessary to use other skin. The downside of this is that it remains not only numb and slippery but will also wear poorly. It also joins to adjacent palmar skin with an unstable junctional ridge, rather like the back of the heel. Palmar [hand] and plantar [sole] skin is very specialised and thickens in a leathery fashion in response to repeated mechanical use. Ordinary skin in these regions becomes hyperkeratotic and brittle. Grafts may look unsightly as their colour and texture match is incongruent. Patients with extensive or complicated skin damage, including full thickness burns, are best referred initially for plastic surgical management. The outcome however, in many cases, may unfortunately still be far from satisfactory.

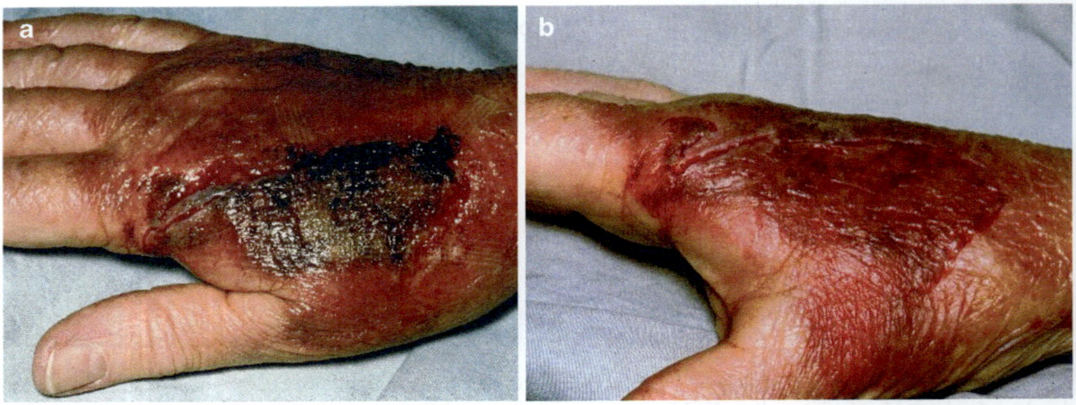

Fig. 12.16 (**a**) 5-day appearance of replaced skin that has confluent haematoma beneath it. (**b**) The changed appearance on the same day after the blood was removed. All fat has been trimmed off and the reapplied skin was then held with tapes. It all survived

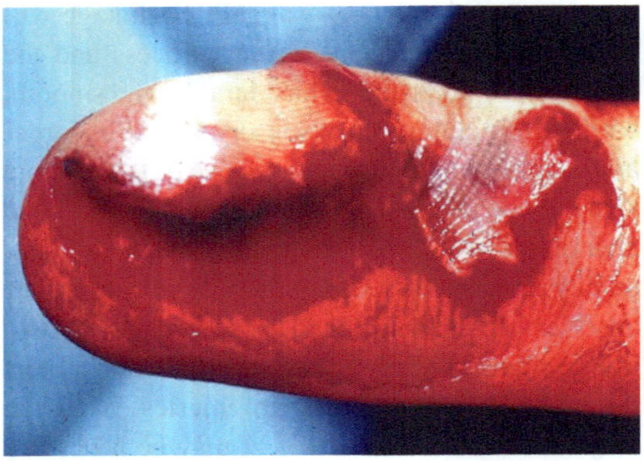

Fig. 12.17 Severely traumatised finger-tip best treated by tulle moulding, not suturing

Finger Injuries

Before making any decision to do anything heroic or complicated with finger injuries, even where there is obviously tissue missing, it is important to envisage the result likely to follow accurate realignment and healing with **a simple dressing regime** [2, 3]. This approach is very safe, most likely to give the best result and must **always be considered first** (Figs. 12.17, 12.18a, b, 12.19a, b, 12.20a–d).

The very worst time to put tissue through the additional stress of complicated surgery is in the 48 h after it has already been acutely injured. Not all operations succeed, even in ideal conditions. Reconstructive operations are best deferred for several days. Patients come to no harm waiting with their wounds cleansed and dressed. The tissues are recovering whilst consultation or referral for further treatment is organised.

Tulle Gras Moulding and Dressings for Fingers

Fingers which have been crushed or damaged with power tools swell markedly and are usually unsuitable for suturing (Fig. 12.21a–c).

Tulle-gras moulding for most finger and fingertip injuries involves the cutting of tulle into accurate strips no wider than the digit and realigning/supporting the wounds with these. Gauze strips and Crepe bandages should also be no wider than the digit (Fig. 12.22a–d). See Chap. 11.

Tube gauze is not accurate enough for first dressings, but it makes a very light, tidy later dressing for digits. There is no need to cover the whole finger if only the tip is injured but it is much tidier to shorten a long dressing by cutting it back rather than trying to do a very small one. Finger dressings are best completed with an Elastoplast cut away anteriorly to allow flexion,

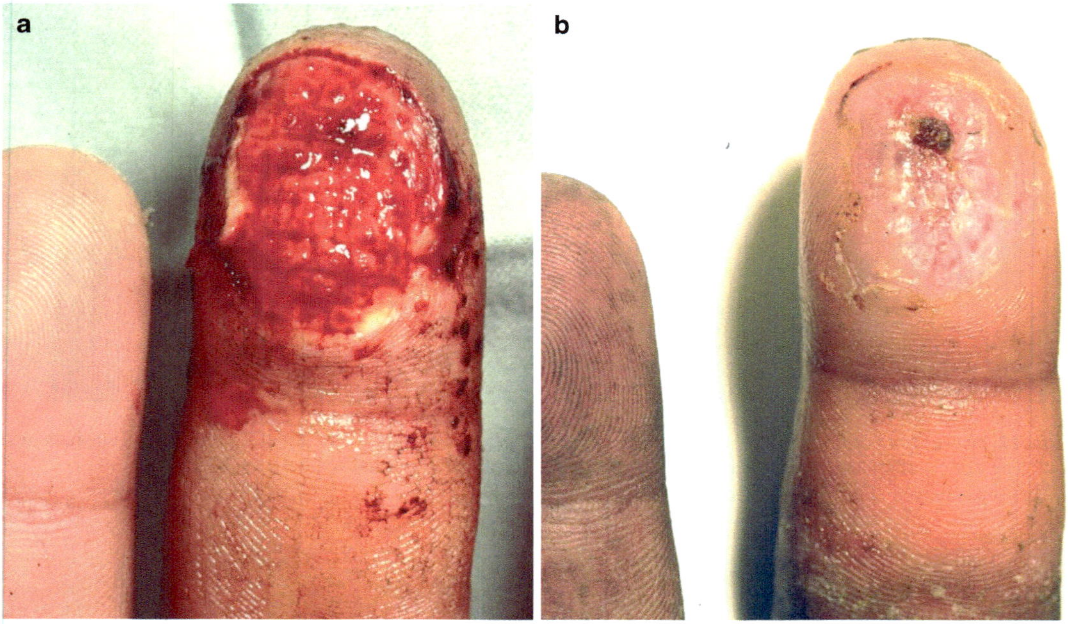

Fig. 12.18 (**a**) Irrecoverable skin loss from finger pulp. A graft from elsewhere would give a poor result. (**b**) 5 weeks later, spontaneous healing with dressings will ensure a much better result than grafting

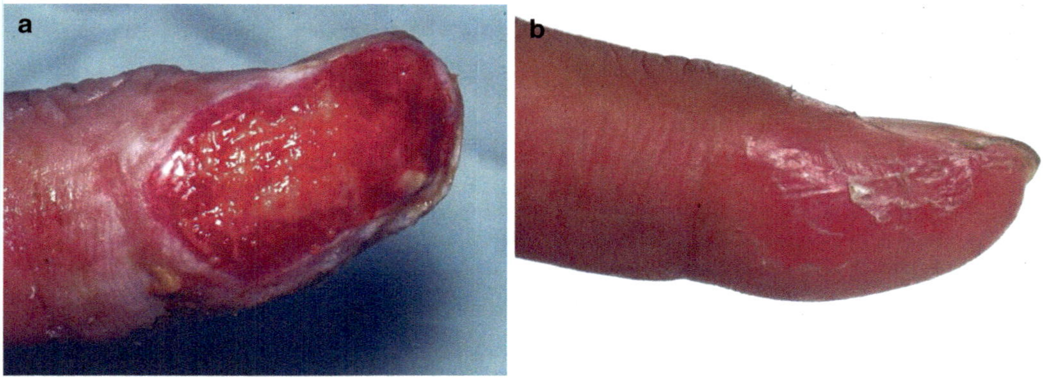

Fig. 12.19 (**a**) Loss of skin from side of thumb tip from a circular saw injury. Skin not available. (**b**) Although this was a sizeable injury, the decision to dress the wound until it was healed was the correct one as evidence by the appearance at 5 weeks

long enough to stick to itself and not applied under tension (Fig. 12.23a, b).

Functional Posturing and Splintage

It is important to immobilise all newly injured hands and digits with the joints splinted in either the ***functional*** position to protect joint function or an alternative position chosen specifically to assist wound circulation for the first few days (Fig. 12.24).

Ordinarily, the patient with an injured hand holds it up to relieve pain. The wrist then flops into flexion, the MCP joints droop into extension and the fingers tend to curl up. In this ***rest*** posi-

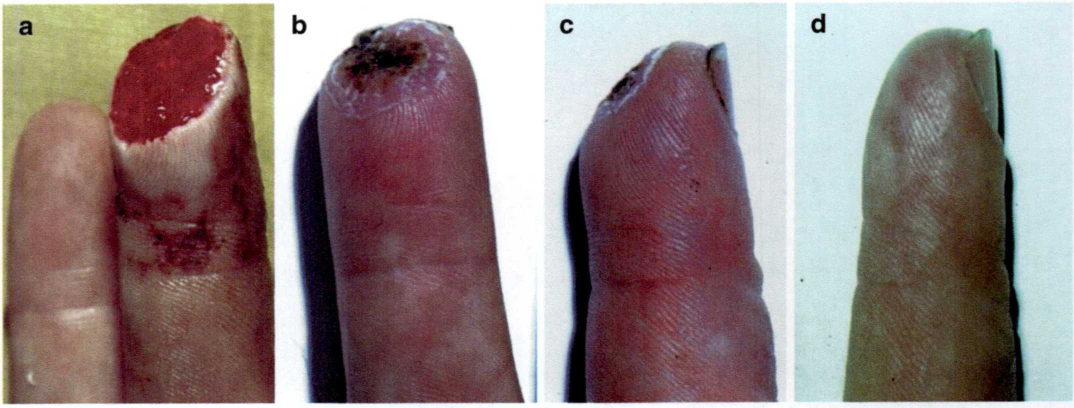

Figs. 12.20 (**a**) Loss of fingertip tissue in a buzzer power tool. The option of spontaneous healing seemed best. (**b**, **c**) Healing achieved after 5 weeks of dressings with some loss of bulk and flattening of the pulp. (**d**) The shape had returned to normal some 3 months later

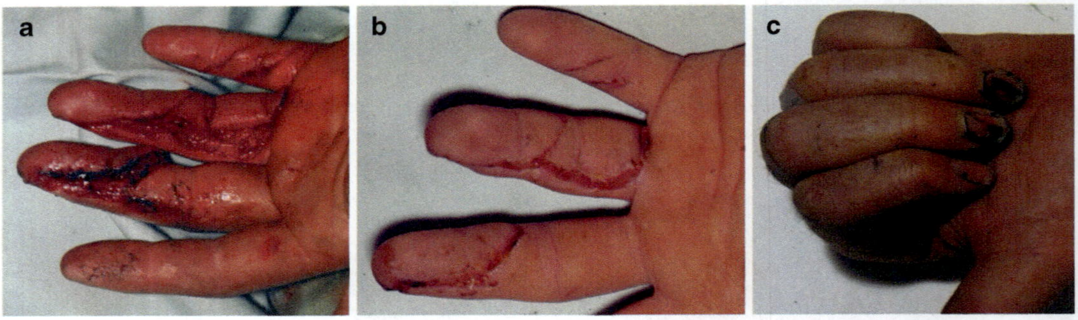

Fig. 12.21 (**a**) Initial appearance of hand caught in pastry rollers. The flaps look viable, but these are burst fingers which will swell. (**b**) The 10-day appearance after tulle gras stabilisation, gauze bandages, and splintage. All tissue is healthy and most of the swelling is gone. The hand has been remarkably comfortable, wounds almost healed. (**c**) At 3 weeks, the patient has made a complete functional recovery and flexion of fingers into the palm is demonstrated

tion, joint ligaments are slack and the tissues accommodate swelling most comfortably (Fig. 12.25).

Unfortunately, in this position, the main ligaments and joint capsules shorten rapidly making it difficult or sometimes impossible to regain full movement. It is therefore important to protect joint function by splinting any painful, injured, or swollen hand in the **functional** position, keeping joint ligaments stretched, preferably before the swelling occurs. **The wrist should be splinted in 15–20° of extension with the MCP joints fully flexed and the interphalangeal joints fully extended (See** Fig. 12.24**).**

Adding a short dorsal slab over the MCP joints and fingers with bandaging to the ventral slab sometimes helps maintain the correct joint posture. The thumb web should be kept expanded with the thumb in abduction and opposition, facing the fingers. This functional position not only prevents ligaments shortening but also happens to be the position in which all digits will be useful even if the injured hand ends up with reduced mobility. The maintenance of this ideal posture also applies in the treatment of acute burn injuries and infections of the hand (Figs. 12.26a–c, 12.27a, b).

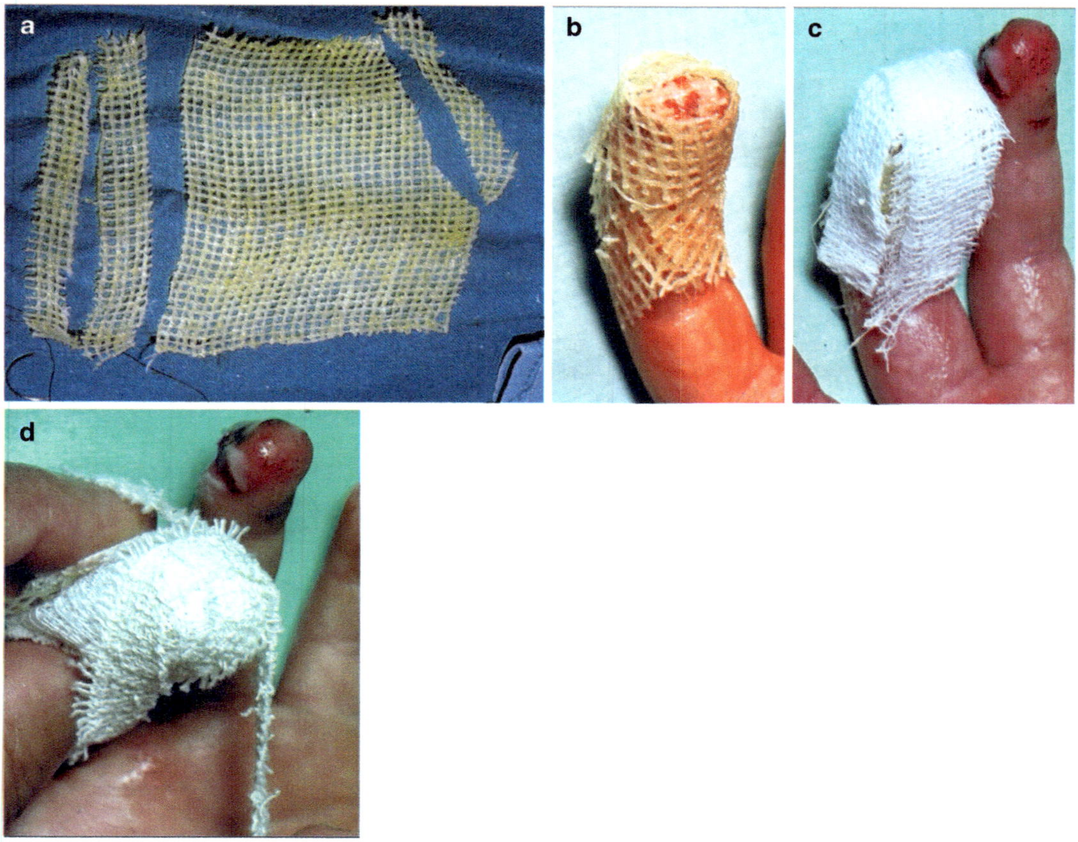

Fig. 12.22 (**a**–**d**) Tulle gras, gauze strips, and crepe bandages for finger injuries. To make useful strips, tulle must be cut parallel to the fibres. Obliquely cut strips just disintegrate. Crushed fingertip after application of tulle strips. Further protection with gauze strips over the tulle strips, then accurate crepe bandaging and finally splinting of the finger

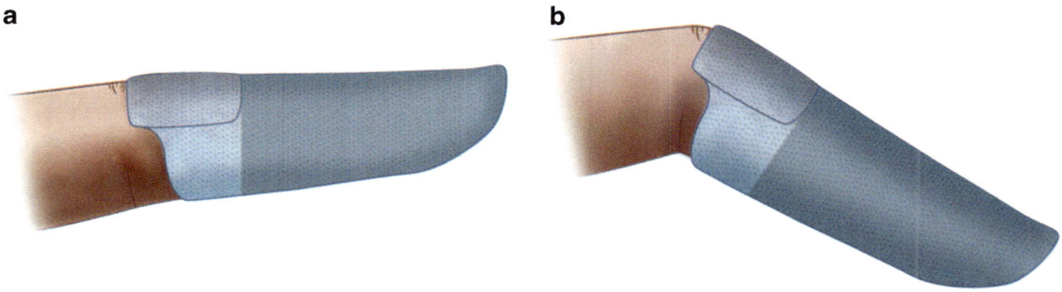

Fig. 12.23 (**a** and **b**) Tube gauze finger dressing which looks tidy. The circumferential basal Elastoplast should not be stretched on, should be cut away to allow full PIP flexion, and be long enough to stick to itself

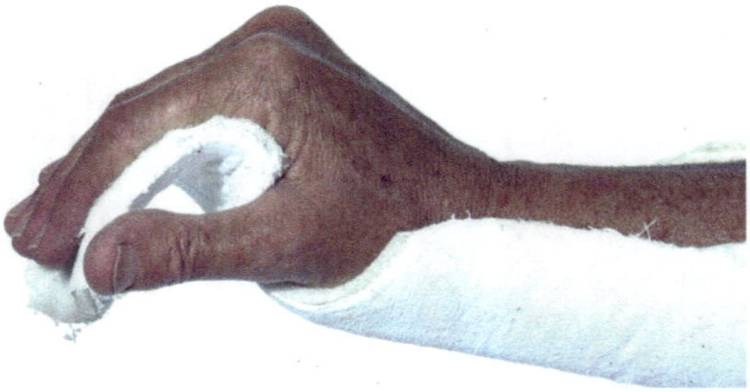

Fig. 12.24 The functional position for hand splintage. This is the functional position for the resting hand and keeps all the ligaments tensed, thus preventing shortening which in turn can restrict later function

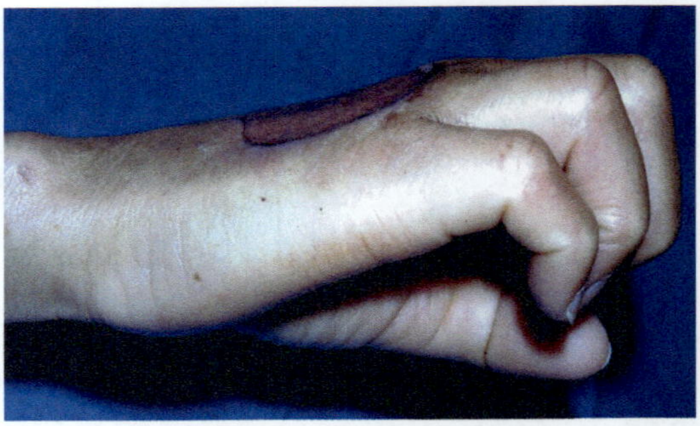

Fig. 12.25 The unsafe 'rest' position of the injured hand

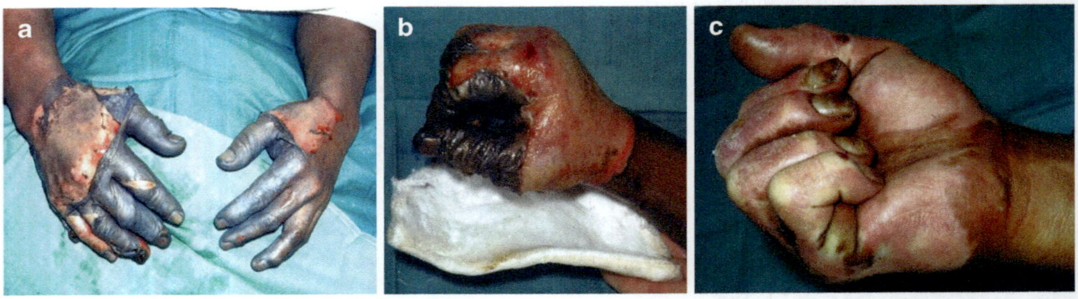

Fig. 12.26 (**a–c**) Partial thickness burns to hands splinted in the functional position with MCPJs flexed and active movement commenced after 5 days. Healed hand with full grip 3 weeks post burn injury. Pigmentation eventually returned to normal

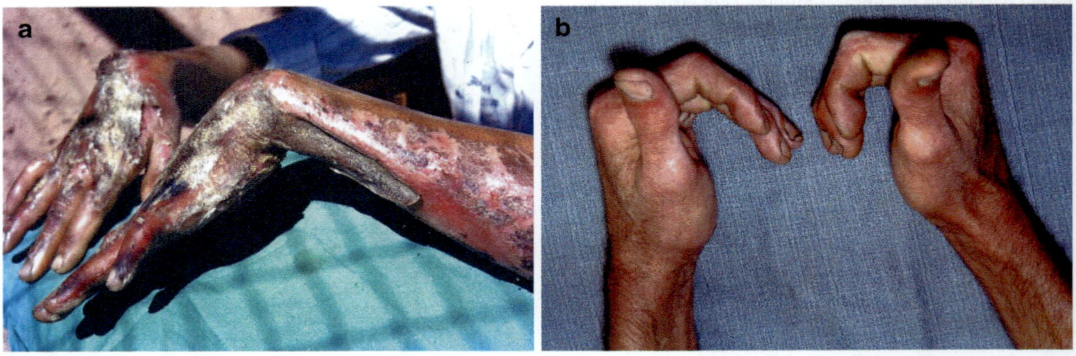

Fig. 12.27 (**a, b**) Partial thickness burns of the hands have been treated for 3 weeks by the exposure method [no splinting]. Without splinting the ligaments have shortened irrevocably and the eventual result is poor with reduced flexion and strength in the fingers causing considerable permanent disability

If the hand initially needs to be in a different posture to safeguard tissue survival, it is very important to retrieve the functional position as quickly as possible. To fail to pay attention to this may be disastrous. Specific different posturing may be needed after some tendon surgery.

Extensor Tendons

Extensor tendons run in subcutaneous tissues, not in tendon sheaths and when only one or two have been severed in a clean laceration, repairing them is a relatively straightforward exercise. It is always wise to review the Anatomy Atlases. With the hand elevated and the wrist extended, tendon ends severed on the back of the hand can usually be produced easily. Extensor Pollicis Longus can sometimes be more elusive but massaging the extensor muscle mass in the forearm downwards with the thumb in extension usually produces it. Keeping the digits extended also greatly assists with the repair process.

Tendon Suturing: The Double Right-Angle Suture

Using a **non-absorbable** synthetic 3/0 suture start by picking up the proximal tendon end with a suture through it vertically from superficial to deep, about 5 mm back from the cut end. Continue by inserting the needle similarly into the distal end from deep to superficial and pull both ends together slightly. The third move goes through the proximal end again, in a plane at right angles to the original stitch and a millimetre or so behind this, taking care not to pierce it. Finally go through the distal end again in this new plane, again in behind the previous stitch and not through it. The knot is then tied with at least two half-hitches across the other thread and gradually pulled up until the tendon ends meet. Once these are approximated nicely, two or three locking knots, tied as running knots are added on top of the previous half hitches. Handling the tendon ends once only and thereafter by way of the suture itself avoids damaging the ends with forceps. Do not cut a tendon suture too short. It is worth threading the needle end up inside the tendon for 5 mm or more before cutting it off and leaving the other end also rather long. This manoeuvre is called **double right-angle stitch,** and it is much better looking in practice than it is in any diagram (Fig. 12.28). It can be used for any tendon that is oval in cross-section rather than flat.

After the skin has been sutured, the hand should be splinted for 3–4 weeks in **full but not forced** wrist extension. This will allow the MCPJs to be comfortably immobilised in about 20° of flexion rather than full extension. This does not jeopardise the tendon repair, but does assist significantly with joint re-mobilisation. What usually happens if no particular attention is paid to the wrist is that it gets immobilised in a more or less neutral position, while the MCPJs get hyperextended by someone holding the fingertips while the splint sets. Both wrist and MCPJs suffer dreadfully from this poor posture and are likely to make a very slow or incomplete recovery.

Beyond the MCPJs, the extensor tendons flatten and are joined by intrinsic tenson slips to function in an elegant and somewhat telescopic fashion down the dorsum of the digit to extend

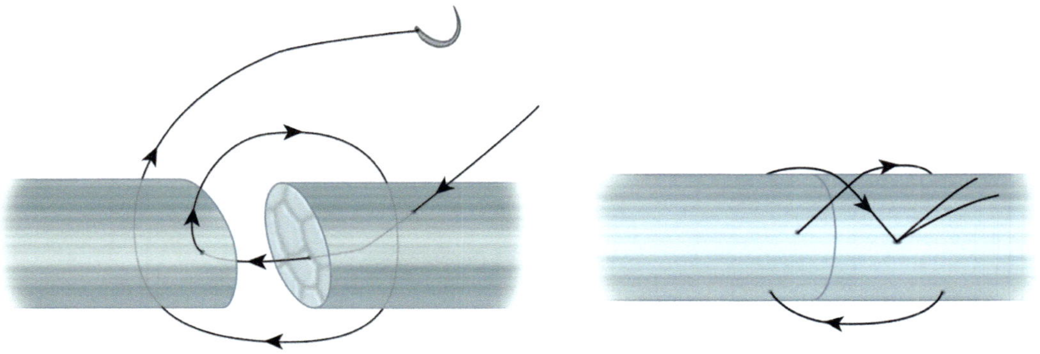

Fig. 12.28 The double right-angle stitch for solid tendons

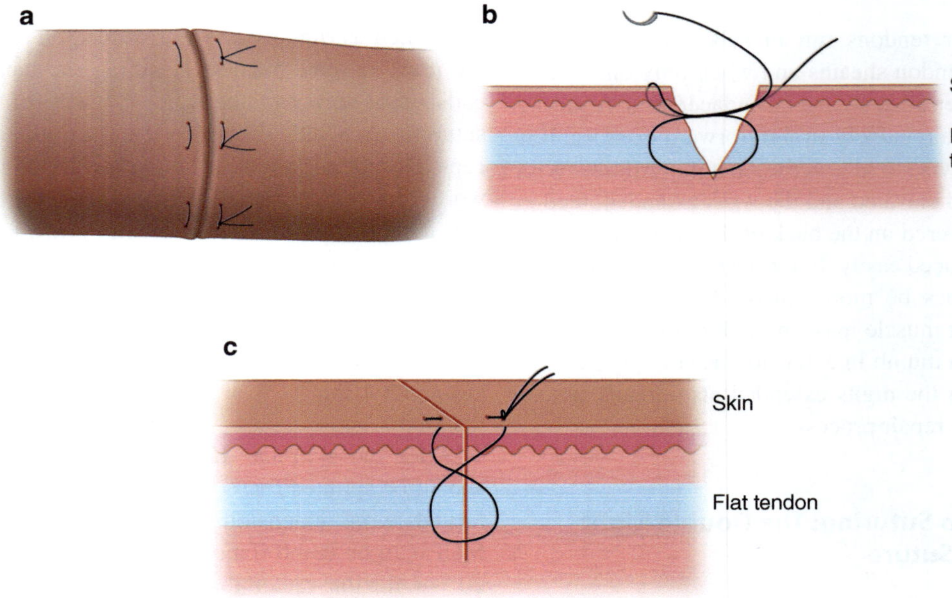

Fig. 12.29 (**a**–**c**) Two alternative suturing methods for flat tendons. (**a**) Interrupted horizontal mattress sutures with non-absorbable 5/0 thread. (**b**) A figure-of-eight suture has been inserted but not pulled together. (**c**) The completed figure-of-eight suture repairs both the tendon and skin. It is left in place for 3 weeks

both IPJs. A synthetic non-absorbable mattress suture or two, or figure-of-eight sutures including skin, is best for repairing extensor tendons in the finger (Fig. 12.29).

Repairs distal to the MCPJs are safeguarded mainly by splintage, which must maintain flexion of the MCPJs and extension of both IPJs for at least 3 weeks. This splint should also maintain wrist extension. The skin over any tendon repair must always be very carefully looked after, particularly if flap lacerations are involved.

Mallet Finger [Drooping of the Distal Segment]

It is essential to X-Ray all digits where mallet deformity of the distal segment has occurred, because there may be a treatable fracture, which should be corrected and immobilised for 4 weeks in extension (Fig. 12.30).

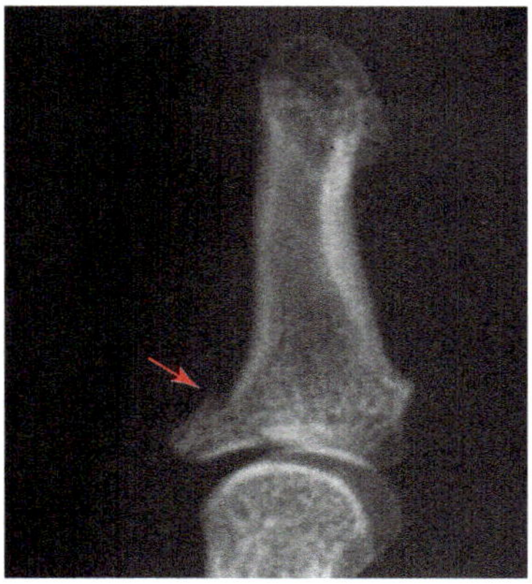

Fig. 12.30 Small fracture of the extensor insertion to the distal phalanx which could lead to a Mallet deformity

Closed Mallet Deformity Without Fracture

This is the most common version with a closed tendon rupture (Fig. 12.31).

The flat tendon insertion has usually pulled apart in the manner of a shaving brush. There is nothing worthwhile to actually suture, so it is not worthwhile trying. It is however worth splinting this injury in a split plastic mallet splint or on a Plaster of Paris slab with the MCPJ flexed and the DIPJ joint extended for a week or 10 days and then discussing further treatment with the patient. Without further treatment, the finger can again be used fully despite its mallet deformity, which will reduce considerably over several months.

For patients who are prepared to make an extra effort, it is probably worthwhile persevering with a small plastic mallet splint which holds the distal finger joint in extension for 6 or 8 weeks so that the frayed tendon can take up maximally. This treatment by no means guarantees full extension. As long as PIP flexion is not interfered with, the patient will regain full strength and flexion of the finger and probably be left with a slight mallet deformity. Later tendon surgery to improve this is much more likely to reduce flexion than it is to succeed in restoring full extension. Arthrodesis is also a poor solution to a mobile deformity because it reduces the ability of a joint to absorb mechanical shocks. In the daily encounters of fingers, a stiff joint is a liability.

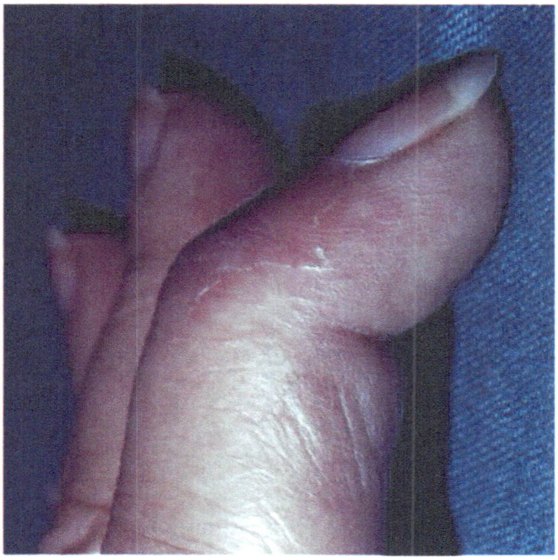

Fig. 12.31 Mallet deformity after closed tendon rupture. These injuries should all be X-Rayed to exclude a treatable fracture

Open Injury with Clean Incised Wound

If the tendon has been involved in a sharp laceration, the tendon ends can be approximated with two 5/0 nonabsorbable mattress or removable figure-of-eight sutures inserted while the DIPJ is pressed into extension (Fig. 12.29b, c). Opened joint capsule is best left to heal itself beneath the sutured tendon, the skin is closed and the wound dressed. The initial splint is a slab, immobilising the MCPJ in flexion and keeping both IPJs fully extended. After 2 weeks, a fitting mallet-finger splint can be used to immobilise just the distal joint in extension for a further 4 weeks. If the repair in a clean injury like this fails, the distal joint can lapse sometimes by as much as 60°

which will urgently need to be treated again, preferably by a specialist. A good result cannot be guaranteed the second time around.

Tendon Crushed or Shredded

In this clinical scenario where the dorsal skin is severely damaged [e.g. in a motor mower blade injury] it is neither possible nor necessary to consider formal tendon repair. Healing is likely to be associated with sufficient scarring to support both the tendon ends and the joint. The wound should be cleansed and dressed and the joint splinted for a month in extension. So long as the joint remains flexible, the long flexor usually retrieves very useful strength and some active extension is often regained mediated through the scar. Deformity is usually slight and there is not usually any disability.

Severe Crushed Joint and Tendon Deficit

When there has been a severe injury to the joint and an inactivated extensor tendon mechanism, the joint is best immobilised in slight flexion while it stabilises and stiffens in this position. Wound dressings can be arranged without having to remove the splint. A mallet deformity will eventuate but there is likely to be surprisingly little disability despite the serious initial injury, mostly because sensation is unaffected.

Rehabilitation

An injured hand can be taken out of the splint to begin active exercises as soon as pain reduces to allow it. This is usually by about 4–5 days. All movements can be encouraged, holding the maximum movement in one direction for 30 s and then changing to the opposite movement for 30 s. Remember the key movements of opposition and rotation of the thumb and also spreading and closing of the fingers. Waggling exercises are instinctive but singularly useless. Squeezing a rubber ball is another over-rated exercise as it builds up muscle strength rather than increasing movement. The ball sits within the grasp, impeding flexion, its elasticity working in the direction of extension but not increasing this either.

The early exercise sessions should be no longer than 5 min several times a day, after which the hand should be returned to its functional position in the splint. By a week or 10 days, the recovering hand can stay out of the splint in the daytime for use and exercises, but remain in at least a wrist splint at night. People naturally curl into the foetal position when sleeping and wrists readily go into the flexed position. MCP and finger flexion exercises are more effective with the wrist stabilised in extension by a short splint or supported in extension by the other hand. Use should be encouraged and additional exercises or physiotherapy should otherwise be limited to about 5 min per hour. It is possible for a person to do too much with the hand too soon. If movement and/or swelling in a hand are getting worse not better and there is no evidence of infection, this is likely to be due to dependency, overly forceful passive exercises or overuse.

Infection

The development of infection can be an important setback and if spreading should be settled as quickly as possible by immobilisation in the functional position and administration of antibiotics, before renewing any mobilisation regime. Infection adds a high protein component to tissue oedema, which gives rise to diffuse and dense scarring. Attempting to mobilise tissue that is still inflamed is particularly counterproductive as this promotes the spread rather than the settling of infection.

The Management of Nail Injuries

Nails grow forwards from the nail matrix lining the nail fold. They then sit on the nailbed and are adherent to it but they must also slide over this as they grow. If a nail is pulled out cleanly, a normal nail will regrow from the nailfold and take about 6 months to form the nail again. It is a complete nonsense to tell patients in this predicament *'Sorry, you've lost your nail'* as if it was a permanent loss. When nailbed tissue has been crushed, there may or may not be an underlying fracture. Clotted blood should be washed out of the wounds using local anaesthetic with adrenaline in a syringe and the tissue moulded back as accurately as possible. Much is made of the meticulous suturing of nailbeds but in Joan Chapple's experience this was rarely needed. In crush injuries and multiple lacerations as inflicted by mowers or buzzers or spindle moulders, the disrupted tissue is very debilitated and particularly likely to be adversely affected by any suturing. Closed haematomata are extremely painful and should be released [see sub-ungual haematoma in chapter on Difficult & Unusual Wounds]. It is sometimes helpful to retain a loose nail or even use a nail that has come right off to fit back into the nailfold so that this heals without adhesions. This will forestall inflammatory and infective complications, which can otherwise occur when regrowth of the nail is obstructed by any soft tissue. Such temporary use of a nail or a tiny silastic template is only necessary for a week or so. When the nailfold and matrix is injured, the new nail is likely to be deformed, even if the original nail appeared intact and there was no nailbed injury. A simple longitudinal cut across the matrix for instance gives rise to a vertical ridge on the nail forever more (Fig. 12.32).

With any major disruption to the end of a digit, it helps to be particularly aware of the nail matrix, which remains capable of growing nail or bits of nail. If the regrowth of part or all of a nail is undesirable, matrix can be looked for and excised at the original procedure. In most cases, a wait-and-see policy will be more appropriate, with a delayed decision eventually being based on *'is the nail or bit of it more use than nuisance, or more nuisance than use?'* (Fig. 12.33).

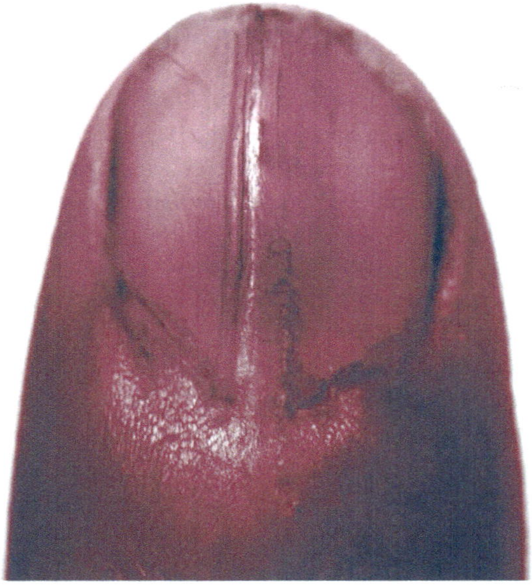

Fig. 12.32 Ridged nail 6 months after a simple longitudinal cut through the nail matrix with a sharp Stanley knife

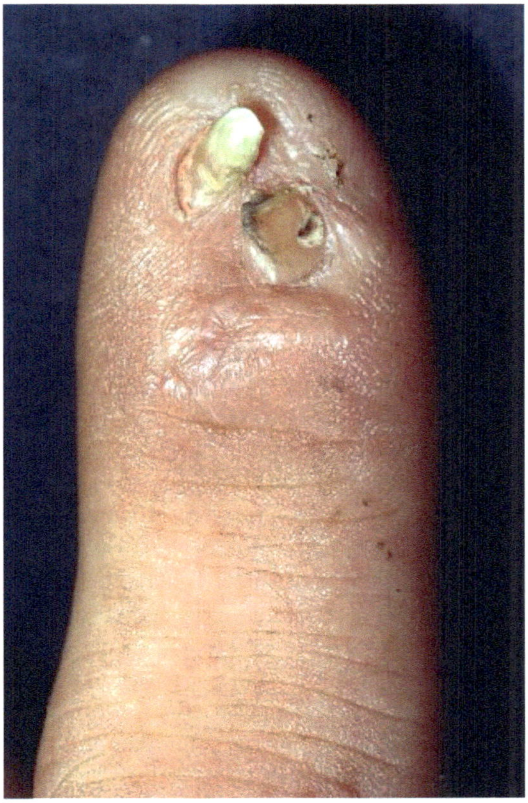

Fig. 12.33 Where nail is involved, it is best to await the outcome of regrowth. These nail remnants were excised

Commentary by Dr Murray Beagley FRACS, Dip Hand Surg [Euro]

Although I didn't ever meet Dr Chapple her teachings were widespread and held as a reference point for dealing with soft tissue injuries of the hand in particular. She ran a soft tissue clinic through Auckland Hospital for complex wounds and her expertise in this area was renowned. I enjoyed reading her account of hand injury treatment. Her wisdom in dealing with difficult hand injuries is evident by the passion in which she describes injuries in general. She then continues with a detailed section on examination, assessment and anatomy which is a concise and thorough record.

Most would agree that sensory evaluation can be assessed with a paper clip rather than a needle. Although Dr Chapple did not assess discrimination, many use two-point discrimination testing as a useful adjunctive test in an attempt to quantify the degree of impaired sensation.

Dr Chapple's notes on Radiology refer to distal phalangeal fractures only and do not cover the full spectrum of hand fractures that are commonly seen in the Hand Unit at Middlemore Hospital today. Indeed, her recommendations are that unstable fractures are referred through to a Hand Specialist. Her comments predate the advent of specialised plating systems for the treatment of hand fractures which are in common use today.

One of Dr Chapple's specialty areas was fingertip injuries and many of her comments on these injuries are as relevant now as they were when she wrote her book. She makes particular reference to crush injuries and those caused by power tools and lawnmowers. Examples are given of suturing such injuries which has led to 'throbbing circulatory pain'. This is often a prelude to ongoing severe pain and tissue necrosis unless the sutures are removed and the tension relieved.

It is the high velocity or crush injuries that need careful assessment as often they do better with debridement and dressing rather than suturing due to the swelling of the tissues and vascular compromise by the sutures.

Fingertip injuries are one of the commonest injuries that we see in our Hand Unit and their treatment remains variable in that there are often many ways to treat a certain injury and different surgeons have different preferences. Dr Chapple does not mention the use of local flaps (or distant flaps for that matter) for fingertips. Hand units worldwide currently use local flaps as an important adjunct for resurfacing and recontouring tissue loss in the fingertip and pulp. This was recognised by Graham Lister, a renowned hand surgeon in the mid-80 s when Dr Chapple was practicing [4].

Dr Chapple stresses the importance of avoiding operating on hands with a tourniquet and also that the worst time to operate on a hand is within the first 48 h after injury. Currently, most surgeons do in fact operate using a tourniquet in such situations and prefer to operate on traumatic injuries within 48 h. Her views on tourniquets are certainly shared by many however, as the trend towards WALANT (Wide Awake Local Anaesthesia, No Tourniquet) continues. This technique has been promoted largely by Don Lalonde, a well-respected Canadian hand surgeon [5]. As for the timing of surgery, most surgeons currently place great urgency on injuries with contamination, infection in a confined space or amputated tissue requiring revascularisation. Maybe the delays in treatment of acute injuries which are being experienced in all of our hospitals secondary to staff shortages are advantageous to our patients.

Suturing techniques espoused by Dr Chapple may be still in use today although I note that comment is only made on extensor rather than flexor tendons. Numerous modifications and configurations of suturing techniques exist today and oftentimes the choice of technique is by surgeon preference. The institution in which the surgeon works may have protocols for repairs of tendons in specific locations in the hand, as is the case in many Hand Units. Dr Chapple's experience with extensor tendons may reflect the spectrum of injuries that she saw, as I expect that in those days most flexor tendon injuries were preferentially sent to the Plastic Surgery Unit at Middlemore Hospital.

The final segment relates to nail bed injuries and Dr Chapple's comments are still relevant.

Drainage of a subungual haematoma is a necessary and appreciated intervention for a crushed fingertip. Replacement of the nail (or remnant) beneath the fold helps to reduce adhesions and allows the unimpeded regrowth of a new nail. Decisions regarding secondary surgery can often hinge on her final question 'is the nail or bit of it more use than nuisance, or more nuisance than use?'

Commentary by Lisa Hansen Dip. Phyt. [Auck], AdvDipMT, Reg HT and Adam White BSc Physiotherapy, NZRP, HTNZ

The current best practice for rehabilitation of hand injuries is to walk the tight rope between protecting the healing structures from forces that will delay or stop the healing process. But at the same time to allow as much early motion and forces that are safe, to allow for restoration of hand function and ongoing brain/hand connection function.

Dr Joan Chapple's principles embody this and the importance of the hand from a biopsychosocial perspective seems to have also been in her consciousness. She understood intuitively that the human hand allows us to work, eat and play, but so much more; it is a vehicle for us to express emotion and connect with others. A handshake, a hug, a pat on the back—the loss of function in a hand has many functional and psychological ramifications.

So many of her key points are still true today including the importance of early motion after injury or surgery where possible, to add to the ability for tendons, nerves and vessels to move on each other.

Specialist hand teams are important for complex hand injury cases and access to them for GPs is so much better, with up-to-date resources available online, and by direct referral. A reminder that information should come from reputable sources is important.

Improved hand dressings are significant, especially Cuticerin™, Jelonet™ and the frequent modern use of Coban™ bandage under no tension to cover and protect hand wounds. Other modern innovations include: better understanding of neural anatomical variants, neural plasticity and central sensitisation, blurring the anatomical boundaries of reported sensory changes. Also, the emergence of Wide Awake Surgery [WAS], supporting not only the exclusion of the tourniquet but also allowing the patient to be able to test the repairs in intraoperative time.

Early motion guidelines define specifically the rehabilitation process for post-operative restoration of function. These have become more proactive and walk the tight rope between protecting the repair and allowing as much early motion as possible [6]. The Norwich protocols, Relative Extension Splinting and the SAM [Short Arc Motion] protocols to mention a few. The concept of little and often still holds true, and now marrying this up with the tissue healing time frames, the inflammatory phase, fibroblastic repair and remodelling, a bespoke management plan can be designed for the individual patient [7].

With respect to immobilisation of the hand in the safe position, one variation to this for the elderly patient or those with severe osteoarthritis or rheumatoid arthritis is to allow a slight amount of flexion at the PIP joints. This is to ensure restoration of a functional flexion grip. For the classic mallet finger deformity, a modern variation is splinting the DIP joint only with either a volar or dorsal splint to allow more tactile use of the injured digit. A PIP joint extension block can be employed in the more flexible patient or with more proximal migration of the ruptured EDC tendon that tends to create a swan neck deformity. A lightweight thermoplastic splint can both support the dip in extension and block excessive PIP joint extension.

Although there is a volume of high quality research for hand therapy scope of practice, there remains a shortage of evidence for numerous diagnoses and activity-based interventions. More evidence is needed for the complex hand cases and activity-based interventions, behavioural and quality of care outcomes.

References

1. Aclandanatomy.com [2003 DVD Atlas of human anatomy series]/Volume: The Upper Extremity.
2. James Quinn, Steven Cummings, Michael Callaham, Karen Sellers. Suturing versus conservative management of lacerations of the hand: Controlled randomized trial. B.M.J. 2002:325, 299.
3. Cynthia M. Illingworth. Trapped fingers and amputated finger-tips in children. J.Pediatr. Surg. 9. 1974:853–858.
4. Lister G. Local flaps to the hand. Hand Clin. 1985;1(4):621–40.
5. Lalonde DH. Conceptual origins, current practice and views of wide awake hand surgery. J Hand Surg Euro. 2017;42(9):886–95.
6. Takata SC, Wade ET, Roll SC. Hand therapy interventions, outcomes, and diagnoses evaluated over the last 10 years: a mapping review linking research to practice. J Hand Ther. 2019;32(1):1–9. https://doi.org/10.1016/j.jht.2017.05.018; Epub 2017 Jun 21. PMID: 28647322; PMCID: PMC5740027, 1.
7. White A, Baldwin R, Stephens F, Shaw H. Extensor tendon repair rehabilitation guidelines—SAM zones III—IV, hand therapy unit. Hamilton: Waikato District Health Board; 2012.

13 Difficult and Unusual Wounds

Summary

Particular sites on the body and certain causes or mechanisms of injury give rise to wounds that are somewhat unique or troublesome. The treatment of several of these wound scenarios is described in this chapter. Other unhealthy wounds may be behaving badly because of underlying diseases or co-morbidities. Not uncommonly, several adverse factors may be combined in the same wound. Modern war wounds have their own specific challenges and are briefly considered by an expert in the commentary. Although Dr. Joan Chapple did not cover this topic in her original manuscript, the co-editors believe it is now a consideration of significant relevance and cannot be ignored, given the mass war casualties of both soldiers and civilians in various parts of the globe in recent times.

Road Grazes and Degloving

Probably because these are so common, they are regarded as less serious than a laceration, dressed to mop up the seepage and covered from view. If they are superficial, they usually dry up quite quickly and peel to leave healed skin. Those that go on discharging are deeper wounds, which often get infected and can be very slow to heal. From the beginning, all grazes are contaminated friction burns — two reasons for them to behave badly. Heat is generated very quickly by friction. The grazed patient usually needs more prolonged pain relief than the usual burned patient, whose pain usually settles down relatively quickly. Grazes damage lots of nerve endings and the tissues often become inflamed or infected. There is quite often an area of 'degloving' where the skin has been separated from the underlying circulation. This area then has to get perfusion from its periphery until it can stick down again. If blood or serum collects in the space, this is a compromise and a tense accumulation will further impair the circulation. In this clinical scenario, incision or vacuum drainage may be very helpful. Degloving and grazing often occur over bony prominences such as elbows, knees, and malleoli, where tears can also involve bursae and ligamentous shredding with open joints.

It is not easy to assess the depth of a graze, even after inspecting it carefully. The centre of a grazed area is usually the site of the deepest damage, because heat is retained here. If central areas are whitish or dark bluish and stagnant-looking, there is probably full-thickness skin destruction (Fig. 13.1).

An accurate pronouncement about depth may have to be deferred and made on the basis of how the wound behaves. This behaviour in turn depends to a considerable extent also on how thick the skin is at the site of the graze. Grazes of the back have to be extremely deep to produce full-thickness destruction, while road grazes on the dorsum of the hands readily expose tendons.

P. Charlesworth, M. F. Klaassen, *Chapple's Principles of Wound Care and Healing*,
https://doi.org/10.1007/978-3-031-53104-0_13

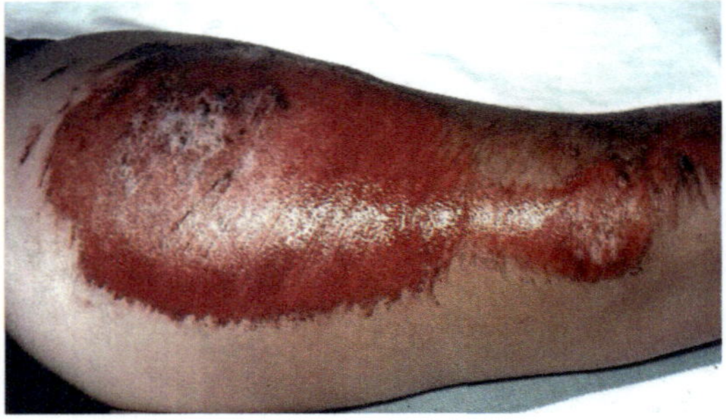

Fig. 13.1 This extensive road graze is a friction burn, with its central area showing the deepest destruction. It took about 6 weeks to heal

Deep grazes sometimes take weeks just to get rid of the dead tissue because collagen fibres pass from living to dead tissue. In most cases, it is usually worth waiting for spontaneous separation, because there are likely to be viable epithelial cells from skin appendages in the deep dermis, which will eventually provide enough islands of epithelium to avoid grafting. Large areas of residual raw surfaces from grazes may require grafting.

Treatment of Grazes

Safe doses of local anaesthetic are 3 mg per kg of plain Lignocaine and 7 mg per kg of Lignocaine with adrenaline, so anaesthetising large or multiple grazes to clean them is not really practicable, and it is also unnecessary. The seepage from grazes is profuse because they are friction burns, and surface dirt generally comes away into the early dressings with the discharge. Permanent 'tattooing' is very uncommon. It is therefore best to use lots of saline in a syringe for irrigation, carefully picking out any remaining particulate dirt with McIndoe's non-toothed dissecting forceps without anaesthetic, and then dress the area with antibiotic ointment on tulle gras.

Where there is a deeper tear, local anaesthetic can be used selectively. Deeper wounds should be thoroughly irrigated and if necessary, more formally explored for foreign material. A degloved space with an open wound will not accumulate fluid or blood as long as gravity drainage is ensured. If the skin is intact over the degloving, the circulation can be so reduced that pressure either from fluid accumulating beneath it or from bandages to prevent fluid accumulating may cause damaging local ischaemia. A small incision can be made through the worst-looking skin to prevent fluid accumulation, and the space obviously does not require cleaning. The central skin rarely has any sensation left, but if it does, local anaesthetic will be required. The patient should then be instructed to spend the next few days with any wound opening postured to drain by gravity. The alternative to incision and gravity drainage is the insertion if a suction drain into the cavity.

Painting grazes with antiseptic solutions that sting is counterproductive no matter how often people are told to *'put up with it, you've got to be cruel to be kind'* or *'it's all in a good cause'*. Exposed living cells are very vulnerable to toxic chemicals, injured ones even more so. They are particularly susceptible to any spirit-based solutions as these denature protein. Hydrogen peroxide oxidises and kills cells as well as bacteria. The slough produced by these applications then has to separate before any healing can take place, and it may get infected.

Grazes need to be dressed with lots of greasy tulle and because of the contamination will benefit from a topical antibiotic cream such as silver sulphadiazine added from the beginning. [Thermal burns are relatively sterile by comparison; infection is much less common and patients with burns don't automatically require antibiotics]. Where there are multiple grazes, it is justifiable to give systemic antibiotics for several days. Early dressings need lots of absorbent material and attention every day or two, but later on, dressings can easily be managed by the patients themselves.

Crushed Fingertips

Tissue injured by high velocity tools and motor-mower blades has sustained invisible concussion in addition to the visible injury. Finger pulps are often burst open by pressure, with cellular damage throughout the tip of the finger (Figs. 13.2 and 13.3).

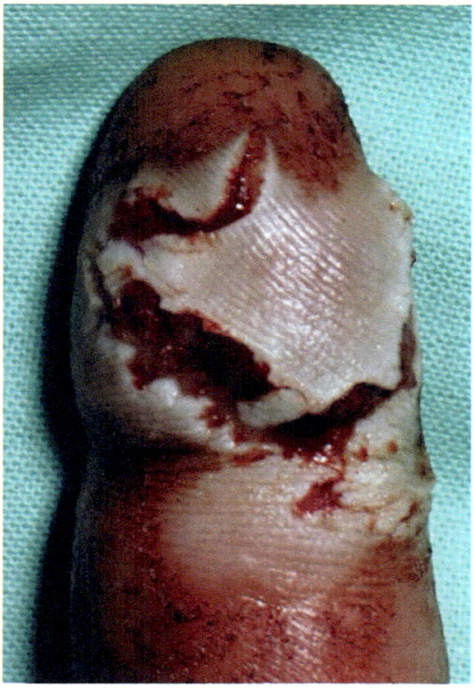

Fig. 13.2 Crushed fingertip treated without sutures. Five day result showing wet [white] but not unhealthy skin flaps. Healing progressed without problems

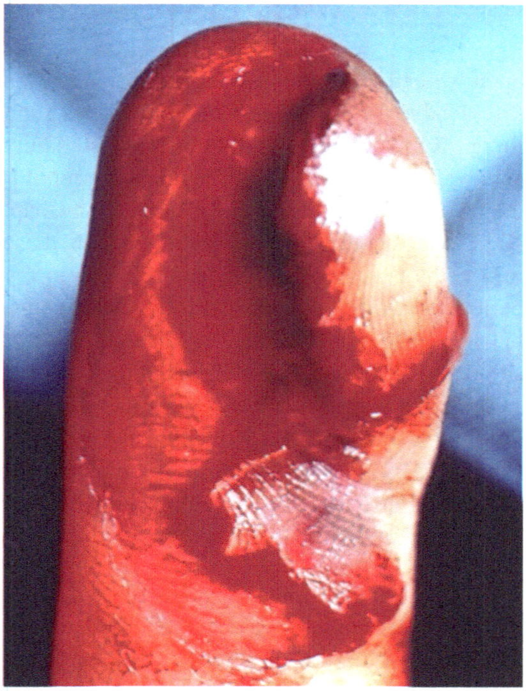

Fig. 13.3 Severely traumatised fingertip, best treated with tulle moulding, not suturing

There may or may not be underlying crush fractures or a flaky injury to the tuft or absent nails (Figs. 13.4 and 13.5).

The treatment of these injuries always needs to take into account the reactive swelling and tension which will inevitably occur for 48 h, permitting the full extent of the process, without any restriction to circulation (Figs. 13.6 and 13.7).

The best approach to injured fingertips, even where there is tissue missing, is usually to clean them, sometimes remove or tidy bone chips, align them, and dress them until they heal spontaneously (Figs. 13.8, 13.9, 13.10, 13.11, 13.12 and

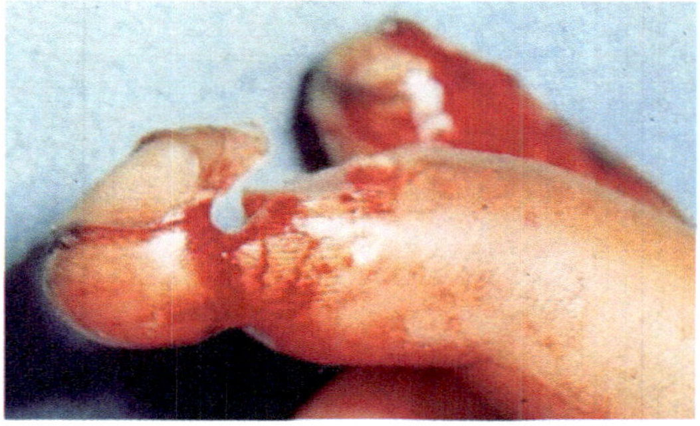

Fig. 13.4 Unstable but healthy fingertip, best stabilised with tulle mould and not sutures

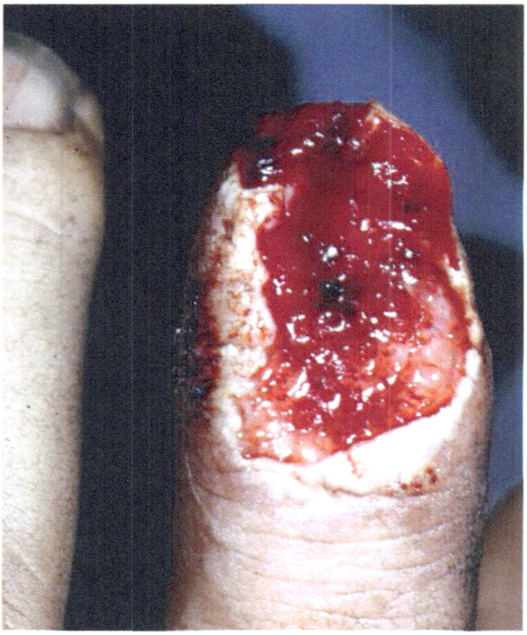

Fig. 13.5 Considerable dorsal tissue loss. Finger pulp was intact and bone not involved

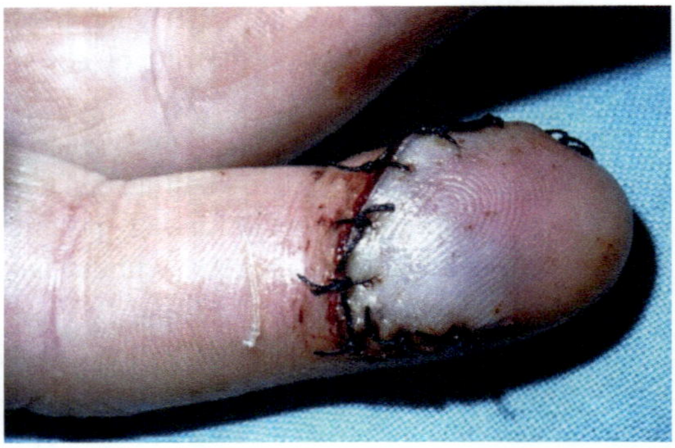

Fig. 13.6 Impending necrosis of a pulp flap on day of injury. The patient returned with severe pain later the same day

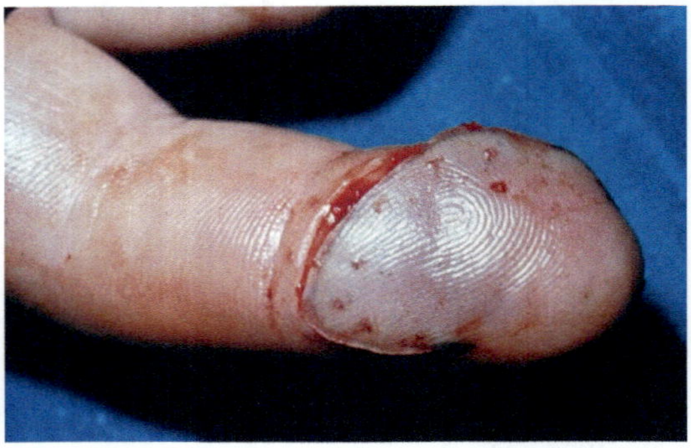

Fig. 13.7 Immediate relief of pain and recovery of circulation followed the removal of the sutures. Same day as Fig. 13.6

13.13). If complicated procedures are required, they are often best deferred for at least 48 h.

Motor-mower injuries or fingers traumatised by other high velocity spinning blades always need anaesthesia for cleaning purposes no matter how clean they look. Grass and grit have often penetrated deeply (Figs. 13.14, 13.15, and 13.16).

Some crush injuries may need anaesthetic for realignment of tissue and evacuation of clots that are displacing tissue or disrupting nail beds, while others do not need this. The presence of

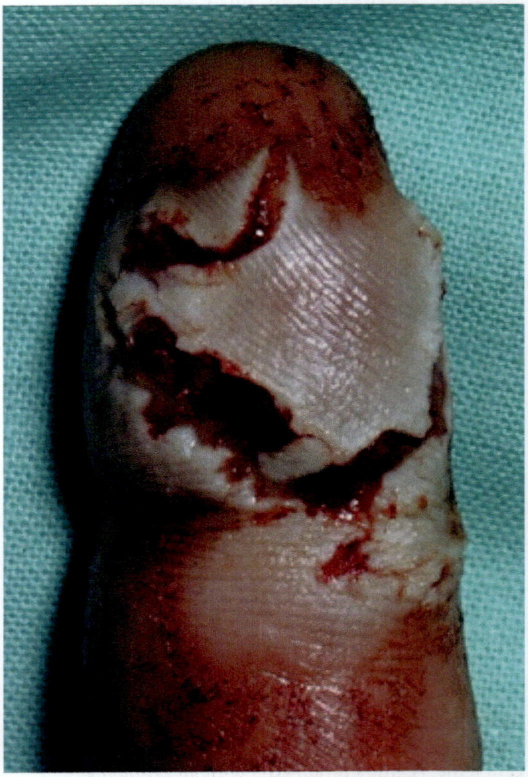

Fig. 13.8 Crushed fingertip at day 5 treated without sutures

open wounds in complex injuries is always a safety valve for decompression and rather a good thing. Repositioning of tissue is most safely achieved in fingertips using the tulle-gras moulding technique. This technique is detailed in Chap. 12. Haemostasis is an important goal in these injuries. It may be necessary to use a temporary period of haemostatic pressure to achieve this, but it is only after bleeding has been absolutely stopped that the tension in the eventual dressing can be reduced sufficiently to allow reactive swelling without reducing perfusion. Decompression by leakage from these wounds is usually profuse and most swelling resolves after

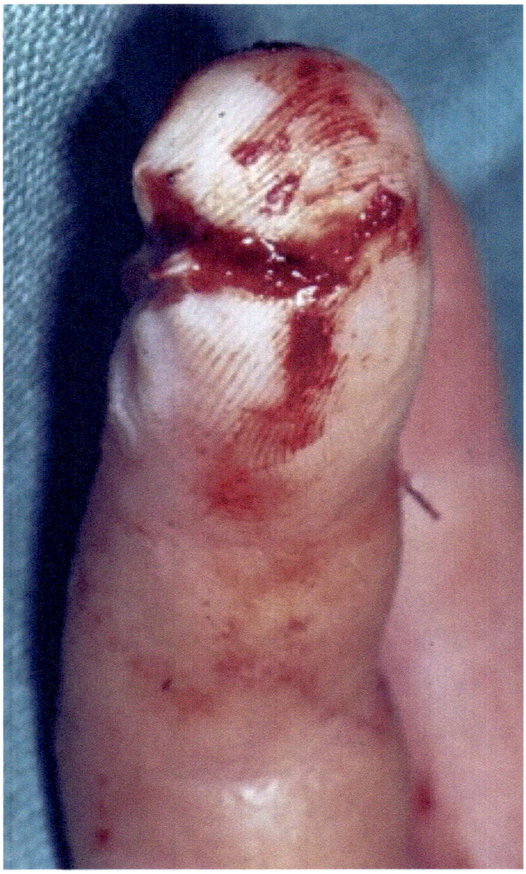

Fig. 13.9 Another crushed/lacerated fingertip unsutured and healing at day 5

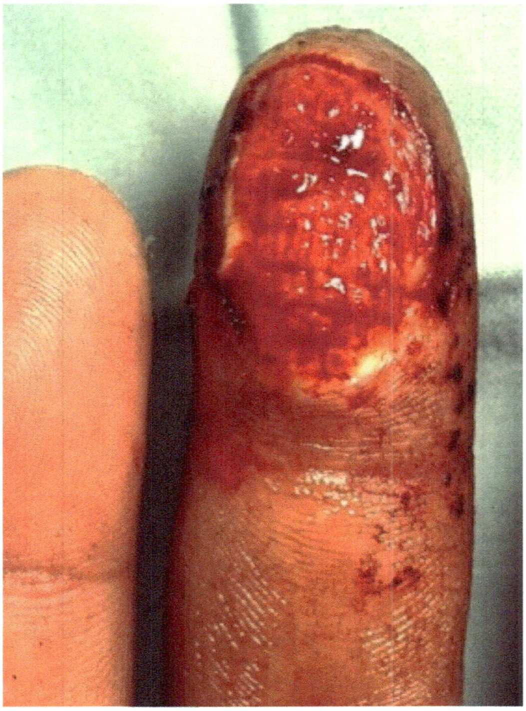

Fig. 13.10 Irrecoverable skin loss from pulp of finger

the first few days. Trying to prevent swelling by applying pressure dressings is inappropriate because it only creates additional circulatory deprivation which will translate into long-term oedema and the atrophies which are characteristic of sickly tissue.

There is no place for pressure dressings in the treatment of acutely injured tissues.

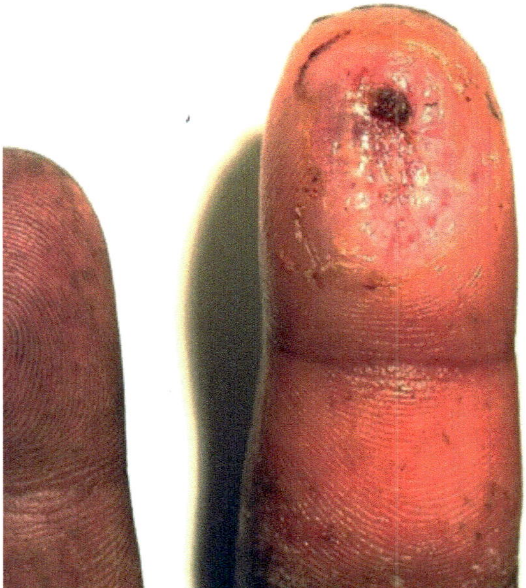

Fig. 13.11 5 weeks of spontaneous healing with dressings ensures a much better result than grafting

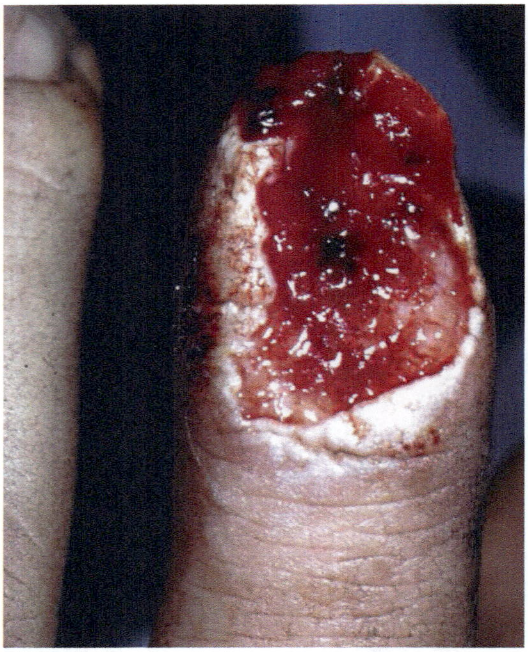

Fig. 13.12 Considerable loss of tissue from dorsum of fingertip, with intact pulp and no bone involvement

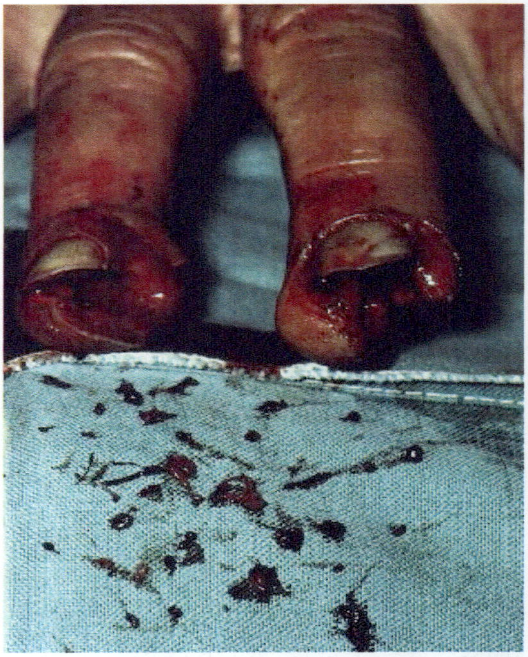

Fig. 13.14 Typical motor-mower injuries to fingertips

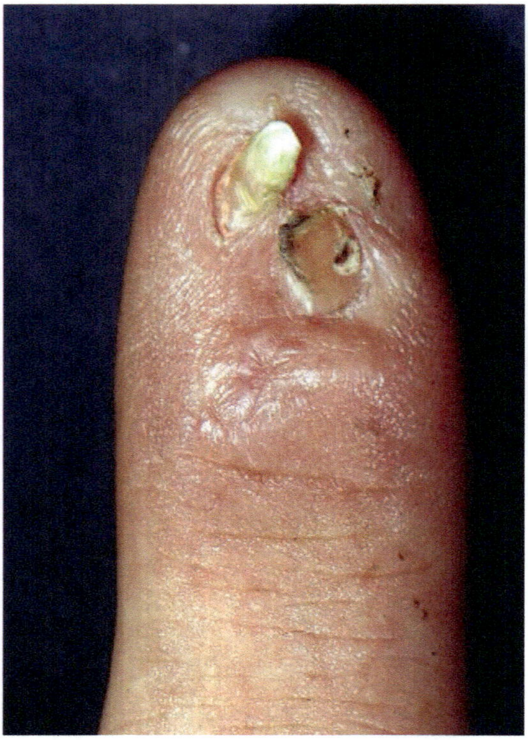

Fig. 13.13 Where nail is involved, it is best to wait the outcome of regrowth. These nail remnants were excised

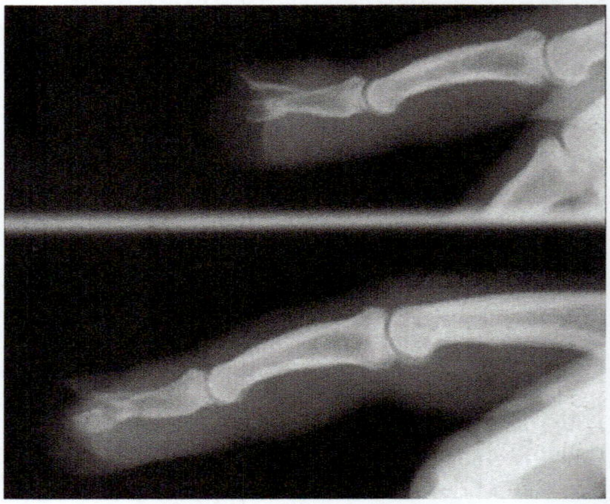

Fig. 13.15 Radiological evidence of damaged phalangeal tufts

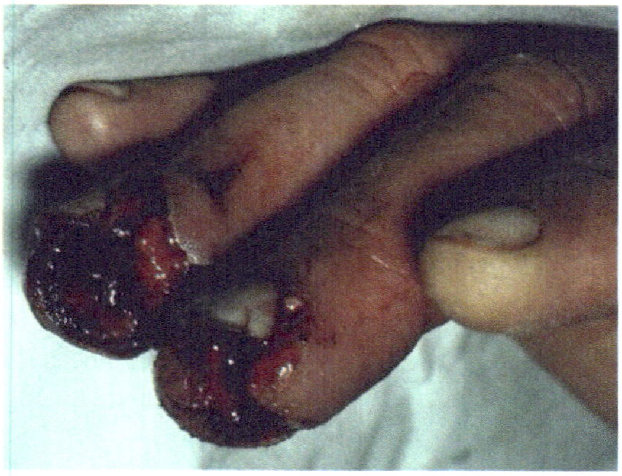

Fig. 13.16 Dirt, grass, and bone chips cleaned out after local anaesthetic blocks. Both fingertips then tulle moulded and healed uneventfully

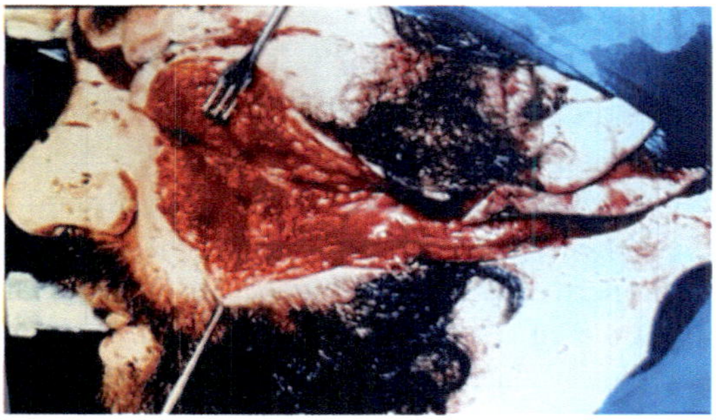

Fig. 13.17 Deep left facial laceration sustained in violent attack with a Stanley knife in the early 1990s, Glasgow City, Scotland. Known as a 'Glasgow Smile'

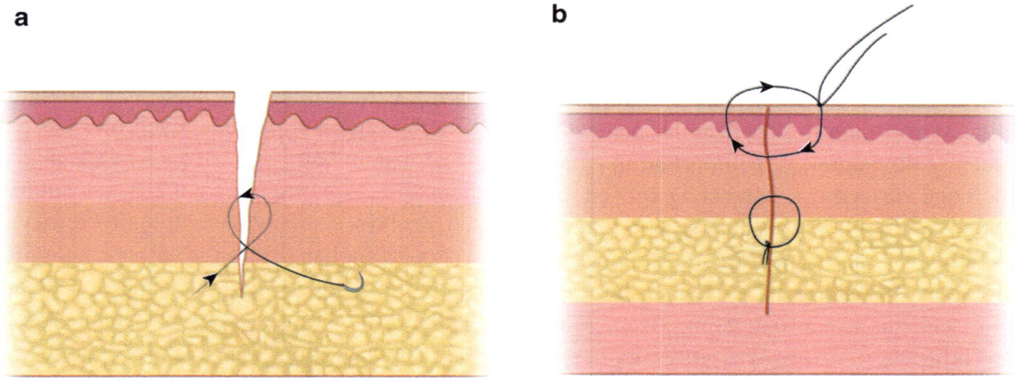

Figs. 13.18 (**a**, **b**) Insertion of sutures in the face. The insertion of absorbable subcutaneous sutures can be done so that their knots lie buried deeply. The superficial skin is then sutured with synthetic removable sutures

Facial Lacerations

Dry blood on the skin is best softened by laying wet saline swabs over the area for 10 min or so, then using wrung-out ones to wipe the skin clean. Lacerations of the face often involve the muscles of facial expression in the subcutaneous tissues and/or the facial nerve fibres plus the parotid gland and Stenson's duct (Fig. 13.17: MFK's experience with Glasgow Smile Stanley-knife facial lacerations in the early 1990s). For this reason [and permissible because of the robust circulation], the use of interrupted 5/0 plain catgut or other absorbable sutures in the subcutaneous tissues is recommended. These should be inserted upside down so that the knots and cut threads face deeply instead of poking up through the sutured wound (Fig. 13.18a). The skin sutures of 5/0 nylon non-absorbable material are then inserted (Fig. 13.18b).

A facial wound sutured with interrupted, non-absorbable skin sutures can have dressings removed after several hours, be greased with Vaseline™ [petroleum jelly] showered on, and have the sutures replaced by tapes within a few days. Unhealed or discharging wounds need dressings of some sort until they heal.

Scalp Wounds

Shave an absolute minimum of hair just along the wound edges. After that, there is the bleeding to contend with. Use a head-up position for the patient, but never work with them sitting unsupported as they may crash to the floor at any time in a faint. A facility to lie patients completely flat needs to be thought about and prepared ahead. Use adrenaline/local anaesthetic routinely and stop bleeders with fine mosquito forceps. Grasping the galeal layer and retracting it outwards is a good tip for controlling scalp bleeders. If this fails, it may be necessary to suture-ligate the bleeders with absorbable material, especially if working alone. Bleeders in the dermis of the scalp can be impressive. Scalp skin is very thick and dense, with hair follicles located deep in the dermis. Deeper still are the fascial layers [galea], in some places, muscles [frontalis and occipitalis] and then the periosteum and bone. In a deep scalp wound, it is important to examine the bone surface if it has been exposed, but do not poke around deeply unless you can see adequately. A depressed fracture may not always show up on a skull X-Ray. If there is a fracture, consult a neurosurgeon. After windscreen injuries it is always worth exploring along the sides of the wound with curved mosquito forceps. There is a characteristic clinking as glass is touched with metal and it is not always palpable to a gloved finger. If hair becomes a nuisance, it can be useful to sponge it flat with saline as you are washing the wound. Tulle-gras sheets [or some paraffin off this] can also be used to control hair during treatment.

It is usually safe to suture the scalp and tapes of course are literally not applicable. If possible, choose a suture different in colour from the hair, a white synthetic for dark hair and black thread for blondes *[Prolene is blue and would do for dark or blondes]*. Finally, put greasy tulle on the wound to grease the hair, the scalp, and the sutures and apply a pad of gauze plus a head bandage for a few hours. Scalp sutures can be left in for up to 10–12 days, with the patient showering over them from day 3 onward, washing the hair and applying cream or Vaseline along the wound so that the sutures become discrete and easier to remove. Complex scalp wounds can be managed accurately with tulle, dressings, and full head bandaging. The ears must always be padded accurately back and front to avoid their deformation. Flattened ears otherwise become extremely painful. Subsequently, an elasticized mesh helmet can be constructed out of tubular material to hold regular dressings in place. This needs to have cut-outs for the ears to avoid distorting them.

Eyebrows

Never ever shave eyebrows as it then becomes impossible for anyone to align a laceration accurately. It is also quite disfiguring for patients to lose eyebrows, which may take months to regrow or not regrow at all. They also look ridiculous during the regrowth process. Eyebrows not only have a range of hair sizes but each hair is aligned specifically with respect to the next. Suturing intact eyebrows involves continually retrieving and extricating hairs from the sutures, but unfortunately this is the only way to achieve accuracy. Alignment sometimes needs trial and error as well as patience (Fig. 13.19). Choose sutures that are a different colour from the eyebrow. As long as sutures are accurately inserted, they do not need to be particularly close together.

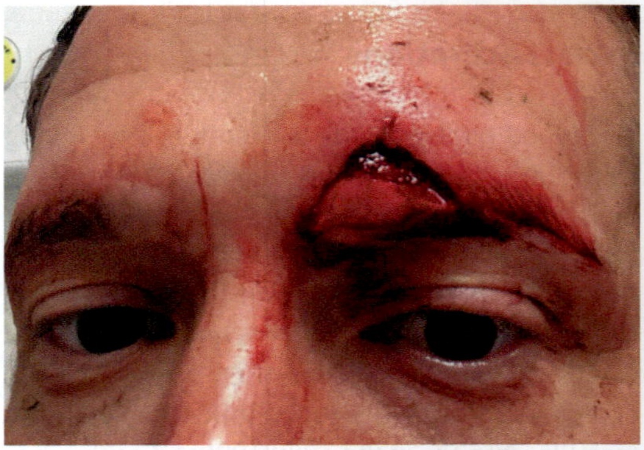

Fig. 13.19 Blunt trauma stellate laceration of left medial eyebrow where accurate alignment is important for ideal repair

Multiple Lacerations

Even if these are incised clean wounds, it is likely that there is some tissue with reduced circulation. This means that there may be a significant risk of further ischaemia from suturing. It is particularly easy to isolate blocks of tissue by suturing adjacent lacerations and produce planes of tension in bridges of tissue which are the last circulatory lifelines (Figs. 13.20, 13.21, and 13.22).

Multiple lacerations about the head and neck usually have a greater margin of circulatory safety and can sometimes be safely sutured. In other parts if the body, especially on the front of the lower leg, the circulation is much poorer and tapes or tulle gras may be the safest form of closure. Secondary suture is rarely needed, as closure is far more safely encouraged by tapes. Even leg wounds heal surprisingly quickly where they are not complicated by debilitated or dead tissue (Figs. 13.23, 13.24, 13.25, and 13.26).

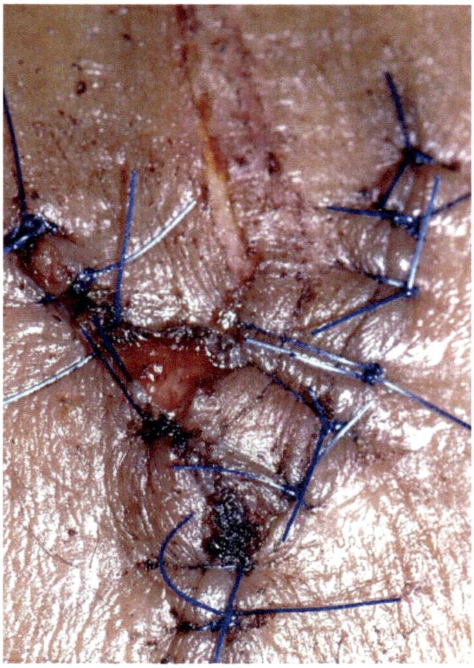

Fig. 13.20 Y-shaped laceration 3 days after routine suturing. Apart from oedema, it is almost looking alright

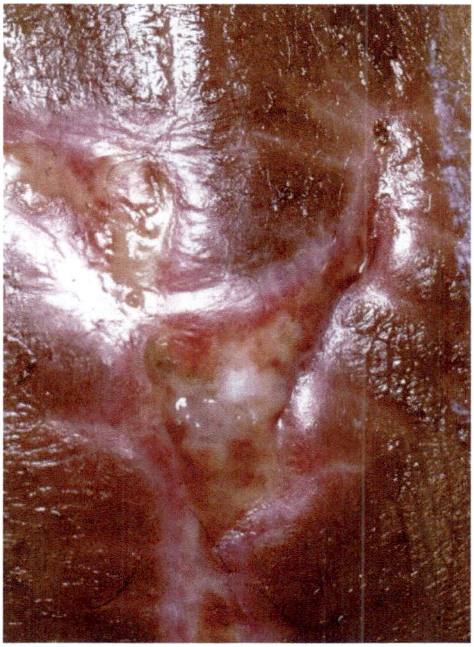

Fig. 13.21 The destructive effects of the suturing are more clearly reflected in the poor result at 6 weeks

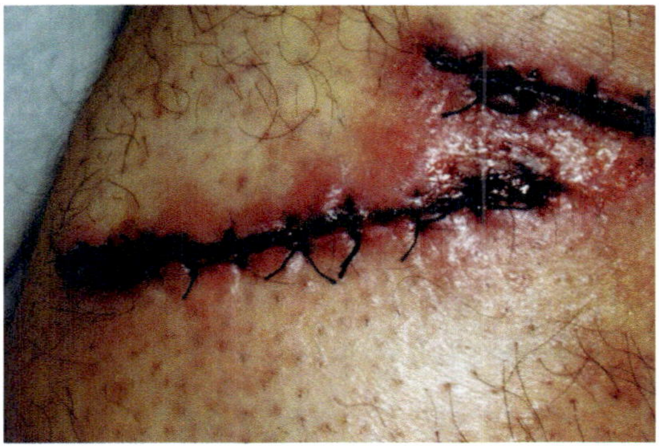

Fig. 13.22 Infection 1 week after the suture of adjacent lacerations. Note that the skin bridge between them is particularly affected

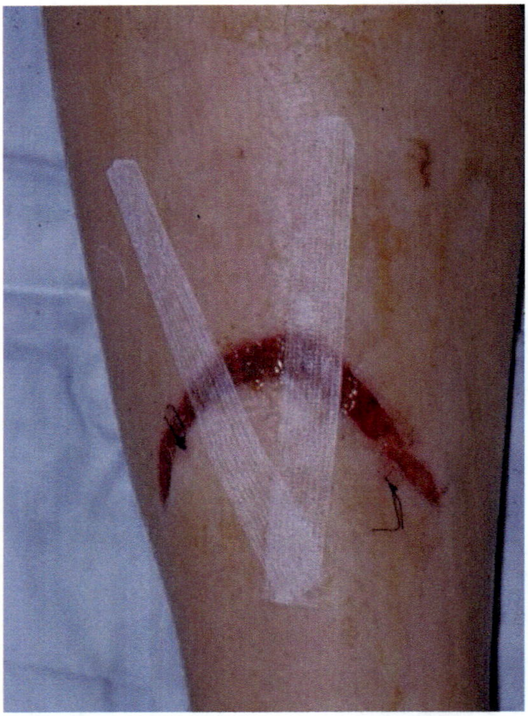

Fig. 13.23 A distally based leg flap has been taped on day 1. Full closure can be achieved by revising the taping in 3-days'-time

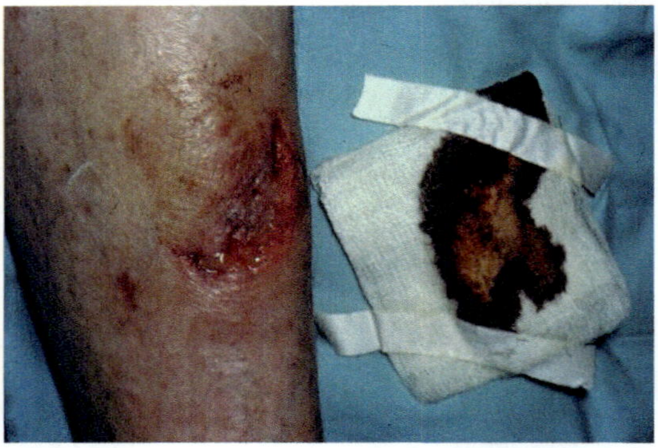

Fig. 13.24 A ragged leg flap has simply been held with tulle gras and dressed accurately. The 5-day result is entirely healthy with all oozing absorbed into the dressing. Healing was uneventful, the filmy skin edges taking largely as a graft

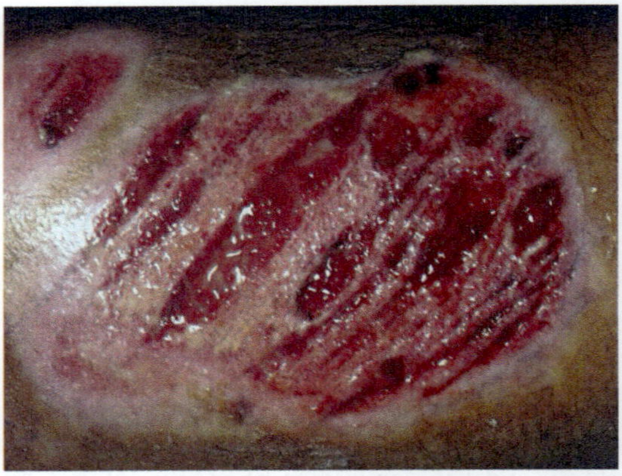

Fig. 13.25 Clean linear raw surfaces 3 weeks after initially sutured lacerations broke down and became infected. Raw surfaces are now healthy

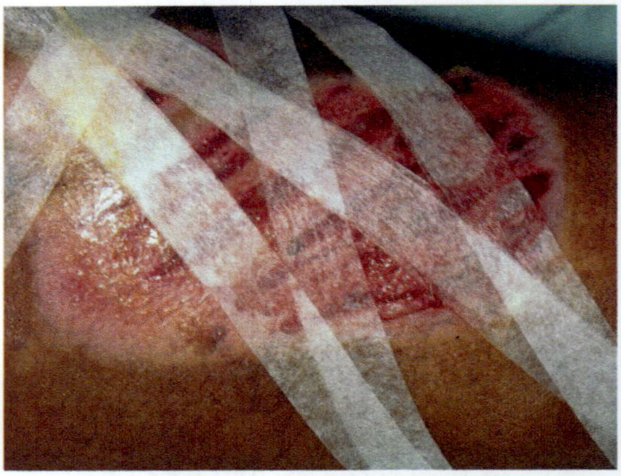

Fig. 13.26 Long tapes were able to reduce the gaps on the same day as Fig. 13.25 and rapid uneventful healing followed

Complete Lacerations Through Ears, Nasal Alae, and Lips

These rather alarming prospects are fortunately not too difficult to repair, using special techniques. Nose and ear wounds have cartilage visible as a central layer and in the lip the orbicularis oris muscle needs to be repaired.

Start away from the free edge, suturing the deepest layer first. In the case of the mouth, this is the mucous membrane. Use small, interrupted mattress sutures and a 5/0 thread of absorbable sutures [chromic catgut or Vicryl]. Start and finish these on the cavity side [as if they were on any surface] and tie several running knots eventually so that sutures don't come undone (Figs. 13.27a–c). Cut the sutures long [at least 10 mm].

If you think the inner sutures are going to be subsequently inaccessible, absorbable suture material is the norm. As the sutures are cut both threads fall through the wound or can be stroked through to lie on the inner surface as quite ordinary mattress sutures. By the time this layer is completed, you will have completed the most difficult part of the repair under direct vision. You will never be faced with trying to look inside the

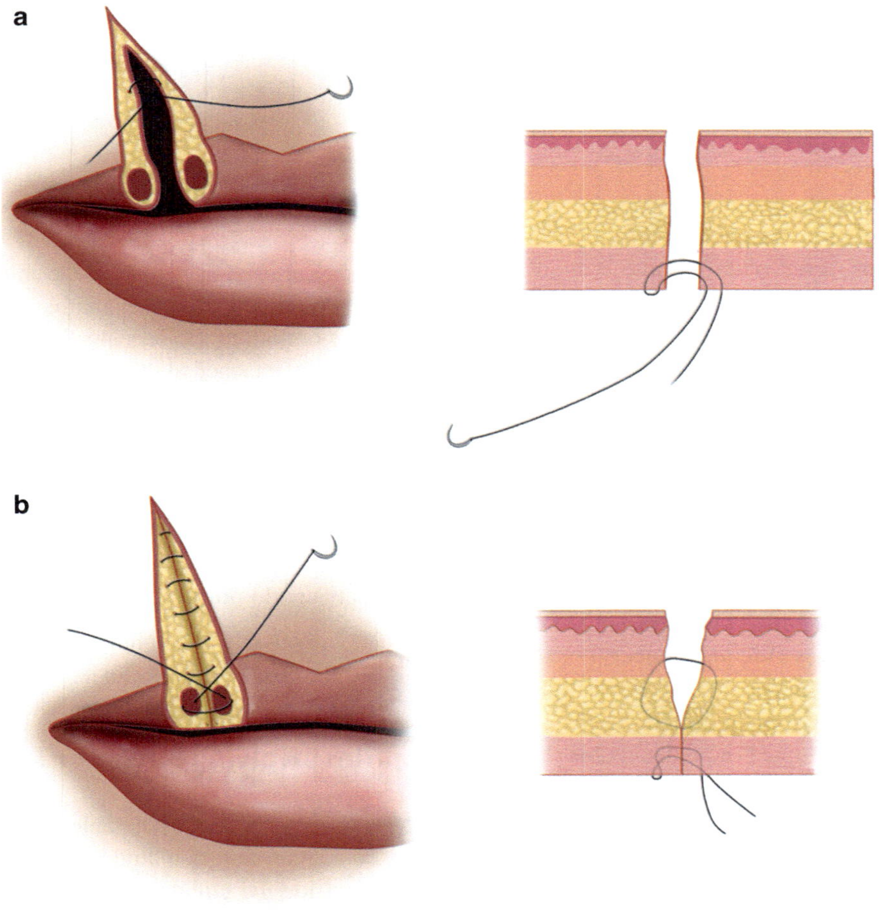

Fig. 13.27 (**a**–**c**) The repair of all layers in a complete laceration to an upper lip. (**a**) The inner layer is repaired first, using mattress sutures that fall through the wound as they are cut. (**b**) The second [middle layer] is repaired next, with upside-down sutures where the knots lie deeply. (**c**) The repair is completed with ordinary skin sutures, having had good conditions for suturing every layer

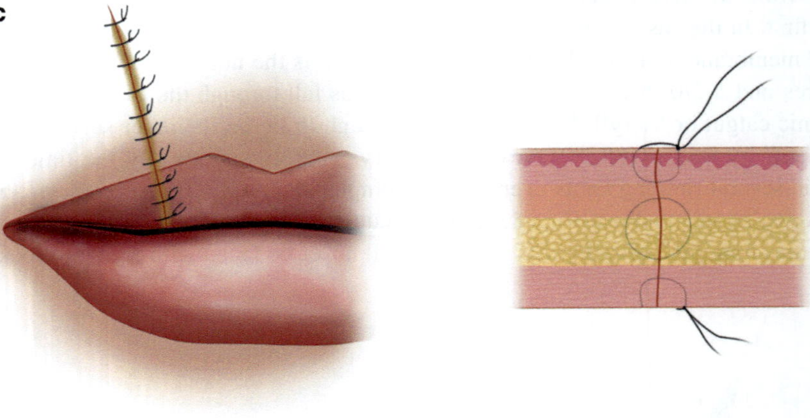

Fig. 13.27 (continued)

nostril or mouth to suture lining after you have stitched the rest of the wound up.

The next layer is the middle section of the wound. Use 5/0 interrupted absorbable sutures into the fibrous perichondrium and cartilage in the case of nose and ear wounds. Sutures through cartilage alone may tend to cut out. It is very important that these sutures align the cartilage without a step. A palpable and sometimes visible permanent ridge will be left if cartilage is misaligned. Use long-term absorbable sutures to muscles, fascia, and subcutaneous layers. In the lip, always locate and suture orbicularis oris muscle, which may initially be retracted out of sight. Synthetic sutures [Vicryl, Monocryl] are best as their strength remains for 3–6 weeks rather than the 5–7 days for plain catgut. Lastly, insert a series of interrupted non-absorbable 5/0 skin sutures, putting several eventual locking knots onto those in the lip itself and cutting these particularly long to prevent them being licked undone. The skin sutures can usually be replaced by tapes at 3 or 4 days, but the lip ones should be left for at least 5 days.

Use tulle gras, gauze, and Elastoplast or a taped-on dressing for 2–3 days, to blot up any seepage. With mouth wounds, advise patients to avoid traumatic food and strenuous chewing for a few days and to rinse the mouth out after eating.

Buccal Tear

Sometimes after a heavy blow to the chin, the soft tissues are pushed off the mandible with a tear along the bottom of the buccal sulcus, where the gum is firmly attached to the bone. There may not be much to be seen, until inspected inside the mouth. It is pretty well impossible to suture this injury, but fortunately the tissue sticks back spontaneously, and the mucous membrane heals without problems. Although the wound is open to the patient's mouth bacteria, infection is extremely rare. Patients do not need anything other than a soft diet for several days, with a mouth-rinsing ceremony after all food.

Injuries Involving Bursae or Joints

These spaces are very vulnerable to infection as they contain protein-rich fluid in a warm environment, outside the circulation. The contaminated cavity needs to be thoroughly irrigated with saline to make sure it is cleansed of all foreign material. It may need further opening, exploration, and sometimes excision to do this properly. The lining layer can then be approximated with a few interrupted absorbable sutures, but it is neither necessary nor desirable to make the closure watertight. It is helpful to arrange a post-operative posture which will encourage fluid to drain out by gravity. The most important features of treatment in these injuries, after initial meticulous cleansing and haemostasis, are the immobilisation of adjacent joint[s] and prophylactic antibiotics commenced immediately. If there is a ragged wound or graze with skin missing, it is a good idea to design a splint with a window, through which dressings can be done without removing the splint.

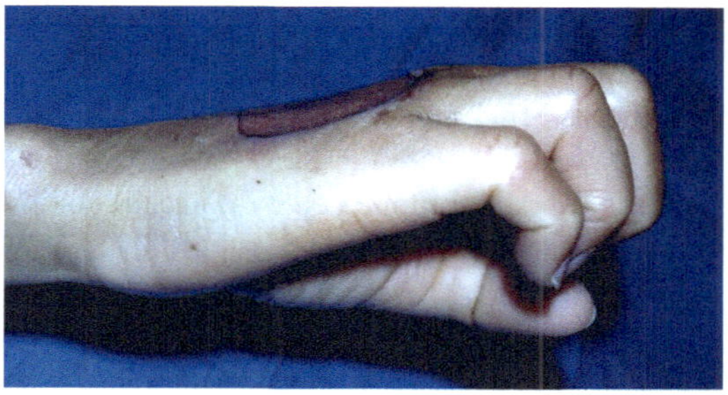

Fig. 13.29 Degloving injury to dorsum hand with MCP joints stiffened in extension after splinting was omitted during the Initial stages of the injury. Patient is trying to grip

Degloving Injuries

Degloving is usually produced by shearing or frictional injury, occasionally by a very severe impact or crush [e.g., wide and heavy bus tyres]. Skin is tougher than the subcutaneous fat and may become separated off the fat and the circulatory attachments in the area involved. Even though there may be no skin wound, this tissue must be regarded as a particularly unfavourable flap, surviving on its peripheral attachments [the so-called closed degloving injury] (Figs. 13.28 and 13.29).

The circulation is usually precarious and as vulnerable to tension from fluid or blood accumulating within the closed space as it is to pressure from bandaging to stop fluid and blood accumulating. This dilemma can be coped with either by inserting a sterile suction drain or by making an incision to assist drainage by gravity. Immobilisation helps the skin to stick down again. Prophylactic antibiotics are usually warranted.

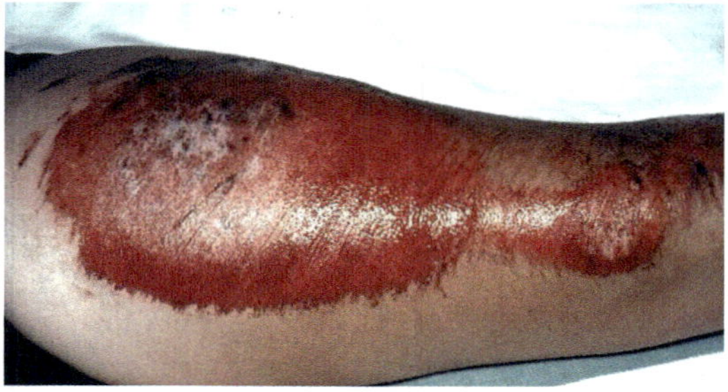

Fig. 13.28 This extensive road graze is a friction burn injury, with its central area showing the deepest destruction. It took 6 weeks to heal

Ear Haematoma

This usually occurs to rugby players involved in scrummaging [Forwards]. Blood collects between the skin and the cartilage of the ear and will lead to deformity if left untreated. An incision should be made under local anaesthetic, at the lower edge of the collection and clot should be evacuated. The wound should not be sutured, and the skin should be very carefully replaced. After applying tulle over the incision, the contours of the cartilage should be carefully followed by building up hollows with teased out cotton-wool, moistened with saline or liquid paraffin and cut into 1 cm strips. Gauze swabs or sponge can be used behind the ear to maintain its relationship to the head. The object of the exercise is to create a dressing which applies gentle even pressure to hold the skin back accurately against the underlying cartilage without deforming it, and obliterating the space so fluid does not re-accumulate. A full head bandage needs to be kept in place for the next 5 days and all scrummaging avoided. The difficult part is to restrain the rugby players from getting back into the scrums too soon. Cauliflower ears, the end result of inadequate treatment for chronic blunt ear trauma from scrummaging, can be seen amongst the male population of New Zealand any day of the week, especially at rugby matches. The condition is practically impossible to treat successfully once cartilage damage has occurred.

Difficult Flaps

The usual difficulties are covered in a previous Chap. 10, dealing with flaps and grafts. Leg flaps of course are all complicated by poor circulation and long flaps or distally based flaps also suffer from particularly severe circulatory disadvantage. In these situations, it is preferable to coax the surrounding tissue in towards the flap rather than pulling on the flap at all. This is best done with long tapes, which can be backed by a piece of the same tape over the flap section, to avoid tape sticking to it. Pressure on flaps must also be avoided and in some situations, it is necessary to go to the extent of building up the level of take-off of the tape with padding, swabs, or plastic sponge until the bridging section no longer touches the flap. Sometimes posturing of an adjacent joint will achieve the same end, and the position then needs to be maintained by splintage. It may be desirable to manoeuvre a flap gently towards that part of a defect which cannot sustain a graft, e.g., exposed cartilage, tendon, cortical bone, or joint space, leaving less important areas to recover by spontaneous healing or grafting. While these manoeuvres may seem complicated, the challenges are real and the solutions logical and practical. Solving them can be critical to the survival not only of the skin flap but also to the function of the far more important deeper structures. Each such situation is unique, with creativity and ingenuity playing an important role in its successful resolution. Flaps that have no circulation are best turned into grafts.

Flaps Over the Tendo-Achillis

These are moderately common and usually caused by something scraping down the back of the leg. The flap is nearly always distally based which makes its circulatory predicament a particularly venous problem. The subcutaneous tissue usually tears downwards exposing the Tendo-Achillis. Very occasionally, the tendon itself is divided and needs an orthopaedic repair. There is almost never any tissue missing, but such flaps tend to shrivel up and look particularly pathetic. The survival of enough flap to cover an intact or repaired tendon is critical to retaining its normal function. Treatment becomes a matter of not doing anything at all which could worsen the circulatory predicament of the flap. Stretching the flap or suturing it are both very dangerous (Figs. 13.30, 13.31, and 13.32).

Occasionally a 'guy-rope' suture or two is helpful to evert a rolling edge, but it is usually most unwise to do anything else in the way of suturing (Fig. 13.33). The flap can sometimes be stabilised with vertical tapes.

The most helpful manoeuvre of all is always plantar-flexion of the ankle. This moves the surrounding tissue to improve closure, tendon cover, and venous drainage without stretching or stressing the flap at all. Complete haemostasis is particularly critical because pressure over the underlying tendon for haemostasis is comparable with that over a bony prominence, where the circulation is particularly vulnerable. All pressure must be avoided.

The area is dressed with several layers of tulle, with gauze swabs, and non-constricting bandages to hold it in place. It is particularly important not to press the flap forcefully against the firm tendon

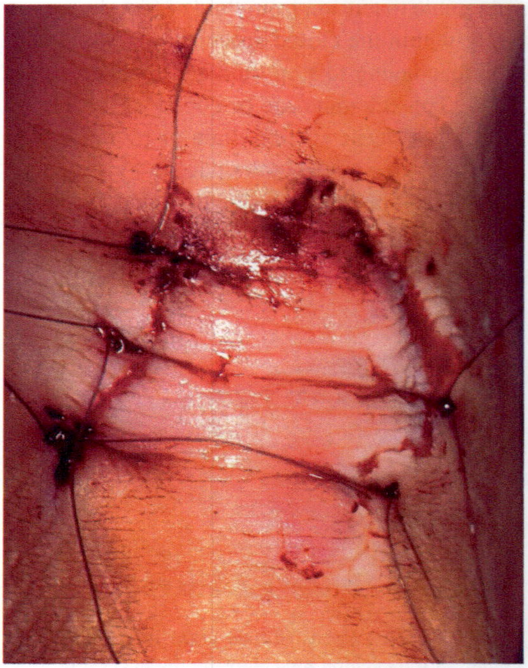

Fig. 13.30 A 3-day old heel flap showing transverse bands of tension caused by ill-advised suturing

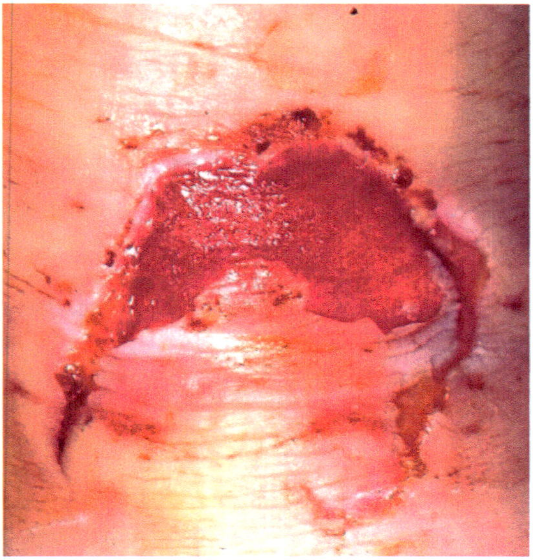

Fig. 13.31 The partial thickness damage was apparent 5 days later. Plantar flexion and tulle would have been safer. Necrosis of this flap would have been disastrous

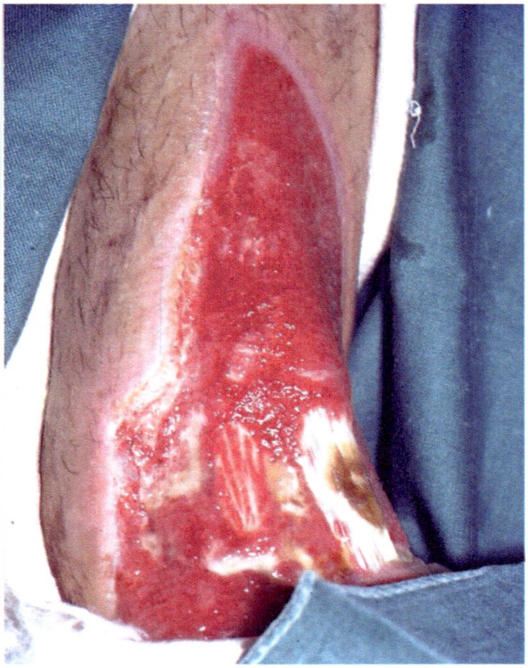

Fig. 13.32 Loss of flap down to Tendo-Achillis. An unsatisfactory flap operation was attempted but below knee amputation was the eventual outcome

beneath it. The ankle is best held in unforced plantar-flexion by a thick padded slab of Plaster-of-Paris from the dorsum of the foot up the front

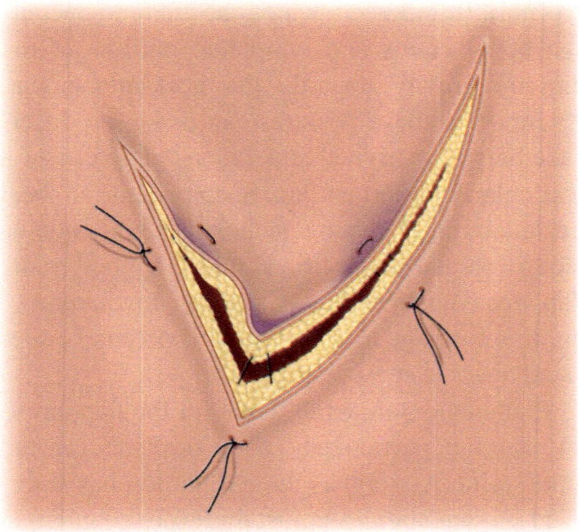

Fig. 13.33 Guy-rope tethering. Small mattress sutures are being used to evert rolling edges. Stretching this flap out to size would worsen its already obvious venous congestion

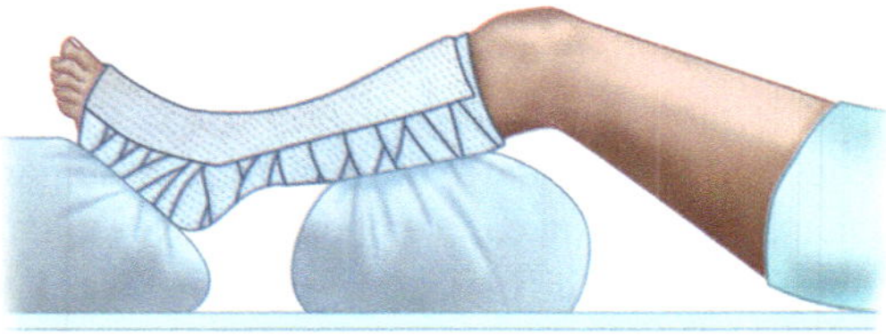

Fig. 13.34 Positioning of the leg after repair of a Tendo-Achillis flap. The leg is elevated generally, with the lower leg slightly dependent to assist with venous drainage from the flap. The dorsal splint maintains plantar flexion and will be bandaged on, avoiding pressure in the flap or heel area. The pillows are endeavouring to avoid direct pressure on the flap or heel area

of the shin. This is bandaged on above and below the flap area, avoiding direct pressure on the flap or the heel. Both the arterial and venous circulation to the flap travel by way of the distal attachment, so direct pressure on or anywhere near this must be avoided at all costs. It is potentially feasible to add a stirrup extension, which makes it possible for the patient to lie safely in bed on their back, but pillows can be used to achieve the same ends (Fig. 13.34).

Simple elevation of the whole limb, while helping venous drainage generally, increases venous pooling in any distally based flap, so the ideal posture is for the thigh to be sloping up about 30–40°, with the lower leg sloping slightly downhill from knee towards the ankle to encourage both venous and lymphatic outflow of the flap by gravity towards the heel attachment. Attention to these postures can make the difference between survival and venous gangrene of a particularly important flap. Such patients are best treated initially resting in hospital. Outpatients require an additional firm bandage applied to the flap area whenever they put the leg down, removing this bandage as soon as the limb can be elevated again [See Appendix].

Plantar-flexion, while great for the flap circulation, is a particularly poor position for the ankle joint. As soon as the circulation has stabilised, urgent attention must therefore be given to progressive restoration of the ideal ankle posture. After 2 or 3 days, the flap can usually be held securely in place by tapes which protect its interests while the ankle posture is being restored to a right-angle. The wound is redressed every few days. Some weight-bearing can usually start at about a week or 10 days with an intact tendon, and this assists the recovery of ankle position and movement. Ambulant patients initially need crutches because a plantar-flexed ankle in plaster is very awkward to manage unless the knee is bent. Once the ankle position has been restored somewhat, commencing weight-bearing is very helpful in regaining full dorsi-flexion.

Serial splintage may be required, with unhealed wounds being dressed through a window in the cast. Once the right-angle position has been achieved, splintage of the ankle at night is still recommended for some time. There is no contraindication to weight-bearing. A bi-valved night-time cast can be removed for dressings, walking, and showering. Walking forward slowly and deliberately onto the forefoot out of cast in the daytime stretches fibrous tissue and helps regain dorsi-flexion. However, with this injury, there is a very strong tendency for an un-splinted ankle to lapse into plantar-flexion again, especially at night. This battle is likely to persist throughout the weeks or months of scar contracture and is even worse if the tendon itself has been severed. Secondary Tendo-Achillis shortening can occur while the ankle is in a poor position. It is a particularly disabling and unnecessary complication and is difficult to treat successfully through the scarred tissues.

*A clinical example of a challenging ankle/Tendo-Achillis region degloving injury, which took nearly a year to rehabilitate with multiple surgeries, wound care, and physiotherapy is illustrated from MFK's database (*Fig. 13.35a–e*).*

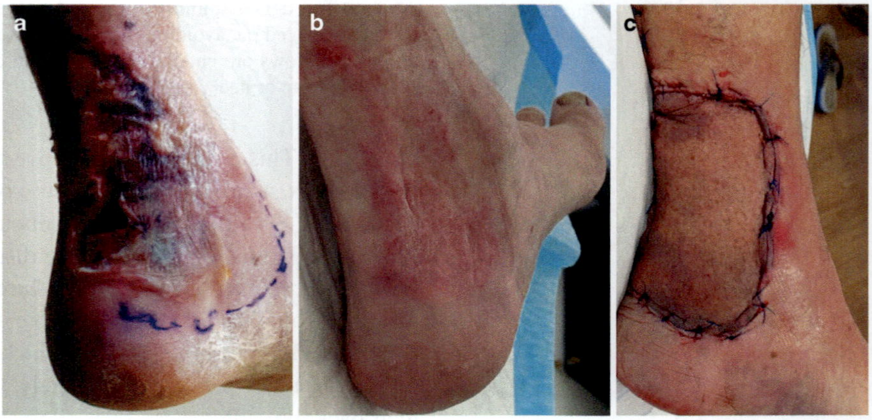

Fig. 13.35 (**a**) 65-year-old male run over by a heavy fork-hoist truck sustaining degloving injury left medial ankle and Achilles tendon region. (**b**) Initial debridement and skin grafting but at 1 year graft was unstable. (**c**) Graft removed and reverse sural artery fasciocutaneous flap used for reconstruction [note early venous congestion at day 1 post-surgery]. (**d, e**) Healed final flap at 10 months post-secondary repair with good range of plantar and dorsal flexion demonstrated

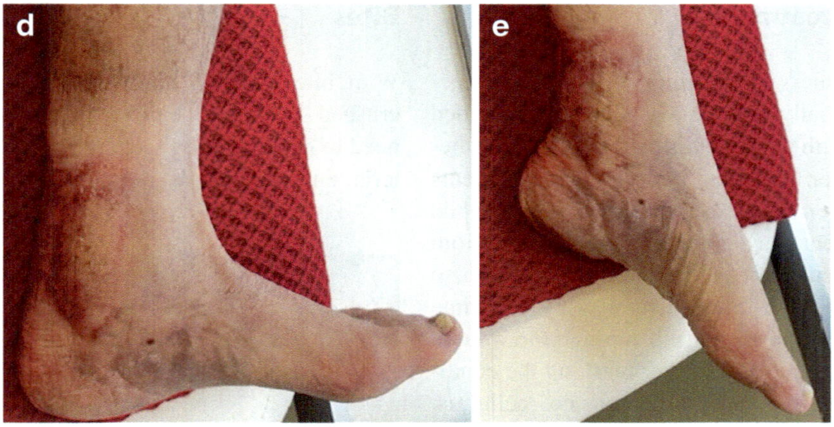

Fig. 13.35 (continued)

Penetrating Knuckle Injury [Clenched Fist Injury]

This important injury is sustained by punching someone else's mouth, forcibly contacting the teeth. With the dorsal tissues of the hand tensed, as in a punching posture, teeth readily open right down onto and sometimes into an MCP joint, usually the fourth, contaminating the wound with someone else's mouth organisms [*including aerobes Eikenella corrodens, Staphylococcus aureus, Streptococci, and Coryne-bacterium species amongst others]*. Patients rarely front up with a truthful history, so it is usually necessary to ask leading questions, stressing the special importance of any injury made by someone else's teeth. A contaminated joint rapidly becomes extremely painful, with severe aching often extending into the forearm. The patient often presents hours later, sometimes unable to sleep because of pain, or the next day, delayed by a hangover and/or the shame of it all. There is often not a lot to see.

There is usually only a small skin wound over the knuckle. Sometimes leakage of joint fluid confirms the diagnosis. The hand is painful and tender locally but without obvious inflammation to explain the pain. The patient is reluctant to move the affected joint. Diagnostic signs include severe pain caused by even slight longitudinal compression of the affected finger from the tip. An initial X-Ray is worthwhile. There may be a chipped tooth or piece of bone present. While a normal X-Ray does not exclude joint contamination, it can be very helpful for later comparison, should cartilage and/or bone become involved.

Treatment

Antibiotics should be started as soon as possible. Two broad spectrum prophylactic antibiotics are required urgently, and it is best if these are given intravenously and until the situation is settling. The wound needs to be immediately anaesthetised and explored. If joint fluid can be seen or produced from a capsular injury, the joint should be syringed out with saline through this opening. If it is not obviously open, the joint should not be entered, and the wound is best left unsutured to drain freely into dressings. The whole hand needs to be splinted in the functional position and elevated. The patient also needs to keep the hand palm-up post-operatively so that gravity encourages drainage from the dorsal wound. The antibiotics/splintage regime should continue for at least 7–10 days, with each of these withdrawn separately once symptoms and signs disappear. At issue is the function of the MCP joint and sometimes the whole hand.

Belated Treatment

The seriousness of this injury is not always recognised initially, and the wound may be regarded as minor, with the patient's pain dismissed as theatrical. When the wound doesn't settle, patients may be given a few days antibiotics, and while this treatment may give them some relief from pain, it often allows the underlying problem to grumble on. The infected joint is by this time usually decompressing itself through the wound, reducing the pain and further masking the condition. There may be little or no cellulitis. Unfortunately, in most of these 'delayed' situations, the whole of the joint cartilage is irrevocably destroyed before the underlying pathology is appreciated (Figs. 13.36 and 13.37).

The collapse of the joint space does not become evident radiologically for 2 or 3 weeks. Belated treatment with splintage and antibiotics should eventually deal with the infection, but unfortunately by then, it is rarely possible to retrieve function.

Bites

With bite wounds, tissue is often ragged and crushed—features which make for wounds which need to be allowed to seep. All bites convey bacteria and should be thoroughly cleaned with

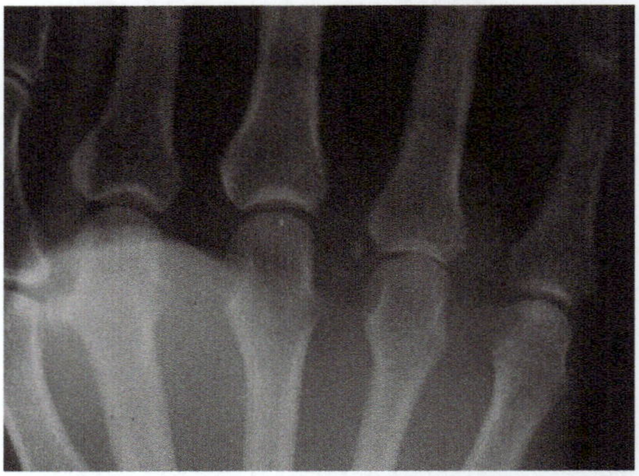

Fig. 13.37 X-Ray of a similar patient, 3 weeks after a 'tooth' injury. Note the loss of space in the fourth MCP joint indicating loss of cartilage

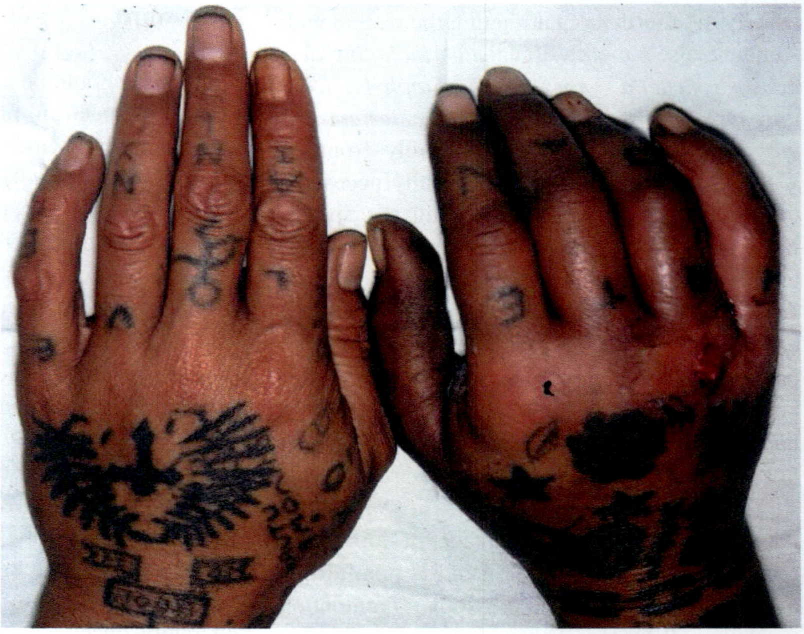

Fig. 13.36 7 days right fourth MCP joint injury from teeth, sustained by punching. Note the whole right hand is swollen and infected

saline. Retrieval of dislodged skin and accurate realignment is important, but sutures are on the whole best avoided. Cat bites are usually puncture wounds, which can penetrate deeply into joints or tendon sheaths. These are likely to be specifically contaminated with Pasteurella multocida. All patients with bites should be managed with appropriate prophylactic antibiotics to prevent infection.

Injected Paint or Grease

Although compressed paint or grease introduced accidentally through the skin is a rare injury, it is always potentially a serious one. This injury often occurs while greasing a cable. The injection site may look trivial, although underlying tension may be obvious and cause extreme pain. An X-Ray may or may not be useful. The presence of injected material can only be excluded by exploration, because it is not always radio-opaque. These are nearly always hand injuries. The operator needs the experience and facilities to carry out an extensive operation, if this should prove necessary (Figs. 13.38, 13.39, and 13.40).

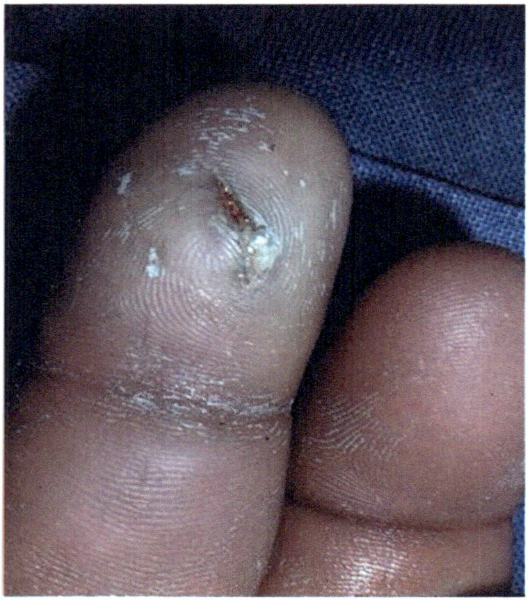

Fig. 13.38 Injury from paint injected under pressure while spray painting. Pulp was pale and extremely painful and tender

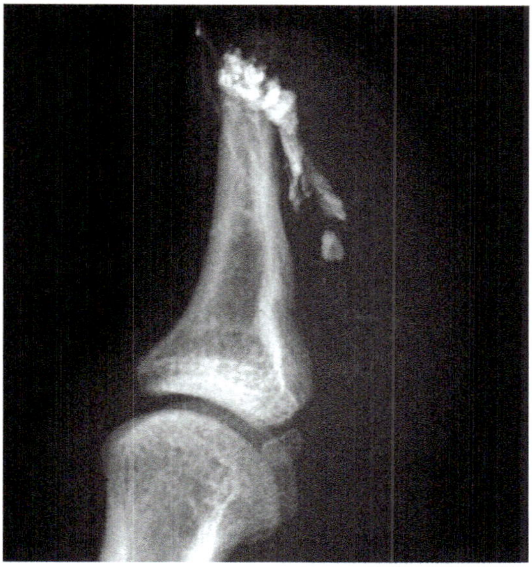

Fig. 13.39 X-Ray of another patient with injected material

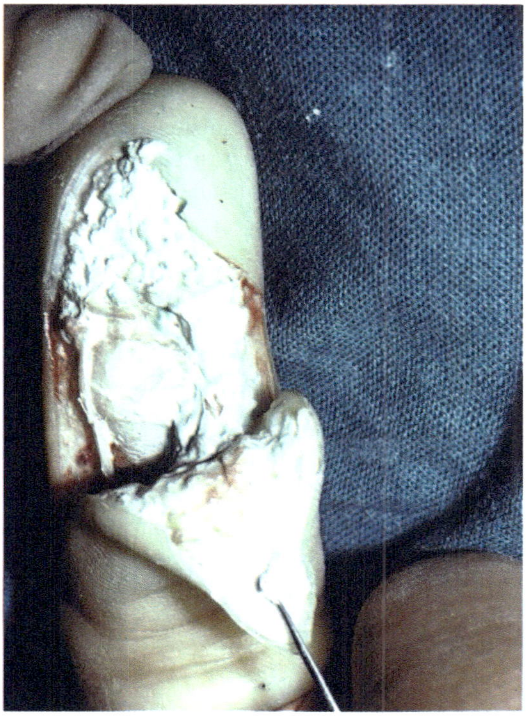

Fig. 13.40 The same finger as Fig. 13.38 at exploration. This finger eventually required amputation

Subungual Haematoma

This is a collection of blood beneath the nail, usually caused by a localised crush injury or a hammer mishap. Usually there is no underlying fracture. When there is a wound to the surface, pain may not be a problem, but the build-up of tension in a closed haematoma under an intact nail rapidly becomes excruciating. Decompression is always worthwhile. This is most suitably done with the blunt end of an unwound metal paper-clip, heated red-hot in a spirit lamp. The heated end is **applied but not pressed** onto the nail surface over the haematoma, where it burns a small dent. It is heated repeatedly and replaced in the hole until it eventually strikes 'oil' and the haematoma is released (Fig. 13.41).

No pressure is needed. Pushing on the clip is likely to increase the pain and also risks poking through suddenly into very sensitive tissue. There is always a surprising amount of blood released and the patient's immediate relief and gratitude after this drainage is remarkable. The main difficulty lies in persuading them to let anyone approach their already exquisitely painful nail with a red-hot implement. An equally effective mechanism is to burn the first dent with the paper clip and proceed thereafter using the tiniest drill bit available and rotating it in the hole between two fingers without any pressure, until it liberates the haematoma. Patients seem to prefer this 'cold' method, given the choice.

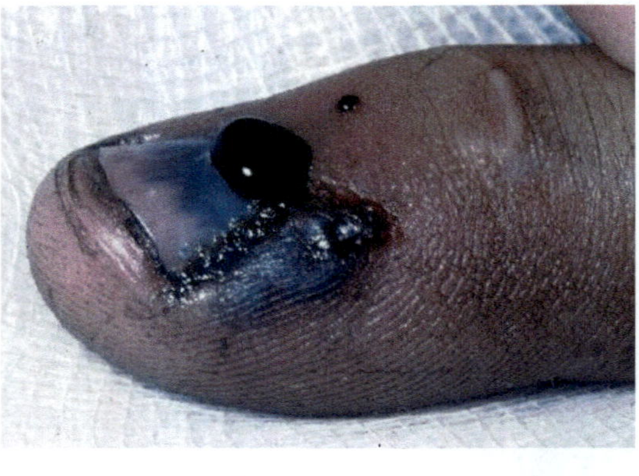

Fig. 13.41 Blood coming out from beneath the nail through a hole bored with a heated paper clip for treatment of subungual haematoma

Commentary by Professor James D. Frame FRCS(Plast)

My, how things have changed over the decades. I don't think many surgeons still use catgut sutures and I don't agree with some of the anecdotes mentioned in this chapter, but there are some rarely discussed management protocols, particularly for high pressure injection injuries and even the management of abrasions.

These days, even complex wounds are surgically reconstructed primarily. Heavily contaminated abrasions are often best cleaned under general anaesthetic, with emphasis on rapid wound healing, restoration of function, and improved aesthetics. Larger centres use vac pumps, electric dermatomes, and a variety of non-adherent antimicrobial dressings that promote wound healing. Clinicians work within multidisciplinary teams.

It is however generally still accepted that blunt/crush trauma causing explosive type-injury within the deeper tissues [as seen from gunshot or shrapnel war injuries] are best debrided and not closed primarily. Healing by secondary intention is now rarely encouraged, especially in patients with skin loss exposing bone, nerve, or tendon. Loss of function and hyperaesthesia are inevitable if these are not promptly repaired.

Finger-tip injuries not exposing bone are possibly an exception for healing by secondary intention, especially in children, because sensate skin can be drawn into the fingertip. The alternative, using partial thickness skin grafts, result in an insensate, non-aesthetic appearance. However, for finger pulp exposure where finger sensation is best retained, innervated local flaps offer the best outcome and avoid the hyperaesthesia often seen in grafted pressure points.

The acute inflammatory phase following injury causes redness, heat, swelling, pain, and progressive vascular impairment. These lead inevitably to progressive tissue necrosis, sepsis, loss of function, and risk of multiorgan failure, especially if crushed muscle is involved. Closing the wound before the acute response is over creates a dangerous situation. However, wounds from sharp mechanisms of injury and some open wounds, especially in the face and hand, can be judiciously managed with aggressive debridement, repair of vital structures, and local flaps, in instances where important structures are exposed and to retain function.

Today it is not just good enough to allow a wound to close through secondary intention; we must retain or regain function and consider longer-term cosmesis. In my view, closure should ideally be achieved within the first 48 h, but certainly within the first week, before the ingress of new blood vessels and fibroblasts. Splinting limbs after tendons have been repaired is now old hat, and this includes acute rupture of the Tendo-Achillis. Early, controlled passive mobilisation of joints is the only way that the fullest range of joint movement, nerve, and tendon gliding can be best achieved. These patients must be managed in specialist centres with adequate numbers of specialised rehabilitation staff.

According to the standard reconstructive surgeon's algorithm, wounds can be closed primarily [Immediate or delayed] using a variety of simple suturing techniques, skin grafts, or tissue transfer. This can involve vascularised composites of tissues using local flaps, regional flaps, or free tissue transfer. It is not good enough nowadays just to get wound closure; it is vitally important that there is an early return of function, with good aesthetic outcome.

Specialist units are vital in these circumstances. Although the surgery is now standard, much emphasis is on rehabilitation, with supervised teamwork between clinicians and the rehabilitation team, including occupational therapy, physiotherapy, and rehabilitation with functioning prosthetic limbs.

Commentary by Mr. Demetrius Evriviades FRCS(Plast) Wg Cdr [Rtd]

Management of Military Blast Injuries

Blast wounds may be distinguished from civilian wounds by their larger size, irregular morphology, and higher degree of contamination with particulate matter 'driven' into tissue by the blast wave. These wounds may affect the entire body.

Debridement is the most important first step in wound management and will significantly affect the end result for the patient. In heavily contaminated military wounds, this is often only achieved with several stages. The first debridement is performed within the constraints of damage control surgery and should be as thorough as possible without being excessive.

A debridement classification as described by Granick and Chehade [1] is a useful model based on the Jackson burn wound model. In the centre of the wound is an area of dead and dying tissue surrounded by a marginal area of injured but alive tissue, this in turn is surrounded by healthy tissue. Granick and Chehade classified wounds according to the level of debridement: Incomplete debridement, where not all of the necrotic material is removed, is to be avoided if at all possible as retained necrotic material will serve as a nidus for infection and inflammation. Marginal debridement—where all necrotic tissue is removed, but where injured and potentially viable tissue is retained—is an appropriate level of debridement at the first operation. The removal at this stage of potentially viable tissue is not necessary as a larger wound will be created, which will require a more complex reconstruction. Providing that there are sufficient resources available for frequent take-backs to the operating room, marginal debridement provides the maximum chance for survival of native tissues.

Before wound debridement, all wounds should be cleaned of particulate matter using soap and water.

A tourniquet should be applied if possible. Large irregular wounds contain crevices into which contamination may be forced between tissue planes. Without tourniquet control, these areas will be filled and obscured with bleeding, making excision of dead and dirty tissue difficult. In addition, blood loss without the application of a tourniquet may be significant. A sterile disposable tourniquet is useful for proximal wounds; the surgeon can apply a sterile disposable tourniquet once the skin has been prepped and draped. With experience, the routine use of a tourniquet helps rather than hinders debridement.

The introduction of negative pressure wound therapy (NPWT) has transformed the management of these wounds as it allows for total exudate capture and also total wound isolation. These dressings are now the standard of care for combat wounds. Our preference is to use dry gauze impregnated with polyhexamethylene biguanide (Kerlix AMD; Tyco Healthcare, Gosport, United Kingdom) and placed directly onto the wound bed. We have not experienced any retained gauze using this technique. Moistening of the gauze with saline, as recommended by the manufacturers, is not required as the dressing soon becomes wet and to do so would reduce the chances of developing a successful vacuum seal. This is then sealed with a semipermeable film, with a 2- to 3-cm border around the wound onto healthy skin. We have found that NPWT, when used in combination with surgical assessment, exploration, and careful debridement, greatly facilitates wound management. It also stabilizes the soft tissues, salvages compromised tissue, reduces oedema, the frequency and total number of dressing changes, and facilitates further reconstructive surgery. NPWT also makes effective hand dressings when used circumferentially. In a hand with multiple composite soft tissue and bony injuries, when functional splinting is required, gauze-based NPWT allows for easily applied dressings that provide optimum conditions for wound healing and functional splinting, negating the need to apply a plaster-of-Paris splint. The ability to use variable intermittent pressure combines the advantages of intermittent therapy without the disadvantages of loss of seal or splinting effect.

The development of infection may also delay reconstruction. Military wounds are prone to infection and in severe cases, fulminating fungal infections may ensue around 7–10 days post-injury. Prophylactic antifungals are appropriate for patients with high Injury Severity Scores with severe wounds that received massive blood transfusions.

Reconstruction should not be performed, however, until the patient is physiologically stable. The patient should be apyrexial, the nutritional status should be optimized, and all inotropic medication should be discontinued. The microbiology profile of the wound should also be understood before attempts at reconstruction. The other consideration is the availability of suitable donor sites for local or free flap reconstruction due to the extensive zone of injury. Reconstruction, which relies on local perforator vessels, should be used with care as the zone of trauma is often much bigger in blast injuries. The primary blast wave is likely to cause damage to the intima of blood vessels beyond the extent of the obvious injury. This occurs where perforating vessels are relatively fixed, that is, where they penetrate the deep fascia. An additional precondition of flap site selection is the potential detrimental effect of the donor defect; commonly used muscle flaps such as rectus abdominis or latissimus dorsi affect core stability, particularly in amputees; harvesting them may subsequently compromise rehabilitation.

Reference

1. Granick M, Chehade M. Surgical wound management. New York: Informa; 2007.

14 Ingrown Toenails

Summary
The difficulties encountered in treating ingrown toenails arise mostly out of a lack of appreciation of the underlying anatomy and the pathology of the problem. Conservative management can sometimes solve the problem, but if not, a reliable minor operation may be necessary. Greater consideration should be given to modern, non-surgical, nail matrix ablation techniques.

The Two Predispositions to Troublesome Ingrown Toenails

These are both inherited traits and include:

1. Congenital short nails
2. Congenital curly nails

Congenital short nails (Fig. 14.1) are nails that sit back within the toe rather than extending beyond the soft tissue. This allows soft tissues to bulge distally.

Congenital curly nails (Fig. 14.2) are nails that curl down at the sides rather than being in one flat plane.

The first sign of toenail trouble is usually pain and redness at a front corner of the nail. On closer examination, the corner itself may no longer be visible. Quite often the patient will have found that they can relieve things for a few days by cutting the corner of the nail down. While this does help for a day or two, it actually encourages the corner to grow outwards even more into the soft tissue (Fig. 14.3).

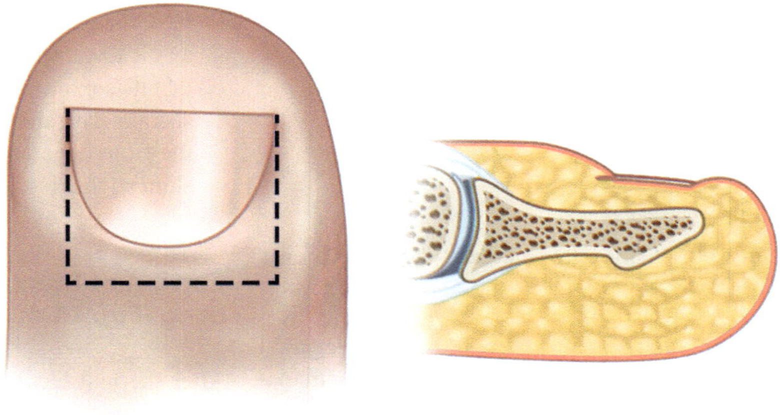

Fig. 14.1 The nail is short and sits back within the toe, somewhat below the level of the soft tissues

P. Charlesworth, M. F. Klaassen, *Chapple's Principles of Wound Care and Healing*,
https://doi.org/10.1007/978-3-031-53104-0_14

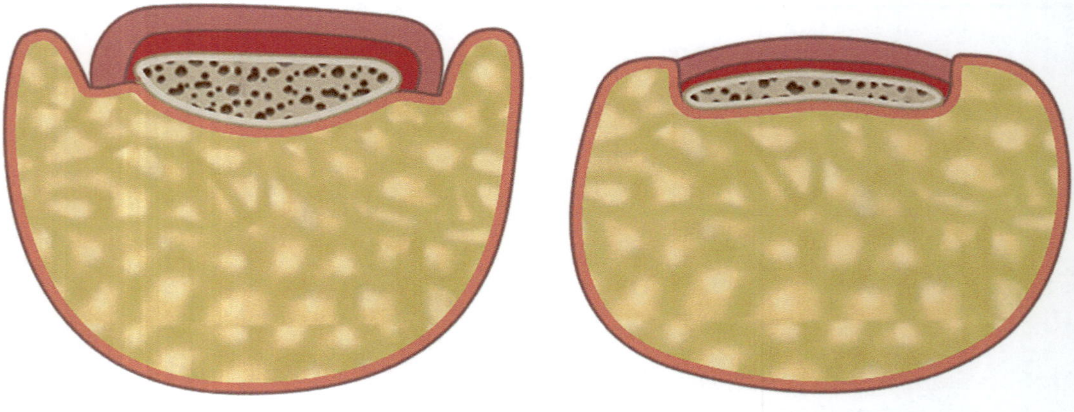

Fig. 14.2 A curly nail is much more liable to grow into tissue than a flat nail. The correct operation simply creates a flat nail surgically by removing lateral matrix

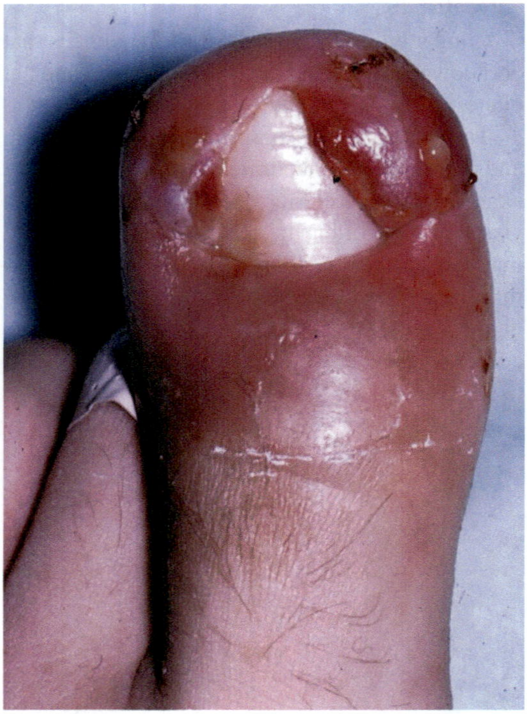

Fig. 14.3 Chronically infected ingrown toenail. Troublesome for 3 months

The condition often flares up whenever tight footwear is worn because this reduces the circulation sufficiently to let infection flourish. Inflammatory episodes are relieved by warm bathing and avoiding tight shoes. Quite often the toe is chronically inflamed rather than acutely so, making it reasonable to wait for a swab result in order to select the most useful antibiotic. If infection is invasive, antibiotics will be needed. While antibiotic treatment may allow healing to occur, it may not be able to prevent recurrence of problems when there is unfavourable anatomy. As a troublesome nail is regrowing it is worth trying the following conservative measures that might pre-empt the problem and permanently avoid operation.

Conservative Management

1. Always take particular care of foot hygiene and soak the feet before cutting toenails so nails do not fracture unfavourably.
2. Do not on any account ever cut or tear a troublesome nail down at the corners, but encourage it to grow. Then cut it straight across, so that its corners become longer than the middle section. The aim is to encourage the whole of the front edge of the nail to lie above healed skin, so that ingrowing can no longer occur.

Cutting of Toenails with Corner Left Long (Fig. 14.4)

After the nail has been softened, by soaking in warm water, cutting a concave piece or a careful shallow scallop out of the nail within the intact corner will encourage the corner up away from the soft tissue. Take great care not to break the corner off.

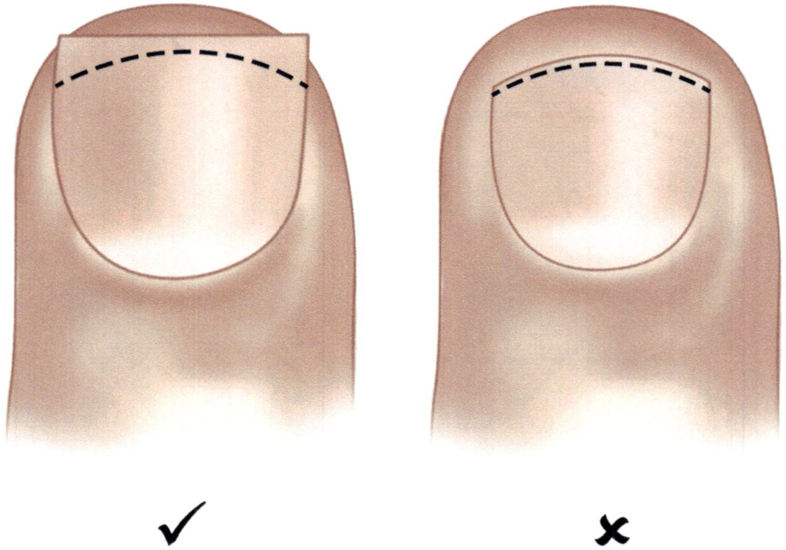

Fig. 14.4 Cutting nails straight across or even slightly convex rather than down at the sides ensures that the corners do not dig into the soft tissue

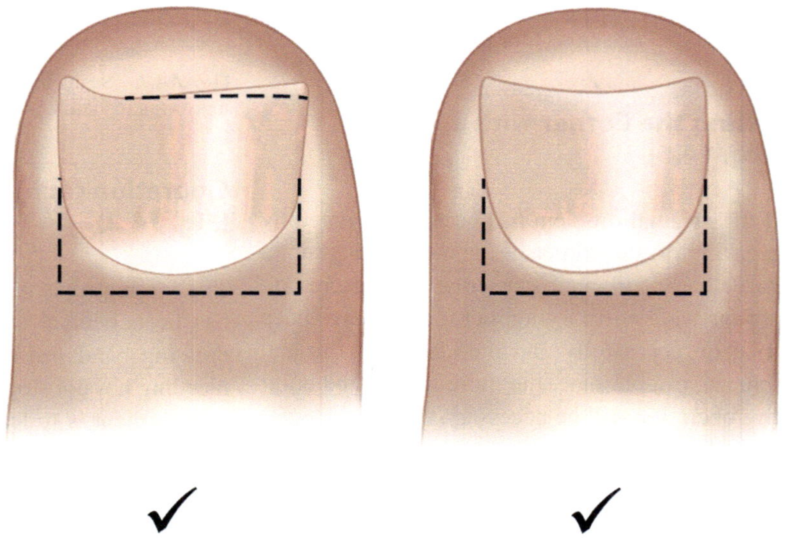

Fig. 14.5 Cutting a concavity or a wedge out of the nail coaxes the corner away from the soft tissue

Cutting the Nail Within the Corner (Fig. 14.5)

It may be possible to lift the corner with a tiny pledget of cotton-wool to coax the soft tissue away or slide a piece of tape or smooth sticking plaster under the corner of the nail to allow healing to occur. Sometimes it may also be possible to achieve this effect using a bisected, short piece of soft plastic, such as from intravenous tubing, which runs along the lateral edge of the nail.

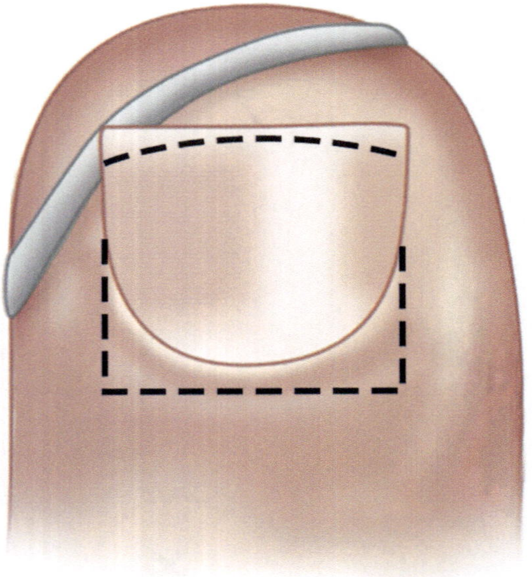

Fig. 14.6 Tape applied beneath the corner prevents the nail digging in as it grows forward

Lifting the Corner with a Tape (Fig. 14.6)

If the original problem has been precipitated by breaking off the corner of the nail and it is not a particularly curly nail, conservative measures are always well worth trying, but if these have been tried unsuccessfully and the corner of the nail remains troublesome, the more formal and curative operation will be necessary.

Operation

The toe should be settled as much as possible before the operation, with the patient started on antibiotics 24 h previously. Under plain local anaesthesia [or local anaesthetic with adrenaline] and with the help of a tourniquet or no tourniquet if adrenaline is added to the local anaesthetic, the side of the nail is removed with a narrow ellipse of nail bed in-continuity with its associated block of nail matrix (Fig. 14.7).

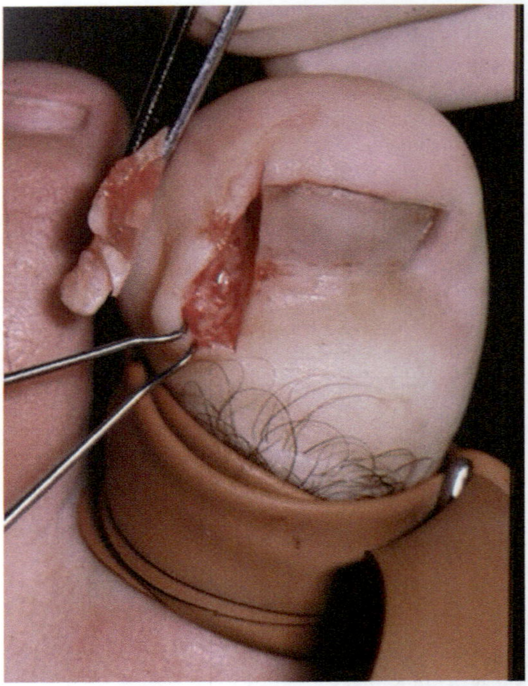

Fig. 14.7 'Segmental' resection of nail matrix for ingrowing toenail. Operation specimen is demonstrated

Operation for Ingrown Toenails (Fig. 14.8)

The tourniquet is released only after the wound has been held closed with tulle strips, with a dressing bandaged on and the foot elevated. If bleeding has not stopped with 5–10 min, the best management is to leave the foot elevated with a firm dressing on the toe for a further 15–30 min, before replacing dressings down to the tulle. There are no big vessels involved in the wound but the toe has been inflamed and the use of a tourniquet creates additional hyperaemia, making the achievement of haemostasis more tedious than usual. The goal of absolute haemostasis is however especially worthwhile, because it means that the ultimate dressing on the toe can be small and tension-free. The patient should be given oral analgesia as soon as the operation is completed, to pre-empt the rebound pain as the anaesthetic wears off. There is actually an even stronger case

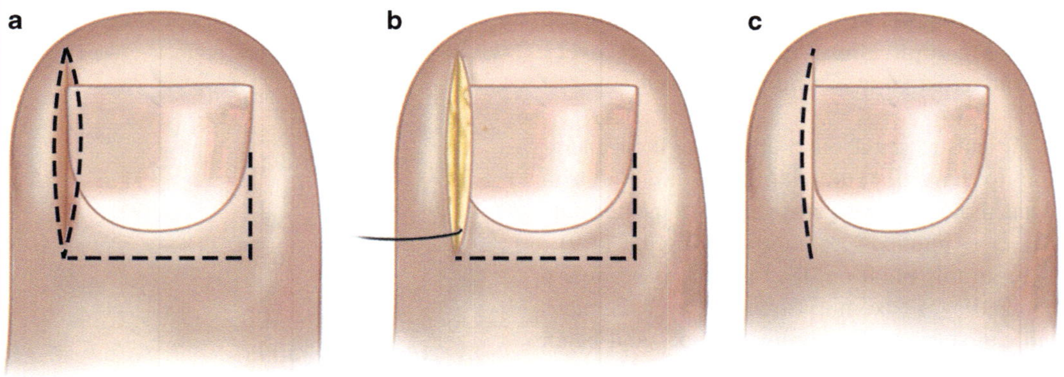

Fig. 14.8 Operation for Ingrown toenails: (**a**) planning of excision, (**b**) the side of the nail, the soft tissue and the matrix related to the troublesome section of nail are excised in continuity, (**c**) the defect is closed with tulle gras strips

for doing this *before* the surgery. This is the most intense pain experienced. Post-operative pain will be dramatically reduced by using the *two bandage regime* described below. See also Appendix.

It is ideal for patients to lie about postoperatively for an hour or so [if clinic space allows this] with their foot elevated, to ensure that haemostasis has been effective and that rebound pain is receding. It is then most essential to apply a second bandage before the patient puts the foot down at all, even if they are going to a vehicle in a wheelchair. This demonstrates what they must do for the next few days. The second bandage allows safe mobility without the risk of haematoma or bleeding, but soon starts to cause increasing throbbing pain indicative of circulatory distress. Patients are thus made aware of the need to put the limb up again so they can safely remove the tight bandage. They are thus able to get to the toilet and back, or move to another room, taking the weight always on the heel and not the toe. They must spend most of the next 2 or 3 days resting with their foot up. While their foot is in level or elevated, there is no possibility of bleeding nor haematoma and no need for a tight bandage, therefore unimpeded circulation to the healing toe and they will be surprisingly comfortable. The Two Bandage method is used and it is helpful to have printed instructions about this [summarised below] for the patient to take home. They also need to be given a prescription for analgesic tablets to cover the next 2 or 3 days and nights, although this may not all be needed. After the third day, the toe usually becomes much more comfortable.

Double Bandage Instructions for Leg and Foot Injuries (See Editors' Comments, Appendix p. 199)

1. **Do not remove the inner bandage. It is holding the dressing on and its end is taped securely.**
2. **BEFORE you put your leg down, always apply a firm second bandage, securing the end with a safety pin. This bandage is to prevent the wound bruising or bleeding when you are upright, but it also reduces the circulation considerably. Your wound will start to throb with it on, reminding you to put your leg up again as soon as you can.**
3. **Once your leg is elevated again it is safe to remove the firm outer bandage, restoring full circulation immediately and dramatically relieving the throbbing pain,**
4. **You should rest up for the first 2–3 days, getting onto your feet only to get to the toilet or to move for a change of scenery. You can safely walk around more after the first few days, as long as the wound is comfortable in a modestly firm supportive bandage.**

5. **This regime will minimise swelling, pain, and complications during your recovery and assist your wound to heal well.**

Patients return about 5 days after their operation to have the dressing removed, the skin cleaned of tulle-gras grease and 2–3 inextensible skin tapes applied across the wound (Fig. 14.9).

From this point on, they usually need only a Bandaid™ or Fixomull Stretch™ over the tapes and can start wearing ordinary shoes and begin showering. Their nail will be slightly narrowed but should hopefully never ever cause any more problems (Fig. 14.10).

Most recurrences and nail spikes follow an operation described as a 'wedge resection of nail bed'. In concentrating on an ellipse of nail bed, inexpert operators leave some or all of the nail matrix behind (Fig. 14.11).

It is not surprising that with the less accurate techniques of wedge resection of the nail bed, the recurrence rate is no better than that achieved by

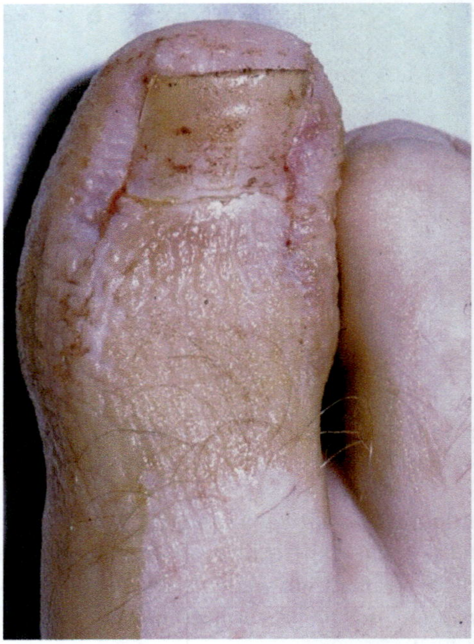

Fig. 14.10 Healed toe, 10 days after a 'segmental' resection on both sides. No sutures were used or needed

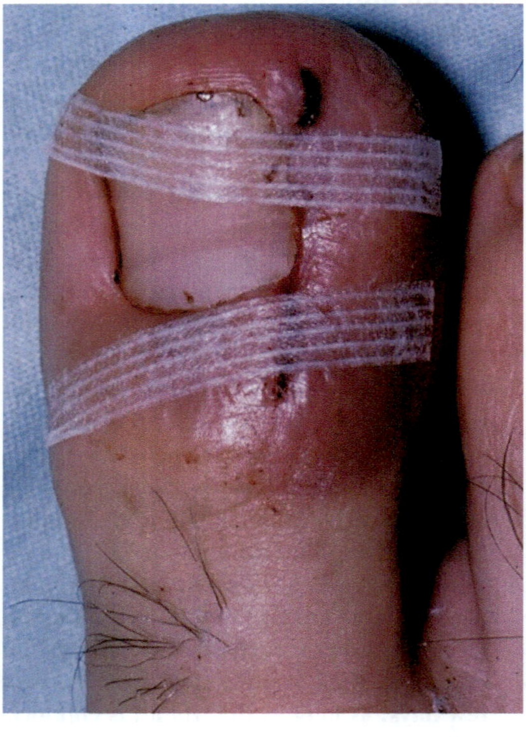

Fig. 14.9 Five-day postoperative result. The original tulle closure has just been replaced by tapes

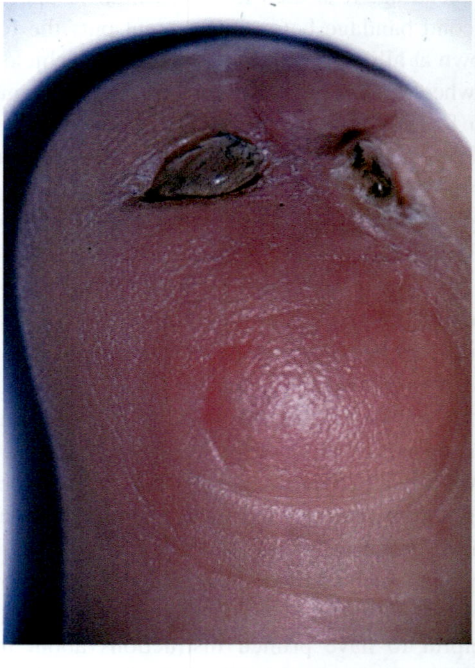

Fig. 14.11 Nail spikes recurrent after nail removal 6 months earlier

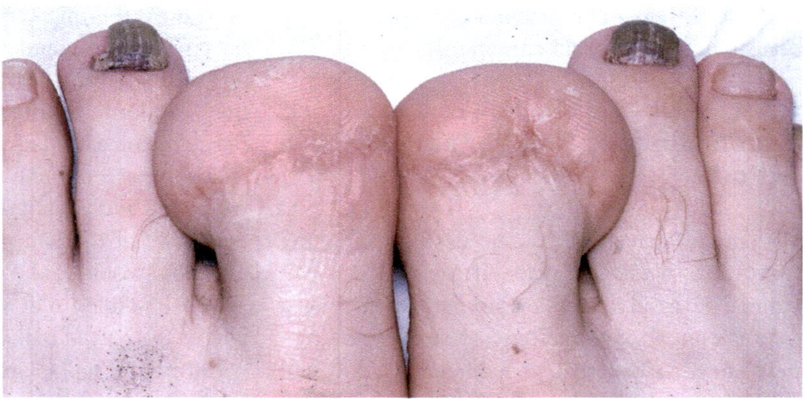

Fig. 14.12 Grotesque result from bilateral partial amputation, carried out as the primary treatment for ingrown toenails in an 18-year-old. The surgeon concerned did not discuss any alternatives with the patient pre-operatively

simply pulling the nail off. That is, approximately 50% of patients do have further trouble. Luckily, recurrences can still be successfully treated by doing the right operation, making it unnecessary to ever do radical or mutilating operations (Fig. 14.12).

After a segmental resection of nail and matrix, it is always possible to leave a normal-looking toe even if both sides of the nail have been treated (Fig. 14.10).

Many podiatrists treat ingrown toenails successfully by anaesthetising the toe, isolating the curled edge of nail on one or both sides and pulling just this section out, after splitting the nail and matrix longitudinally. They then insert a small 89% phenol swab into the empty segment of the nail fold for about 3 min to obliterate its germinal lining. The wound generally requires a small dressing for about 3 weeks and the narrowed nail never digs in again.

Commentary by Dr. Peter Charlesworth FRACS—Co-Editor

Personal dissatisfaction with the treatment of ingrown toenails observed during my surgical training led me to explore the phenolisation technique used by podiatrists. Subsequently, I used that method exclusively during my specialist career, with the virtually complete exclusion of surgery for the condition. This seems a counterintuitive approach for a surgeon, but I was convinced that the results of chemical nail matrix ablation were demonstrably better. Therefore, with rare exceptions, I believe that the modern primary treatment of the ingrown toenail should be by chemical nail matrix ablation and not surgery.

Notwithstanding the congenital conditions emphasised by Dr Chapple as causes of ingrown toenails, a much more common factor is the practice of cutting toenails inappropriately short or tearing them in an uncontrolled fashion into the lateral nail fold. This predisposes to the formation of an entrapped in-growing nail spike and a cycle of pain and infection. This introduces an important patient behavioural education aspect, as part of any follow-up to treatment.

Once an ingrown toenail is established, the presence of the increasingly obtrusive lateral nail spike means that any associated infection is most unlikely to resolve, either spontaneously or with a course of antibiotics usually prescribed by primary health carers to 'see if things settle down'. Antibiotic therapy is often already on-going when patients are referred for 'specialist' treatment. However, whether or not this is the case, immediate removal of the offending lateral nail segment, even in the presence of significant local inflammation, is almost always dramatically successful. This approach also has the benefit of saving the patient the potential cost and disruption of a second visit for definitive treatment, following an initial consultation.

Unless there is extensive or spreading infection in the toe, the need for post-procedure antibiotics is also moot. Naturally, there is a strong case for preliminary and/or continuing antibiotic treatment in high-risk groups, such as diabetics or those with digital ischaemia and other possibly contributory premorbid conditions.

Commentary by Natalie Tanner FCPodS

Podiatrists have been successfully treating ingrown toenails for years. If the ingrown nail cannot be resolved with conservative methods, then chemical matrixectomy or surgery are recommended. Conservative methods include nail cutting techniques, the use of cotton wool, thin gauze or Steristrips™ at the distal nail fold, to discourage the nail from growing into the toenail skin.

The main stay of Dr Chapple's principles were to cause as little soft tissue trauma to the affected area as possible and therefore she did not use any sutures in the closure of her partial incisional matrixectomy and advocated the use of steri-strips and compression bandaging. In current practise, podiatric surgeons often use dissolvable sutures such as 4/0 Monocryl in order to close down any dead space and to reduce the risk of haematoma.

Most podiatrists will perform a chemical matrixectomy either with phenol 89% or in some cases sodium hydroxide 10%. Commercially available Phenol EZ swab or Phenol Swab-it (Podopro, UK) make the application of the Phenol more precise and safer. Three minutes of application on the nail matrix is recommended. Longer application times risk tissue damage [1]. A disadvantage of using phenol is a long post-operative healing time (2–4 weeks). The prolonged healing time of the necrosed tissue has also been noted to increase risk of post-operative infection [2]. Phenolisation is contraindicated for pregnant patients as well as patients with peripheral vascular disease.

Sodium hydroxide (10%) is a strong basic salt which causes tissue destruction and produces a liquefaction necrosis in contrast to phenol which causes a coagulative necrosis. Chemical ablation of the nail matrix with sodium hydroxide (10%) is known for quicker healing times. This has become a more popular treatment in recent times due to the advantages, however, more studies on the long-term results with regard to regrowth rates are currently lacking in the literature.

The most common surgical technique is partial or full avulsion of the nail plate depending on the shape of the nail plate. Note that a full nail avulsion would only be recommended with a severe involuted nail with gryphosis. The main aim of the partial nail avulsion is to decrease the width of the nail plate of the troublesome nail border to relieve pain and pressure. For a more permanent solution, this would include removal/destruction of the nail matrix by either chemical or surgical excision to cause long-term narrowing of the nail plate.

A partial or total nail avulsion with chemical matrixectomy is widely accepted as an effective form of treatment for ingrown toe nails. It is a quick and simple procedure which is easily performed in the clinical outpatients setting or clinical room. As mentioned, the Phenol 89% has been the main agent used to achieve effective chemical destruction of the matrix. Sodium Hydroxide is emerging as an alternative chemical ablation with lower complications.

Future trends may include the non-surgical Onyfix correction system which uses a hardened composite to control nail growth, increasing use of Sodium Hydroxide instead of Phenol and alternative surgical tools such as the Winograd, Carbon Dioxide LASER, electrocautery, and radiofrequency treatment of the nail matrix [3].

References

1. Muriel-Sanchez JM, Cohena-Jimenez M, Montano-Jimenez P. Effect of phenol application time in the treatment of onychocryptosis: a randomised double-blind clinical trial. Int J Environ Res Public Health. 2021;18:10478.
2. Vlahovic TC. Current concepts in nail surgery. Podiatry Today. 2016;297.
3. Aung B. Are there emerging alternative treatments for ingrown toenails? Podiatry Today. 2020.

Burn Injuries

15

Summary
Both the prevention of burns and their immediate first aid are extremely worthwhile endeavours. Splinting plays an important part in protecting joint function in burns of the extremities. The severity of the burn is dictated by the skin thickness, the surface area burned, the anatomical site, the temperature or chemistry of the burning agent, and the efficiency of any subsequent cooling. Additionally, any pre-existing disease or disability and the depth of burn injury contribute to the outcome. Burns are unhealthy wounds associated with dead, dying, and inflamed tissues. Prolonged hospitalisation and an extended recovery period are inevitable after massive burn injury, usually with resultant long-term deformity and disfigurement, with a chronic psychological impact. Infection is a common complication. Dressings need to be devised for the convenience of the patient and caregiver, but apart from keeping cells moist, absorbing discharge and treating infection, they do not change the outcome.

Dr Joan Chapple's early experience of treating burn trauma at Middlemore Hospital in South Auckland was under the mentorship of William (later Sir William) Manchester [1913–2001]. He had WWII experience of burn management at East Grinstead and St Albans in England, Helwan in Egypt and subsequently, at the Burwood Military Hospital in Christchurch. This was almost 50 years before the establishment of a National Burn Centre at Middlemore in 2006. Manchester's wartime experience of managing severe burn injury was considerable, and he had learned the key principles of burn management from the early plastic surgeon pioneers Gillies, McIndoe, and Mowlem. The destructive nature of deep burn injury was anathema to Dr Chapple's reconstructive sensitivities and principles of wound healing, so ***she viewed prevention as a key strategy*** *in the big picture of Burn Trauma Management. She also believed strongly that only experience of managing burns leads to real expertise in assessment and appropriate decision-making. As well as burn prevention, Dr Chapple was very aware [back in the 1960s & 1970s] of the presentation of non-accidental injury [particularly in young children] as unexplained burn injury.*

Burns and the unhealthy way they behave is not really a mystery. Heat damages and kills living tissue, which makes all burns particularly unhealthy wounds that are liable to infection. The most immediate initial assessment is

P. Charlesworth, M. F. Klaassen, *Chapple's Principles of Wound Care and Healing*,
https://doi.org/10.1007/978-3-031-53104-0_15

of the total impact on the patient and their blood volume. The fluid loss, proportional to the area of the surface burned, is conveniently estimated using the **Rule of 9's** (Fig. 15.1). The rule of 9's has since been refined to take into account the disproportionate anatomical ratios between children, adolescents, and adults (Fig. 15.2).

Patients with burns involving more than about 10% of their body surface, especially children, need to be hospitalised to monitor their general state. This will be unstable for at least 48 h, as the fluid loss diminishes blood volume and toxic breakdown products are dealt with. Patients with large or wetter burns may need to receive intravenous fluid replacement.

The very next important assessment is to determine whether or not the full thickness of the skin has been destroyed, in other words deciding how deep the burn is likely to be. If any epidermal cells survive, even from sweat glands, sebaceous glands, or hair follicles, the area can regenerate skin from its depths and be able to heal itself (Fig. 15.3).

Conversely, if all the skin elements have been killed, the burn can only heal from its periphery and will probably require grafting (Fig. 15.4).

In deeper burns, after separation of the slough, the underlying tissue has to produce a healthy raw surface upon which skin cells can migrate in continuity from the epithelium at the periphery. Producing granulations after burns is always slow as the tissues adjacent to the dead tissue are always debilitated. Sizeable residual raw surfaces may be helped by skin grafting.

Skin grafts, although they expedite healing, are always a poor substitute for normal skin. They lack protective surface sensation, rarely have a smooth surface, may remain dry/scaly, and may be a poor colour match (Fig. 15.5).

Scarring and contractures are a feature of deeper burns and further surgery, although it can improve some things, is quite often disappointing in terms of appearance. There is always a lot of blame, shame, and guilt associated with burn injuries, particularly those sustained in childhood. Many families, as well as the patient are never the same again.

Head and neck	9%
Each upper limb	9%
Front of trunk	18%
Back of trunk	18% (not shown)
Each lower limb	18%
Perineum	1% (not shown)

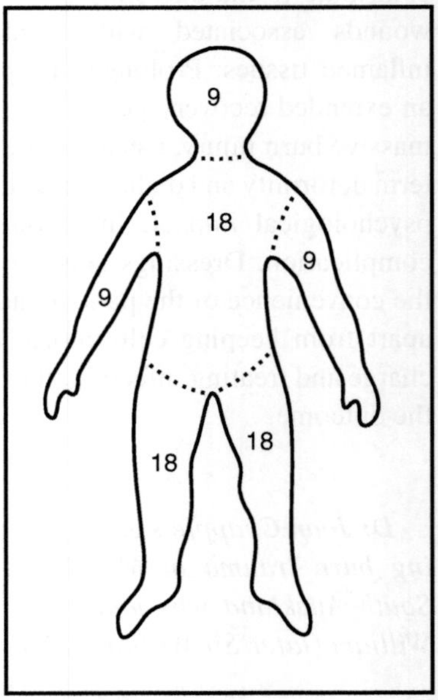

Fig. 15.1 Estimation of burned area by the Rule of 9's

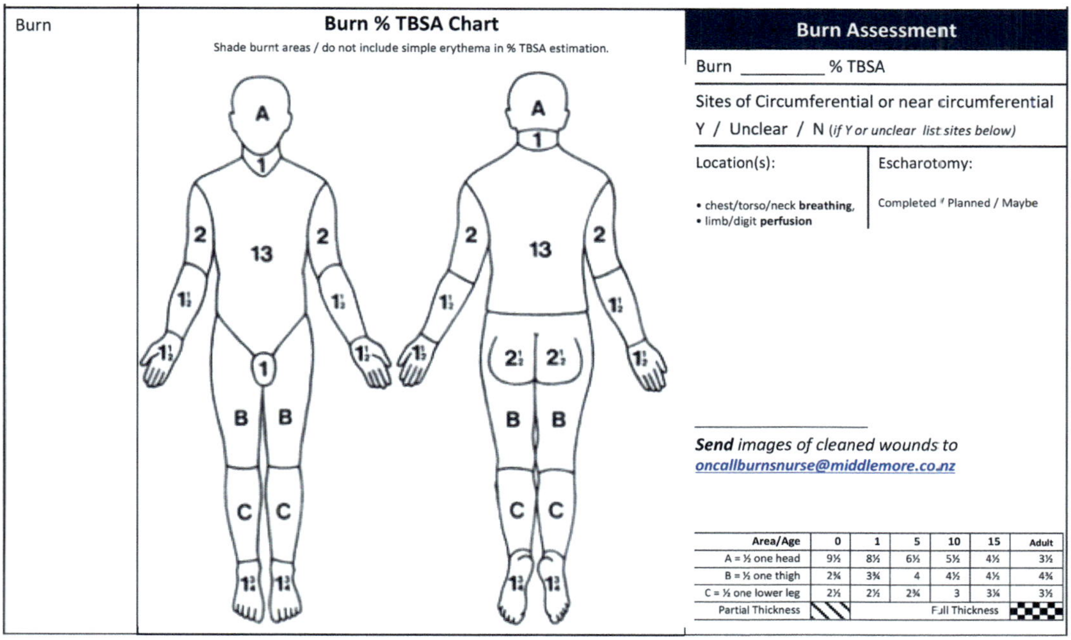

Area/Age	0	1	5	10	15	Adult
A = ½ one head	9½	8½	6½	5½	4½	3½
B = ½ one thigh	2¾	3¾	4	4½	4½	4¾
C = ½ one lower leg	2½	2½	2¾	3	3¼	3½
Partial Thickness		Full Thickness				

Fig. 15.2 Modifications of the Rule of 9's in total burn surface area [TBSA] charts as currently recommended by the National Burn Centre at Middlemore Hospital, Auckland, New Zealand

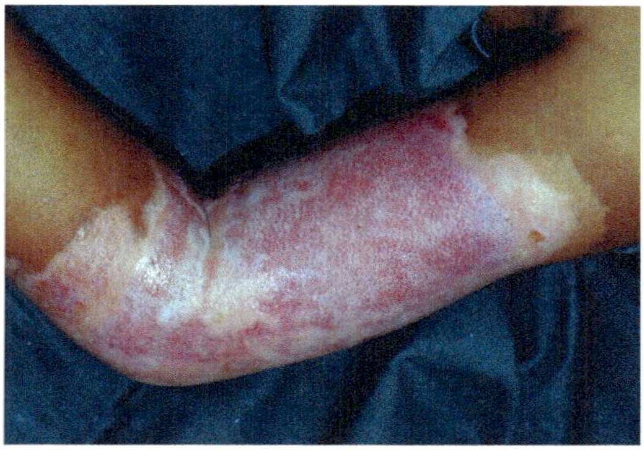

Fig. 15.3 Spontaneously healed partial thickness burn 3 weeks after hot water jug scald. Prompt cooling has made a huge difference to the depth of the burn

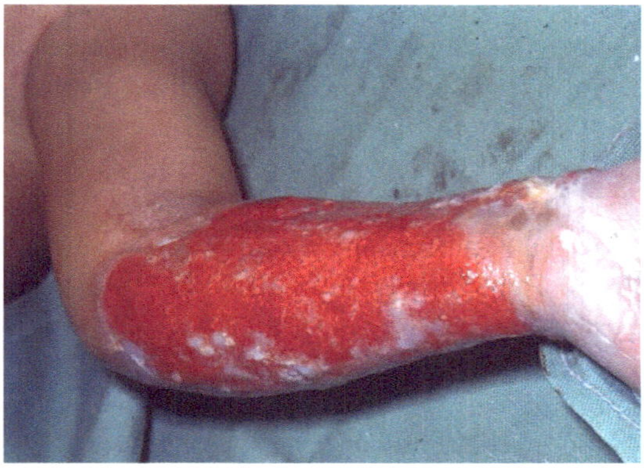

Fig. 15.4 Full-thickness burn of a child's forearm from jug scald. The clothing was not removed and the burn was not cooled. Appearance of the forearm at 1 month. These raw surfaces required skin grafting

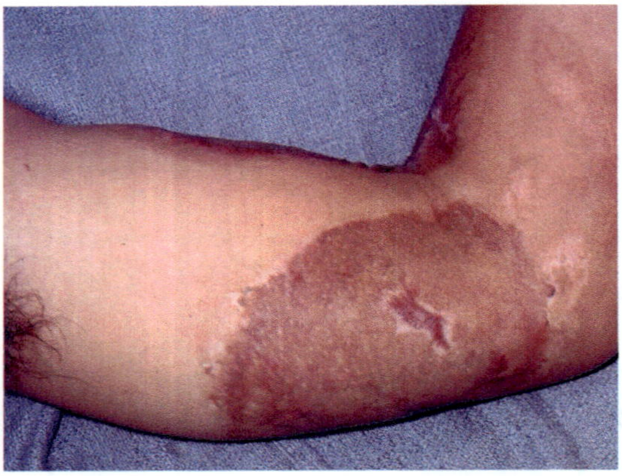

Fig. 15.5 Permanent hyper-pigmentation of a skin graft in a person with brown skin

This Case Study Is Illustrative of the Social Challenges of a Paediatric Burn Injury (See Fig. 15.4)

A 2-year-old boy, in the kitchen, pulled on the dangling cord of a hot-water jug which had recently been boiled and it spilled down his left arm. He screamed, which brought his mother in from the washing line. She could not immediately see where the heat was because he had a skivvy and thick woollen jersey on, but when she grasped his arm, she realised that he had been scalded. She couldn't think what to do and ended up phoning 111, who told her to cool the burn under running water. She took her screaming son to the bathroom, taking his clothes off after she ran cold water down his arm, as initially his clothing was too hot to touch. He stopped crying. She could see that redness and some surface blisters were appearing before her eyes. Some skin was peeling, and he wanted more water on his arm every time she turned the tap off. Finally, leaving the tap slightly on for him to use himself, she telephoned the local health clinic, and they advised her to bring him down immediately.

The child was transported with his mother by ambulance to the hospital 50 km away and admitted. The father came there straightaway from work, having been phoned by his wife. The doctor told them that their boy was not in immediate danger but might need some skin grafts later on. The child became very upset when they had to leave.

The parents got into an argument on the way home about the accident. The mother had not stopped blaming herself and could have done without the bitter accusations from her husband. After regular visits by the family to their son over several weeks had sapped their energy and income, his burns eventually needed extensive grafting (Fig. 15.4). The boy had split-skin grafts taken from both his thighs, which took a further 2 weeks to heal and left red itchy donor surfaces. The grafted skin kept blistering and bleeding if he knocked or scratched it, despite the application of creams and Calamine™ lotion.

When he came home from the hospital, the child was very tearful and anxious, waking with nightmares through the night and suffering from itchy scars for several months. He was very demanding, and the two older children and their father felt quite neglected. The mother felt guilty, depressed, and exhausted. She felt tearful herself, every time she undressed him. He wanted his baths nearly cold and wouldn't let her out of his sight. She kept bandages on his forearm and lower extremities mainly so that they could not be seen, especially by his father. The father kept wanting to know whether even the donor site scars would ever match his normal skin again. *'How would she know? She wasn't a doctor!'* The father started drinking heavily, shouted at everybody and he left the family altogether when the boy was nearly 5.

The child went through school hating it because other children were forever making fun of his scars and grafts. He never went swimming and never learned to swim. His older brother and sister resented him because of all the attention he got. The mother often found herself thinking that all their lives would have been very different if only the jug had not been left full of boiling water or it had a short cord or if he had not managed to pull it over himself. This accident affected all of them for the rest of their lives.

Prevention

After years of treating burn victims, the only appropriate conclusion one can come to is that burns are so awful that prevention must be the best approach to them. Burns have to be the most preventable of all injuries. We know almost without exception where the hot things and hot places are, especially around the home. It is important that prevention, first-aid, and action plans are talked about in homes. The only additional thing to realise is that young children do not automatically link hot things or even the caution *'hot'* for any potential for harm until they have experienced this for themselves. They must therefore be taught this as early as possible, in a controlled environment. Otherwise, they are destined to join a large group of children that learn the hard way in some uncontrolled and disastrous situation, ending up scarred for life. The most important lessons must be with hot fluids, matches, stoves, heaters and fires, and through careful demonstration, allowing the heat to be unpleasant but not damaging. Young girls should be dressed in pyjamas rather than nightgowns. This simple measure alone would immediately reduce the incidence of serious body burns to girls, which is presently six times that of boys. This would significantly reduce the numbers of children requiring admission to hospitals for deep burns and their sequelae. It is also important to be aware that burns are not uncommonly a form of child abuse (Fig. 15.6).

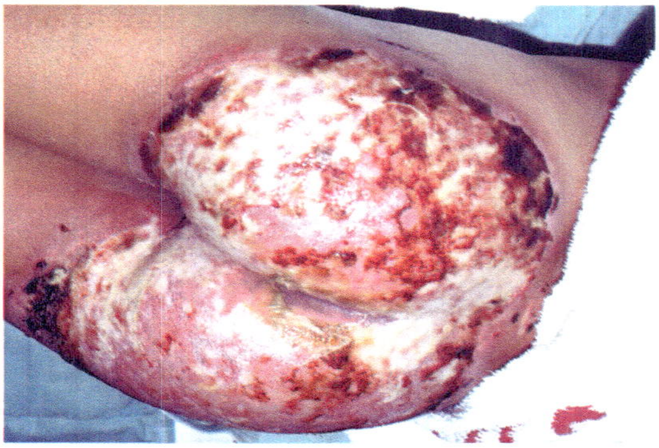

Fig. 15.6 Deep burns to the buttocks of an 8-year-old girl. This injury could only have been inflicted by another person holding the child forcibly in hot water and should have been recognised instantly as a non-accidental injury. Unfortunately, it wasn't

First Aid

The only treatment which can limit the injury is immediate first-aid cooling with cold running water, which is effective in reducing both the temperature and the time for which the heat acts. It is worth doing this until the excess heat is removed which may take 15–20 min, or more. A comparison of the burn injury appearances in Figs. 15.3 and 15.4 clearly illustrates the value of first-aid cooling. Following the initial cold water, continuing cooling will reduce the searing pain of the acute burn but if continued in extensive burns can lead to hypothermia. Any skin that peels during cooling was never going to survive. Burn creams, butter, and spider-web applications do nothing worthwhile. Analgesia or sedation is often needed for the first few hours, after which the burns are usually much less painful than mechanical injuries, unless they become infected.

Depth Assessment

The depth of a burn determines both its local behaviour and the final scarring. The only possible way to improve one's accuracy in the assessment of depth is to attempt to predict it in every case. This will then create a particularly focused interest in the behaviour of each burn. Also known as experience, the retrospective correlation of the behaviour and outcome with the initial history and appearance is the only possible way to develop expertise for use on another occasion.

Superficial burns heal quickly without permanent scars, despite looking dreadful initially. Confident reassurance based on clinical experience can in these cases be a very important part of the initial treatment. Patients are much better dealing with bad outcomes if they expect them and are happier to find things turning out better than anticipated, rather than worse. If in doubt about the depth, it is therefore best to err on the pessimistic side in making a forecast.

The depth of a thermal burn is related to three things.

1. The temperature of the burning agent
2. The time for which the heat acts
3. The thickness of the skin at the burn site

History

The detailed history of a burn is much more useful in predicting the depth of a burn than any of the other features. The temperature of the burning agent and time for which it has acted are usually obtainable. When the person really does not know how they got burned, it is important to inquire about altered states of consciousness such as can occur with drugs, strokes, alcohol, or epilepsy. It is also key to be aware of reduced sensation such as in paraplegia, peripheral neuritis associated with diabetes or alcoholism, nerve damage, or anaesthesia. When the patient, particularly a child, is too anxious or frightened to say what happened, has an unlikely story or evidence of previous burns or mechanical injuries, particularly a child, there has to be suspicion that abuse may be going on (Fig. 15.6).

It is important to know how quickly cooling was carried out. Cooling reduces both the time of heat application and the temperature effectively, but only if carried out straight away. Unfortunately, some people panic or try to phone someone just to be sure and waste precious cooling time. Others cool burns belatedly when they find out that they should have done so, reducing the effectiveness of it considerably, or altogether.

Encounters with and experience in treating burns make it possible to fairly accurately predict the depth of a burn from the history. A scald with water on exposed skin, even without cooling, is rarely a full thickness burn. With instant and effective cooling, the damage can be very superficial indeed. A scald with a cup of milky tea or coffee which is cooled immediately is also likely to be superficial. Further up the scale, scalds from a boiling jug or steam, with heat retained by clothing and not cooled, is capable of destroying the full thickness of the skin, particularly where this is thin, as on the front of the forearm in a child (Fig. 15.4). Assessments using the history thus becomes a matter of squaring off the different features. Soup and fat are hotter and linger for longer and always cause full thickness burns if not cooled quickly. Porridge, coffee, tar, or molten wax burn more deeply still but, even these benefit greatly from cooling, as involvement of deeper structures may be reduced. Direct flames on skin from burning clothing or bedding usually cause full thickness burns, but the damage may be limited to skin if the burn is cooled. When this has not been done, flame burns may be much deeper, as they are unfortunately in many house fires.

Liquid chemical burns should be washed instantly and liberally. Corrosive powders should be dusted off first. A small electrical burn is often deeper than a contact burn and the electrical damage can sometimes track beneath intact skin, with extensive and serious consequences. Cooling cannot retrieve this damage.

Skin Thickness

Skin thickness is a somewhat imprecise clinical evaluation. Dorsal skin is generally thicker than ventral skin, that on the scalp and back being very thick. Palm and sole skin is also very thick, but skin on the top of the foot and back of the hand is particularly thin. Skin is thin in babies and young children and becomes progressively thinner in old age. These differences can often make a profound difference to the outcome. The determining factor in any burn's behaviour is never its depth in millimetres, but whether or not epithelial elements remain alive to provide reservoirs within the burned area to enable it to heal from the depths, rather than from the edges.

The Appearance of the Burn

The appearance usually reinforces the depth assessment made on the basis of the history and the site. A red but unblistered burn is likely to be very superficial. Sunburn for example often does not blister immediately and usually peels several days later. Blisters coming slowly or remaining intact after several hours nearly always means a partial-thickness burn. Blisters appearing rapidly and bursting indicate a deeper burn. The colour of the base of ruptured blisters then becomes a good guide to the depth. A uniformly pink sticky surface may be a partial-thickness burn, but whitish, blotchy, bluish, grey, or brown stagnant-looking areas, usually in the middle of a burn indicate full-thickness skin destruction. Burns sustained in flames will be deepest at sites from which the heat cannot escape, such as beneath the chin or on the margins of nostrils or ears. These features often indicate from which direction the heat has come. Dry, contact, or electrical burns are not so impressive to look at initially as a blistered burn but are usually much deeper. These deep burns may not need a dressing at first, but will do within a week or so, gradually exposing the full extent of injury.

Local Treatment of Burns

Occlusive dressings are the most appropriate way to manage burned patients at home. It is important to posture and splint burned hands in wrist extension, metacarpo-phalangeal flexion and inter-phalangeal extension, while pain and swelling is present. Deep hand burns should probably be managed by hand specialists. Burns are mostly sterile injuries and until or unless they become infected, patients do not need antibiotics. Superficial burns will be well on the way to healing within a week. Intact blisters don't have to be drained, but unwieldy ones can be decompressed with an incision, with the surface skin then pressed flat and retained.

Partial-thickness burns are much more comfortable during recovery if the blistered skin is retained initially. Eventually of course the surface layers will peel, leaving a thinned pink but healed skin surface. If the blister fluid at any stage becomes turbid, or inflammation and pain increases after the first day or two, draining the infected blisters is clearly necessary and at this stage treatment includes trimming all the skin debris away as well, to expose the burned surface to dressings with antibiotic cream (Fig. 15.7a, b).

Burns need redressing every few days until the dead tissue separates. Burns discharge to help get rid of the slough, but this is not synonymous with infection unless there are associated symptoms and signs of this as well, namely, increasing throbbing pain and inflammation. Deep burns are more liable to get infected, so vigilance and repeated swab-taking are an on-going and important part of their care. Antibiotic creams are very useful for local infection within the burn. Systemic antibiotics will be needed whenever invasive sepsis develops. Most herbal remedies with a good reputation for use in burns do not have antibacterial properties, perhaps apart from certain types of honey.

Raw areas remaining after separation of slough indicate full-thickness skin destruction and if sizeable may be helped by skin grafting (Fig. 15.4). If a burn is relatively small but clearly a full-thickness one, it may be well worthwhile referring the patient to a plastic surgeon for consideration of excision and grafting within the first few days, to avoid the weeks of dressings preparing the areas for the inevitably necessary grafting (Fig. 15.8a, b).

Burn Scars

Burn scars are typically bulky, red, and itchy [hypertrophic] for several months. Pressure dressings in the early months after healing can help minimise this. After several months, burn scars begin to soften and relax, reduce their bulk and they lose their redness and itchiness over the first year. They continue to improve further over several more years. While grafts contribute epithelium and expedite surface healing, they also become part of the 'scar' to most people and may be very unsightly if they end up a different colour from the surrounding skin, as they do in dark-skinned people (Fig. 15.5). Donor areas should

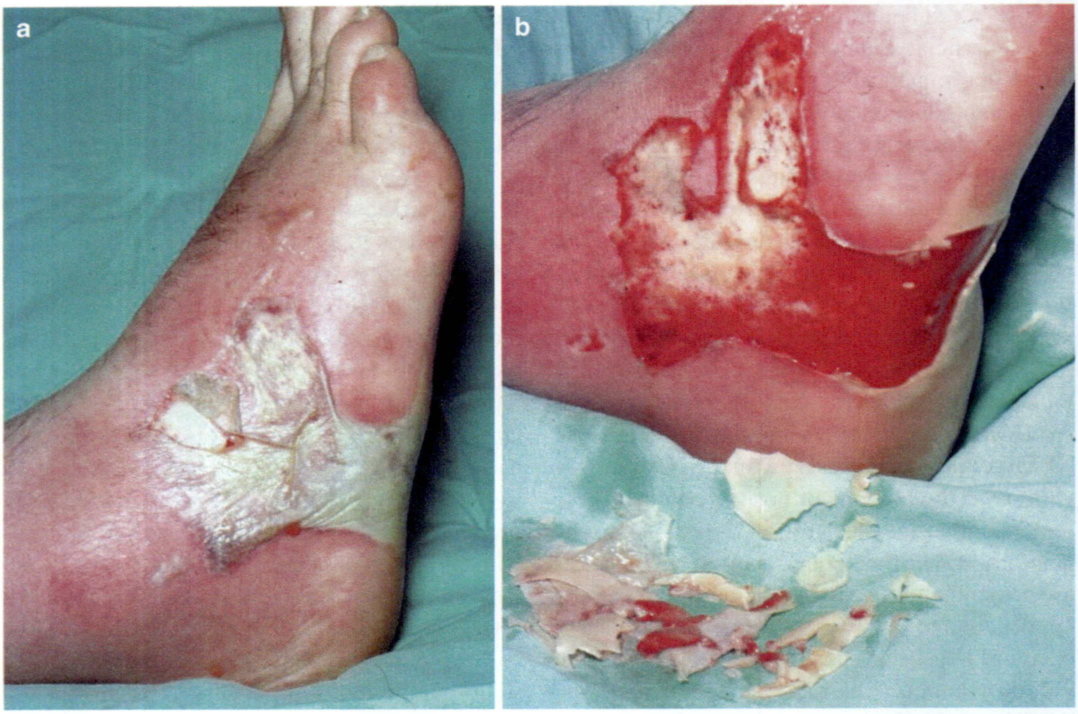

Fig. 15.7 (**a**, **b**) Full-thickness burn 5 days after molten metal had run inside a boot. It is already infected. Drainage of the blisters and excision of debris was done the same day and the infection settled promptly with antibiotics

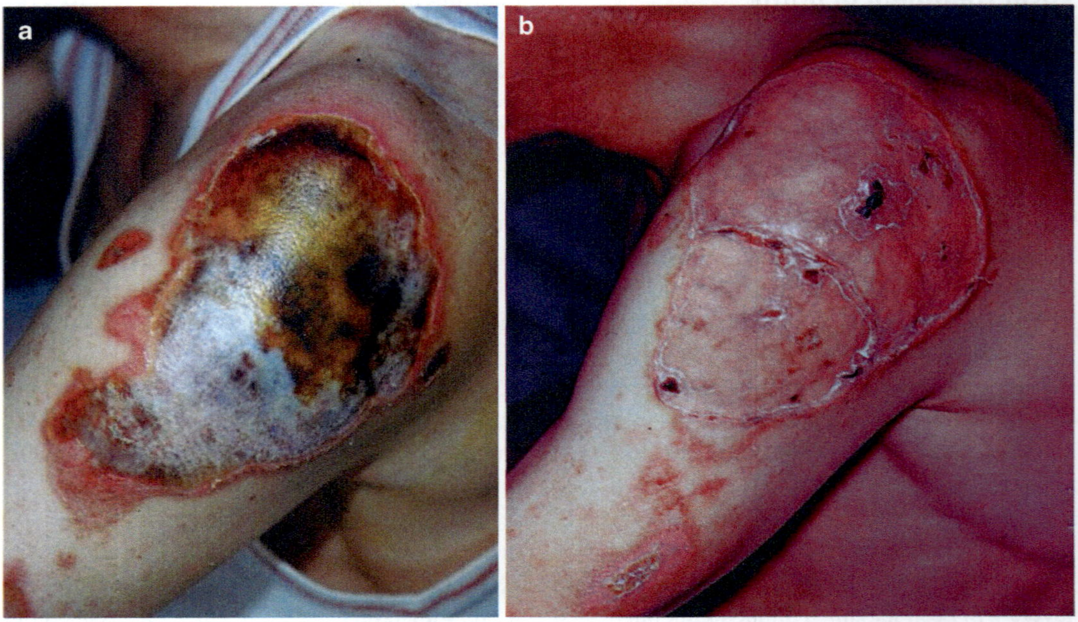

Fig. 15.8 (**a**, **b**) Deep contact burn left shoulder. Patient fell onto a hot metal plate. Referred at 4 days for early excision. This burn clearly full-thickness was managed by excision and grafting at 5 days, bypassing several weeks of dressings. Healed 1 week later

never make palpable scars unless they have been far too deep, but they can remain permanently different in colour or texture. Unstable burn scars or those producing contractures of joints can be helped by plastic surgery, but improvement of the appearance of the scars themselves can only ever be relative. Surgery for burns scars is often relatively disappointing.

Five Point Summary for Burns

1. **Help prevent burns and educate everyone about prompt cooling.**
2. **Patients with more than 10% of their body surface burned may need to be hospitalised initially for intravenous therapy. Always make an initial attempt to assess the burn depth from the history, thickness of skin at the site of the burn and clinical appearance. Be prepared to modify this prediction according to the behaviour of the burn wound. Most burn wounds are best looked after with tulle gras and creams with occlusive dressings changed every few days until healing occurs. Burned hands and feet usually need splintage. Sizeable residual raw surfaces may need skin grafts.**
3. **Burns, because they are associated with dead tissue, are always innately unhealthy wounds until the slough is removed and they are granulating. Increasing pain after a few days indicates infection. Burns then require swabs, drainage of blisters, excision of debris and sometimes systemic antibiotics.**
4. **With deeper burns scarring is inevitable and permanent. Scar contractures can usually be relieved surgically. Improvement in the appearance of burn scars by surgery is usually only relative and often disappointing.**
5. **The damage done to patients, their psyches, and their families by burn trauma seems to be worse than that from mechanical injuries and persists long after the skin heals. The only satisfactory approach to burns must be to prevent them.**

Commentary by Dr Richard Wong She CNZM, FRACS

There is so much of Dr Chapple's principles which is still relevant today and the insights and weighting of these insights remain relevant.

Prevention is key and the best 'treatment'. Prevention programmes are an integral part of every burn service and burn association. As is eloquently stated 'burns have to be the most preventable of all injuries'.

Following a burn injury, the next most important step is accurate assessment which takes into account multiple factors (history, anatomical site, and clinical appearance). Importantly, the dynamic nature of a burn injury where the reader is advised to 'be prepared to modify this' remains true today.

Also relevant is the observation that the injury affects more than just the patient—it affects their entire family and that this injury, to both patient and family 'seems worse than that from mechanical injuries and persists long after the skin heals'. Acknowledgement of the psycho-social impact of a burn injury, particularly for paediatric patients, is important. Referral criteria for a burn injury are well established and agreed upon. Burn size is not the sole determinant for the appropriateness for referral or admission.

The threshold for fluid resuscitation remains debated, as does the composition of the optimum resuscitation fluid to use (crystalloid vs. colloid). Although there have been those proposing greater use of oral rehydration, intravenous resuscitation remains the standard in burn centres, utilising 'balanced salt solutions' and with maintenance fluids (with glucose) for paediatric patients [1].

Burn depth is the major determinant of whether a burn wound will heal within the time limits expressed above. Clinical assessment of burn depth remains as described in the text. Despite advances in technology and proponents of technology such as laser Doppler imaging to accurately and objectively diagnose the depth of a burn injury, clinical expertise remains vital in determining optimum burn care. The explanations given in the text about interpreting the mechanism of injury, as well as the guides to clinical assessment of burn depth remain accurate and useful for clinicians.

The role of burn first aid in limiting tissue damage is well recognised and perhaps the most important development is the recognition that the benefit of cool running water for 20 min is effective even 3 h after an injury [2].

Whilst the assessment of a burn injury and initial cooling remain relevant and accurate, the management of burn injuries has advanced and changed significantly.

Advances in burn care have centred around minimising scarring and maximising functional outcomes and taking a more proactive approach to debriding necrotic tissue and closing the wound. The risk of scarring increases exponentially, particularly after 14 days, which drives the current mantra of grafting paediatric burn wounds which have not healed (or predicted not to heal) within 14 days and 21 days for adults.

Wounds are no longer dressed until necrotic tissue separates and blisters are not left intact. Active removal of necrotic tissue and blistered epithelium is encouraged to allow both accurate assessment of the burn wound and removal of potential bacterial growth media. In children, this may require a general anaesthetic to achieve good wound care without traumatising the child (and their family). Modern burn dressings typically incorporate some antimicrobial properties and can be left intact for several days and surpass blistered (dead) epithelium.

The concern around the quality of skin grafts is genuine but outcomes today are improved by grafting before scarring is established, as well as surgically preparing the wound bed as opposed to relying upon granulation tissue. Advances in the development of dermal substitutes allows current plastic and burn surgeons the luxury of being able to 'reconstruct' the lost dermis and create a better foundation for skin grafts which more closely mirrors what was destroyed in the burn injury.

Whilst burn injuries will forever be life-changing for an individual and their family, they need not result in unsatisfactory outcomes, and surgery is no longer the treatment of 'last resort', but rather a proactive form of minimising scarring and functional limitations from a burn injury.

Commentary by Professor James D. Frame FRCS(Plast)

I agree with Dr Richard Wong She and would go even further and say that this chapter is essentially stating the management of Burn Injury in adults and children in the period before 1980. Extensive published evidence from The Shriners Institutes in the USA and from the larger global Burn Units is that with treatment in highly specialised, well-staffed units in state-of-the-art facilities, both survival figures and outcomes for burns improve. An established principle is that the faster a burn wound heals, the better the scar quality and appearance, the better the functional gain and the better the psychological outcome, whether the injury be in children or adults [3]. The key to the latter is to identify vulnerable burn-injured patients of any age, then emotionally and psychologically support and treat them at an early stage, initially in hospital and continuing after discharge, when they are most vulnerable. These individuals need support, since they will often consider themselves as victims, rather than the lucky survivors of burn injury.

Delayed healing means a longer inpatient stay, many painful operative or dressing procedures, missing of school and interaction with peers, and a life in a very protected environment often lasting for months. Introversion and fears of appearance can lead to suicide.

Secondary surgery is commonly required after delayed healing, to improve both cosmesis and function. The optimum time to perform it for children is always in school holiday time, so that they can continue to interact with their peers and keep up with their education at School. (Victims to Survivors Multidisciplinary, International Symposium, Essex, 1992).

Small burns in children can still kill and having personally witnessed fatality in minor 3% deep dermal scald injuries in children caused by using a delayed approach, I was swayed by the data and research to favour immediate surgical intervention, including grafting wherever indicated [4]. With a thermal injury, the immediate surface has, by definition, been heat-sterilised. However, the deeper adnexal structures contain normal gram-positive commensal organisms that quickly erupt onto the burn injury surface within the first week. Later, about 2 weeks after injury, a mixed microbial soup develops, including gram-negative and possibly antibiotic-resistant organisms mainly due to opportunist nosocomial pathogens, some of which can be nasty. Toxin-mediated illness can be fatal within the first week of burn injury. A massive release of toxins is due to the inflammatory process, in an environment shown to be dependent on a critical low value of magnesium. This promotes massive and sudden release of toxins from a number of gram-positive Staph. Aureus or Streptococcal strains, that may be on the burn-injured surface or in the surface dressings.

Burn injuries will always occur, despite best efforts to reduce the incidence. However, I also feel that the future of burns treatment is dependent on promoting better ways of reducing the harmful aspects of inflammatory response to burn injury. This can be achieved by preventing the inevitable deepening of injury that occurs in the zone of stasis over the first hours. Personally, I think that nitric oxide topical therapy has much to offer, but current delivery systems are proving painful and harmful to the host, because of the uncontrolled conversion to nitrous acid. A direct gaseous delivery system is available and looks more promising. The advantage is the improvement of tissue oxygenation, using the vasodilatory effects of nitric oxide and also the highly effective biocidal activity of nitric oxide plasma. If a deep biofilm is contributing to hypertrophic scars, subcutaneous calcification and poor functional movement with contracture deformity, then nitric oxide is an obvious advance in the therapeutic management of burns resulting in less scar deformity and less need for secondary surgeries.

The Holy Grail of burn injury is to return the injured person to a pre- injury appearance and function. We are nowhere near achieving this yet, but we must advance our thinking and continue to research these heinous injuries, because surgery is only part of the answer.

Commentary by Professor Fiona Wood AM, FRCS, FRACS

This chapter resonates with the essential basic principles of burn care. It is clear that Dr Joan Chapple's training that led to this philosophy was at the hands of those who had learnt the craft of burn care in the most austere of conditions, in the theatre of war. To this day, we absolutely know that prevention is better than cure. The emphasis on a clear, well taken history and clinical examination to guide clinical patient care is a message that should never be lost.

Using the assessment of the injury in terms of the depth and surface area, linked with the patient condition, remains at the centre of modern burn care. The excision of the burn tissue as a priority remains the challenge when planning skin repair. The emphasis on infection control and multimodality treatment of infection, including the role of surgery, are sound teachings.

Those of us who treat burn injuries know all too well the profound psychosocial impact on the affected individual and their families. As Dr Chapple makes clear in this chapter, we need to consider all aspects of the trauma to provide the best environment for holistic healing.

The concept that all deep burns will scar is a concept we need to interrogate into the future. Is scarring inevitable? The inflammation associated with the burn has lifelong impact in many burn survivors physically and physiologically. The early excision of the burn will reduce the inflammation. Advances in tissue engineering and cell-based therapies provide opportunities for scar minimisation in the future.

This chapter provides clarity around the essential steps comprising the foundation stones from which we can build, by fostering research and innovation, to improve the burn care of the future.

References

1. Cartotto R, Burmeister DM, Kubasiak JC. Burn shock and resuscitation: review and state of the science. J Burn Care Res. 2022;43:567–85.
2. Jeschke MG, et al. Burn injury. Nat Rev Dis Primers. 2020;6:11.
3. Slator R, Frame JD. Management of burn injuries in children. Eur J Plast Surg. 1996;19:207–12. https://doi.org/10.1007/BF00176281.
4. Frame JD, Eve MD, Hackett MEJ, et al. The toxic shock syndrome in burned children. Burns. 1985;11:234–41.

Bleeding, Haemostasis, and Tourniquets

16

Summary
The control of bleeding is best achieved by elevation and focal pressure, not by the application of a tourniquet. Complete haemostasis, accomplished progressively during treatment, is a specific goal, because achieving it means that the final dressing tension no longer needs to be haemostatic. Only with total haemostasis can bandage tension be reduced sufficiently to maintain maximum perfusion of tissue during the critical period of reactive swelling.

Stopping bleeding is always a priority, to be attended to as soon as possible. No wound in which bleeding has stopped needs to be explored further until both anaesthetic and surgical facilities are available. Bleeding can usually be controlled by elevation and pressure or stopped by dealing with an identifiable, troublesome bleeder. Major vessels needing specialist repair must be controlled as soon as possible by accurate pressure, forceps, or temporary ligation.

At operation, with the patient at rest and the wound elevated, dressings are gently removed, picking up bleeders with mosquito-forceps as they occur. These can be tied off with fine plain catgut or synthetic absorbable sutures or stopped with a series of forceps left on for several minutes (if there are enough forceps), after which only about one in five small bleeders will eventually need tying off. Controlling the bleeding in this way takes place progressively as the wound is being cleansed and assessed. It is usually helpful to have an assistant. When working alone, dealing with bleeders is easier using an absorbable suture on a curved needle. Occasionally, bleeders which are hard to find, or retracted within cut muscle, are best located with curved mosquito forceps, used somewhat serially as retractors until the offending bleeder is located. Troublesome bleeding can also arise from a partially cut vessel, which hasn't been able to retract and clot. Unless this is a sizeable vessel requiring vascular repair, it will usually require clipping each side of the leak, complete division between the two clips, and ligation of both ends.

The blood clotting mechanism obviously plays a huge part in normal haemostasis. However, this is not usually obvious until or unless a patient with a bleeding disorder or taking anticoagulants is encountered, when every tiny bleeder keeps right on trickling. If there is a known bleeding diathesis, it is always worth seeking the advice and assistance of a haematologist before commencing. Whenever untoward bleeding or bruising is encountered, underlying clotting difficulties should be considered, and specialist advice is always worthwhile. Orthodox and absolute haemostasis still has to be patiently and painstakingly carried out in these patients, and their management is likely to incorporate elevation, some pressure, and close supervision for several hours.

P. Charlesworth, M. F. Klaassen, *Chapple's Principles of Wound Care and Healing*,
https://doi.org/10.1007/978-3-031-53104-0_16

Tourniquets

A professionally applied pneumatic tourniquet may occasionally be needed temporarily, where a major vessel has been involved in a wound and needs to be inspected before repair or ligation. The traditional use of a tourniquet during surgical procedures is otherwise for the convenience of the operator and always at the expense of tissue sustenance. Tourniquets can be justified when looking for a difficult foreign body, locating nail matrix, or dissections in scar tissue, but are not necessary for most acute wounds or straightforward procedures. The use of a tourniquet automatically deprives the tissue of circulation and always complicates the process of achieving haemostasis.

Tourniquet use is particularly contraindicated in: the management of severely damaged tissues; anyone who has a bleeding problem; and elderly patients whose tissues and vessels are very fragile.

Prolonged use of a tourniquet can be associated with post-tourniquet oedema for several days and sometimes cause injury to peripheral nerves.

The application of a tourniquet to perform ischaemic blocks by venous infusion is a far from ideal technique. One of the major disadvantages is that anaesthesia is always lost immediately following the tourniquet release. Faced with post-tourniquet hyperaemia and bleeding there is neither time nor opportunity to achieve proper haemostasis, so dressing pressure is often hurriedly applied. The recovery environment thereafter is likely to be both painful and hazardous for the injured tissues. It is a 'snatch and grab' technique and is unsuitable for children because of dosage limitations. It is also a technique which adds the risk of haematoma to closed injuries such as fractures.

Arguments Against the Use of a Tourniquet in Surgery

1. The use of a tourniquet requires prior anaesthesia of the skin it is going to be applied to. In the case of an ischaemic block, a second tourniquet is applied after the intravenous infusion of local anaesthetic, onto insensitive skin below the first one, which is then removed [Double cuff tourniquet required].
2. Tissue vitality can no longer be assessed once a tourniquet is on.
3. Tissues are absolutely deprived of circulation for the duration of the tourniquet application, hardly encouraging at a time when what they are most in need of is the establishment and maintenance of maximum circulation.
4. Irreversible thrombosis can take place in damaged vessels, during the time that the circulation is at a standstill.
5. The hyperaemia after tourniquet removal usually produces brisk bleeding for some time and can cause additional bruising in already-injured tissues. The standard management of this problem is to apply firm bandaging before removing tourniquets. The downside to this is a reduction in circulatory throughput, which worsens as tissue subsequently swells. Complicated deep repairs to muscles, tendons, and nerves can be severely disrupted by bleeding after a tourniquet is released. This can affect outcomes, whether or not there are external visible signs on the surface.

Diathermy

There are also always additional risks when fluids and electricity are in close proximity. The use of any alcohol or spirit-based skin preparations is incompatible with diathermy. The use of diathermy to stop bleeding is acceptable only if the bleeders are tiny and the diathermy is used as a precise instrument. It is best reserved for stopping small bleeders in neurosurgery, liver surgery, and scar tissue, where conventional methods of haemostasis can be particularly difficult. To 'ziz' around with diathermy in the vicinity of a larger bleeder simply leaves unacceptable quantities of dead tissue for the body to have to deal with subsequently. Even when this technique appears to stop bleeding, vessels often bleed secondarily from the coagulated mess, as dead tissue discharges and separates.

Adrenaline Use in Haemostasis

It is sometimes useful to irrigate a still-oozing wound with a dilute adrenaline solution at the end of a procedure. The simplest manoeuvre is to use local anaesthetic with adrenaline in a syringe and drip it on topically, with a tiny injection here and there, sometimes right onto a bleeding point. While stronger solutions are very effective, the absorption levels may be undesirable and rebound bleeding can also be a problem when the adrenaline effect wears off. Whenever adrenaline has been used, it is sensible to apply a supportive dressing for several hours.

Stopping the Last of the Bleeding

The re-approximation of wound edges and their stabilisation with sutures or tapes or tulle-gras has a helpful effect in bringing about final haemostasis, probably by encouraging tiny bleeders to clot off against another tissue surface. If oozing persists at this stage, the ultimate way to stop it is the use of **temporary** local pressure applied over tulle-gras by means of a gauze pad and a crepe bandage. This can be left in place for 10–20 min before re-bandaging at a reduced tension. If bleeding has still not stopped completely, pressure can be tried again for 30 min or so or the wound may have to be reopened and the bleeding source searched for and dealt with. **The aim of the whole exercise is not to have to use haemostatic tension in the ultimate dressing, thereby allowing for a range of swelling to occur without ever jeopardising the circulation.** This technique also allows patients to re-bandage their own wounds if the bandages feel tight, knowing that they can do this without starting bleeding again. It also makes it possible for the operator to inspect the wound at any time without encountering bleeding. When dressing pressure has been used definitively to stop bleeding, the loosening of bandages to relieve pain and improve the circulation may start the bleeding again and/or start off the development of a wound haematoma. Immobilisation and continued elevation assist with the maintenance of haemostasis. For lower leg and foot wounds in outpatients, the double-bandaging technique is essential to ensure an ideal recovery. [See Appendix].

Haemostatic Technique Summary

1. **Elevation**
2. **Local focal pressure**
3. **Clipping of bleeders**
4. **Tying of bleeders**
5. **Suturing of bleeders**
6. **Adrenaline irrigation**
7. **Tissue apposition**
8. **Temporary pressure**
9. **Time and the clotting mechanism**
10. **Dressing support**
11. **Immobilisation and continued elevation**
12. **Two bandage technique for leg and foot injuries** [See Appendix]

Commentary by Dr Michael F. Klaassen ONZM, FRACS Co-Editor

In this useful chapter, Dr Joan Chapple considers the important clinical aspects of bleeding and bleeding control.

Surgery could be so much simpler if surgeons did not have to worry about bleeding and haemostasis. This becomes obvious when practicing flap-raising in applied anatomy labs using thawed cadaver material. Bleeding is an everyday reality and many of the practical techniques of surgery are a balance between controlling the inevitable bleeding and minimizing the risks of complications, like haematomata, which threaten a successful outcome. Circulation is a key physiological function, but we need the blood to stay within the circulatory vessels.

Any doctor having experienced the clinical situation of uncontrolled bleeding will remember the stress and sense of urgency this evokes. At times like these, a simple pragmatic approach out-trumps textbook idealism. For extremity surgery, packing and pressure, combined with elevation of the involved limb, will buy you some time.

Dr Joan Chapple was quite dismissive of the pneumatic tourniquet, but I believe it can be used safely depending on the pressure **[<250 mmHg for upper extremities in adults, or 100 mmHg above systolic pressure in paediatric patients**] and strict observance of duration **[< 60 min**]. For accurate, anatomically congruent limb and hand/foot injury repair, I have always found judicious use of limb tourniquets to be very helpful, remembering that safe compression pressures and limited ischaemic time [<60 min] should be followed. Delicate traumatised structures such as tendons, nerves and vessels need to be accurately dissected and identified for precise repair. In this situation, appropriate regional anaesthesia is very beneficial for safe and continuous anaesthesia.

Ischaemic (or Bier's) blocks have been the norm for the closed reduction of displaced common wrist fractures like the Colles' fracture. Increasingly, modern emergency departments are utilizing the haematoma block, which is simpler, effective and reliable for manipulation of the fracture fragments into alignment before the cast is applied. Dr Chapple was critical of the ischaemic block, but for guidelines to the modern application of the technique, see [1].

Increasingly, surgeons are faced with more patients who are prescribed a wide range of anticoagulants for their cardiac conditions, post coronary artery stenting and arrhythmias like atrial fibrillation, which can lead to intracardiac thromboses and strokes. These drugs include Plavax, Clopidogrel and Rivaroxaban, which should be stopped before elective surgery. Some modern innovations which may aid the surgery in these patients at high risk of bleeding include the use of Tranexamic acid perioperatively, topical 1: 10,000 Adrenaline, and calcium alginate dressings (like Kaltostat™) for raw bleeding surfaces.

Innovative specific haemostatic devices include the Codman Raney™ + Codman Leroy-Raney™ haemostatic clips and clip applicators,

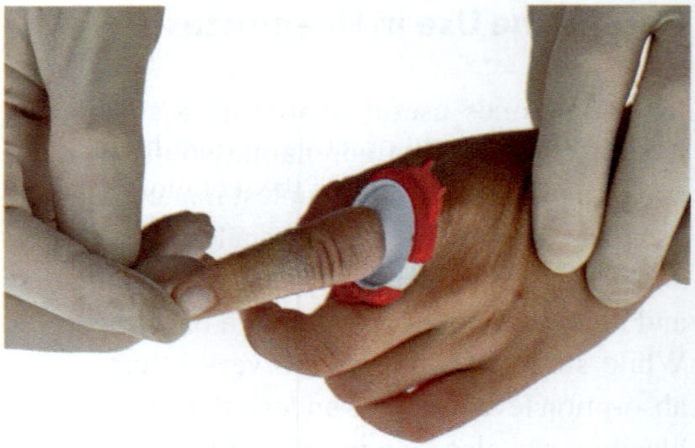

Fig. 16.1 The T-Ring™ Digital Tourniquet Device [available from SheffMed NZ Ltd./E: sales@sheffmed.co.nz]

used for controlling the very vascular scalp flaps in craniofacial and neurosurgery. Alternatively, a good trick for haemostasis is to grasp the exposed galea with several mosquito haemostats and retract the galea.

For digital surgery, I favour the physician-designed T-Ring™ digital tourniquet (Fig. 16.1). It looks like a brightly-coloured casino chip, so as not to be left on, and one size fits all. The brightly-coloured [red] outer plastic ring surrounds a flexible disc containing a hole into which the digit fits. Two cutaway sections allow for the two halves of the device to be pulled apart [see T-Ring.com]. The T-Ring™ device produces a reliable low pressure on the digit needing surgery of between 150–165 mmHg. This is much safer than the alternatives e.g. rolled surgical glove with clamp or a Penrose drain, where measured pressures were consistently > 300 mmHg [2]. If the T-Ring™ is not available, then the unclamped rolled glove is safer than the Penrose drain or rolled glove with clamp.

Further Commentary by Dr Peter Charlesworth FRACS Co-Editor

The principles of Dr Chapple's philosophy on bleeding and haemostasis are axiomatic, but they are rarely found so simply or logically explained in standard teaching or textbooks. She expresses very negative opinions about the use of pneumatic tourniquets and ischaemic local anaesthetic blocks, but the strength of her antipathy may well have been influenced by the relatively restricted range of her clinical practice. While the majority of her specific criticisms of the techniques cannot be denied in principle, the fact remains that both have a valuable selective role in modern surgery and trauma treatment. As Dr Klaassen has stated, the possibility of negative sequelae from pneumatic tourniquet use can be reduced by careful attention to optimal inflation pressures and application times. In the case of the ischaemic local anaesthetic block, purpose-designed newer cuff devices and new local anaesthetic agents have essentially eliminated the issues that Dr Chapple found unacceptable [3].

References

1. https://www.nysora.com/techniques/intravenous-regional-anesthesia/intravenous-regional-block-upper-lower-extremity-surgery.
2. Lahham S, et al. Comparison of pressures applied by digital tourniquets in the emergency department. West J Emerg Med. 2011;12(2):242–9.
3. Kraus GP, Rondeau B, Fitzgerald BM. Bier block. NCBI Bookshelf, StatPearls; 2022.

Case Studies 17

Commentary by Co-editors Peter Charlesworth and Michael F. Klaassen

Summary
This chapter includes five clinical case studies, with commentaries by Joan Chapple, illustrating key principles of her evaluation and treatment philosophies. Some of the cases are also referred to in the relevant individual book chapters.

Case Study 1
In the early pages of her original book, Joan Chapple described, in a lengthy parable which she entitled 'The Tale of Two Toenails', a case study illustrating many of the potential clinical challenges faced in the treatment of ingrown toenails. Paraphrased, the parable is presented as the case study below:

A young man suffered recurring problems with ingrowing of a great toenail (Fig. 17.1), symptoms from which interfered significantly with his quality of life. Over a period of several years, the toenail was treated by his general practitioner with a variety of unsuccessful methods, including antibiotics and avulsion of the whole toenail. Eventually, formal excision of the ingrowing edge of toenail was performed by a surgeon.

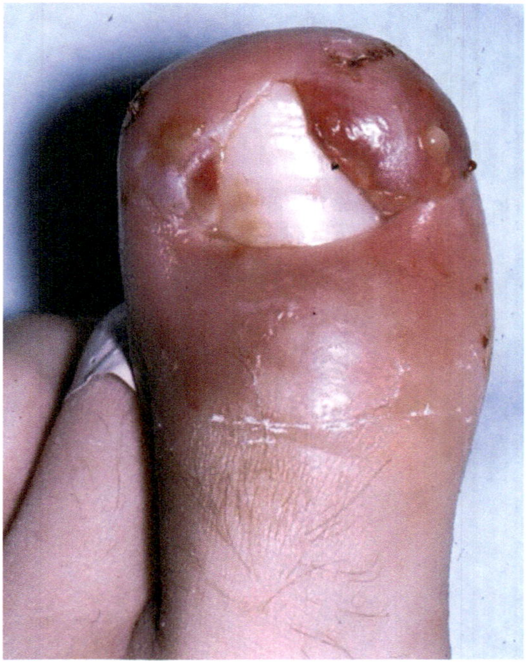

Fig. 17.1 Ingrown toenail

A few months later, the man developed further infection in the same toe, caused by re-growth of a symptomatic 'spike' of nail remnant (Fig. 17.2). This required another surgical procedure, which resolved the problem. However, his overall experience with the toe over an extended period had been complicated by significant pain, infection, disability, and in addition, gastrointestinal symptoms probably attributable to the side-effects of repeated courses of antibiotics and analgesics.

Unfortunately, problems recurred with ingrowing of the contralateral border of the same toenail, and the man consulted a **second** surgeon, who performed a radical removal of the whole

P. Charlesworth, M. F. Klaassen, *Chapple's Principles of Wound Care and Healing*,
https://doi.org/10.1007/978-3-031-53104-0_17

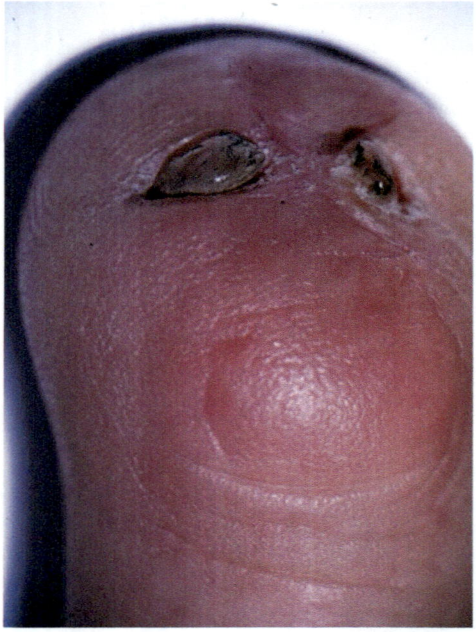

Fig. 17.2 Recurrent nail spikes

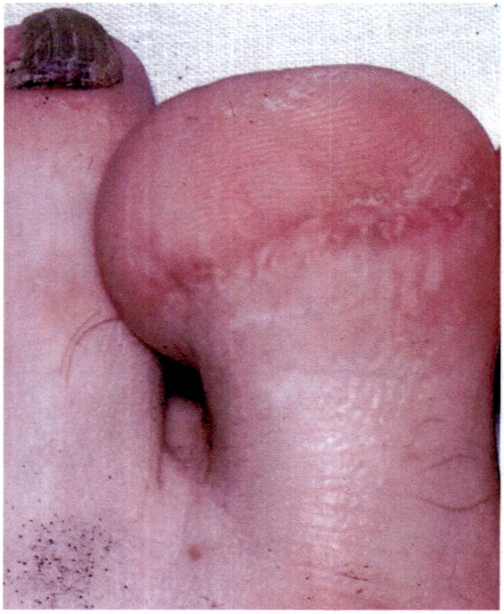

Fig. 17.3 Grotesque local flap repair

nail and matrix with an unsightly flap repair, the appearance of which caused the patient subsequent on-going embarrassment (Fig. 17.3).

Some years later, when the man developed ingrowing of the **opposite** great toenail following trauma, he consulted a **third** surgeon. However, on this occasion, the problem was treated with surgical removal of only the very edge of the nail and associated nail matrix with wound closure using tulle strips, not sutures. He was given a clearly explained postoperative regimen of elevation and bandaging to help alleviate discomfort [See Appendix], with a short course of antibiotics and analgesics. His disability was minimal and healing rapid. He considered this treatment experience to be revelatory, in comparison with his previous ones for the same condition.

Commentary

In using as an example, a seemingly trivial, common medical condition which is nevertheless responsible for considerable human misery, the outcome of Joan Chapple's 'Parable' of the ingrown toenail well encapsulates the general philosophy of her craft. In particular, it illustrates her holistic method of treatment, combining a sympathetic approach to the patient and consideration of the personal and social effects of his pain and disability. In addition, she strongly advocated the gentle handling of tissues, close observation of tissue circulation, and a very conservative approach to surgery.

The case study also allowed Dr Chapple to express her often cynical view of the standard of medical/surgical practice of the day and the perceived inadequacies of the health system as a whole. Sadly, many of her criticisms still remain pertinent, especially in these straitened times of increasing pressure on healthcare systems with a critical shortage of health professionals.

Unfortunately, it seems that many patients with recurrent problems following failed treatment for an ingrown toenail do not consult the original care-provider. One factor may be their loss of confidence, due to the disappointing outcome. However, a potential issue within the framework of public hospital institutions is that treatment of this nominally 'trivial' condition often devolves to the most junior member of a surgical team, who may have had the relevant minor operation demonstrated only once, perhaps by a more marginally experienced colleague. By the time recurrent problems occur, the surgical resident may have moved to another rotation, never having had the salutary opportunity to reflect on the vagaries of the toenail condition or the possible inadequacy of their own technique. Subsequently, difficult recurrent cases may eventually come under the purview of a more senior surgeon, who perhaps would be inclined to a more radical treatment approach, because of the previous failure(s) of 'simple' methods. In the context of the health system, even senior surgeons are unlikely to see negative results of these cases that do occur, and therefore unlikely to modify their own treatment philosophy.

The accurate technique for a very conservative lateral matrixectomy and non-sutured closure described by Dr Chapple in Chapter 14 should be universally adopted, where a surgical approach is deemed absolutely necessary in this condition. Her key associated principle is the better understanding of the 24–48-h interval of temporary reactive swelling after surgery or trauma, which is part of the normal physiological response.

The non-surgical technique of chemical matrix ablation for ingrown toenails should now be more widely accepted and promulgated outside of the podiatry fraternity. Only one or two semi-specialised instruments are required to perform the procedure well, and newer chemical ablation agents may promise greater efficacy and fewer side-effects than traditional phenolisation.

Case Study 2

A 40-year-old viola player musician had a heavy briefcase fall on his left wrist from an overhead luggage rack during a turbulent international flight. His wrist was deformed but there was no broken skin, so the airline steward bandaged his wrist onto a plastic splint and gave him some analgesia.

On landing a couple of hours later, he had X-Rays at a local hospital which confirmed displaced fractures of both distal forearm bones. Under an ischaemic arm block, the fractures were reduced and a padded complete below elbow cast applied. Although the splint felt tight he was allowed to continue on his next flight.

Twelve hours later at his next destination, he needed to attend another urban hospital because of increasing severe pain in his forearm. By now his fingers were extremely swollen and painful to move. The attending doctors were reluctant to remove his splint, because the post reduction X-Rays looked so good. He was instructed to keep his hand elevated and continued on his journey.

By the time he landed in New Zealand, 36 h after his initial injury, hand swelling and intense pain were significant. The fibreglass splint was removed at the orthopaedic department of the nearest hospital which improved the pain considerably and also the dusky colour of his hand. There was extensive bruising in the palm and forearm which was explained as due to bleeding from the fractures. He was placed into a plastic slab similar to the original one applied by the airline steward.

He returned to the hospital 24 h later with an inability to move his fingers and a tender swollen forearm. Under general anaesthetic, his left forearm was explored. When he woke from his anaesthetic, he was told that the surgeon had to remove not only a sizeable haematoma but also quite a lot of dead muscle from his forearm. The surgical wound had been left open and was closed secondarily several days later.

Although the fractures healed well as confirmed by X-ray, he never regained full flexion nor extension of his left fingers despite months of hand therapy. Eventually he had to give up his music career.

Commentary

The dangers of a compartment syndrome in closed limb fractures are illustrated here.

The risks of tight complete casts which have not been split to allow for the profound swelling and oedema of traumatised bone and soft tissues in the first 24–48 h may result in the devastating effect this may have on circulation to muscles, nerves, and other soft tissues.

The danger of flying in pressurised cabins at high altitude is also stressed.

Better early treatment of his simple closed wrist fracture may have resulted in a better functional result for this musician.

Case Study 3

An elderly woman slipped in her garden, damaging her shin on a ragged stony wall. She managed to put her leg up and wrapped it up with her cardigan to stop the bleeding.

About 30 min later, she was able to alert her neighbour, who called for an ambulance and she was transported to hospital. She was treated in the Emergency Department by a specialist, who stopped the bleeding carefully, turned all the damaged skin into a graft, dressed and bandaged the leg, and admitted her to the ward.

Strict instructions were given for her to keep her lower limb elevated and only to be allowed up to the bathroom after a firm additional bandage had been applied. Once she was back in her bed, the second bandage was to be removed. This is the double bandage method summarised in the Appendix.

Unfortunately, the surgical ward was full so she was transferred to an Aged Care ward. Because she did not have a fracture, she was 'mobilised' the next day, walking around on crutches and allowed to sit in a chair with her leg dependent. No double bandage was ever applied.

At day 5 when her initial dressings were changed, there was a massive haematoma with diffuse bruising of the underlying tissue. She required surgical evacuation of the haematoma and debridement of damaged skin.

It took another 3 weeks of dressings to prepare her wound for skin grafting. There was only a partial take of the skin graft and she was discharged unhealed from hospital to the care of community nurses 6 weeks after her original injury.

The damaged leg took another month of dressings to heal and it was a further 2 months before she was able to do everything for herself again at home.

Commentary

The Gillies fundamental principle 'the aftercare is as important as the primary treatment' is clearly the issue here and despite initial appropriate management of this elderly woman's degloving leg injury from a garden fall, the aftercare was completely inappropriate.

Should we blame the primary specialist for not ensuring that the patient's aftercare was followed according to the proper plan, should we blame the nurses on the Aged Care ward for not following instructions or should we blame the whole system that let this patient down?

Attributing blame seems such a pathetic exercise in the face of systematic failure. Knowledge is power and the aim should be obvious; educate all hospital staff into the basic and fundamental principles of safe and effective wound care.

The priorities are understanding the physiological process of healing, defining the exact diagnosis and how this then guides the management plan.

How to achieve this in a broken state hospital system is the challenge, and many would argue an impossible goal. But why?

Case Study 4

A 25-year-old motor-mechanic who had healed well and recovered full strong flexion after a small penetrating hand wound was referred a month after injury because he complained that he still couldn't use his hand properly.

The hand looked normal apart from a small, healed scar in the central palm. He could flex and extend his fingers fully, grip strongly and had no pain or numbness. 'I just can't do my work', he said. When questioned about what he couldn't do he replied without hesitation, 'For a start, I lose

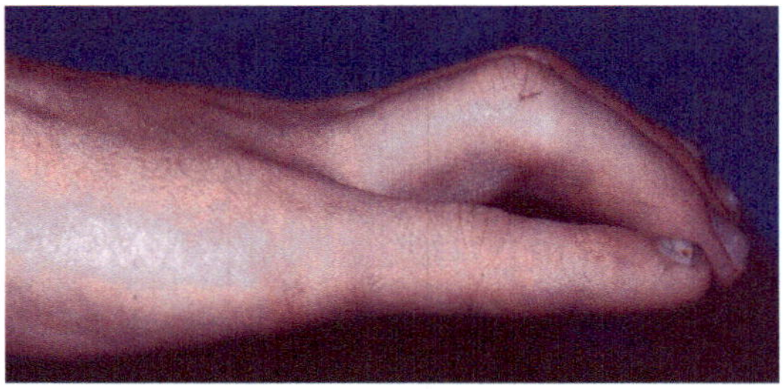

Fig. 17.4 Intrinsic muscle function loss can't make a flat hand

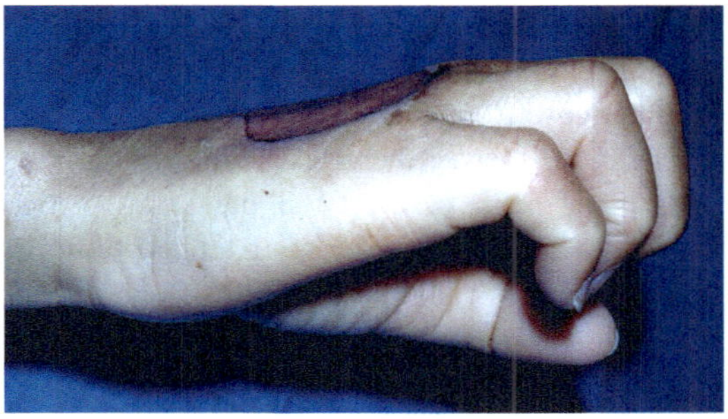

Fig. 17.5 Stiff MCPJs after splinting was omitted for a severe dorsal degloving injury

change through the gap', 'I can't make a flat hand to get into my pocket or down in amongst engines without knocking skin off my knuckles, and I can't position my fingers ready to do anything'.

This is a classic description of intrinsic muscle function loss (Fig. 17.4).

Basically, he could not stabilise the middle and ring fingers strongly in MCPJ flexion and IP extension, which is the position from which one sets out to do most things.

Fortunately, he recovered full function after another month of waiting for the nerve fibres to grow down again into the interosseous muscles.

Commentary

This case is included in Chap. 12.

The interosseous muscles of the hand are supplied by the ulnar nerve [C8] and include the first dorsal interosseous muscle which activates strong radial deviation of the index finger and also abducts the ring and little fingers away from the middle finger. The palmar interosseous muscles are adductors of the fingers. The interosseous muscles alone are capable of flexing the MCPJs with extension of the IPJs and this is defined as the intrinsic plus position.

The detailed techniques for assessment of motor function of the human hand are found in Chap. 4 of Tubiana's excellent Examination of the Hand and Wrist.

[Ref. 1996: Tubiana R., Thomine J-M, and Mackin E. Publisher Martin Dunitz].

Case Study 5

A young woman caught the back of her hand against a belt sander and sustained an area of friction burn with a closed degloving of dorsal skin.

The skin initially looked white and was simply dressed by the local doctor. Both her hand and fingers were swollen for several days and by day 5 the skin was looking darker. There was no haematoma and she was instructed to mobilise her fingers.

The margins of the damaged skin began to discharge and a month post-injury she was finally referred to the Hand Clinic. There was a sizeable area of dead skin to be excised and repaired with a split skin graft 2 weeks later.

Although the hand eventually healed her MCPJs had all stiffened in extension and her wrist could not be actively extended from the neutral position. She was left with severe and permanent disability of her left hand despite prolonged hand therapy and was never able to play her guitar again (Fig. 17.5).

Commentary

Another case from Chap. 12.

This emphasises the critical role of splinting an injured hand or digits in the safe position [cobra position] with wrist extended, MCPJs flexed, and IPJs extended (Fig. 17.6).

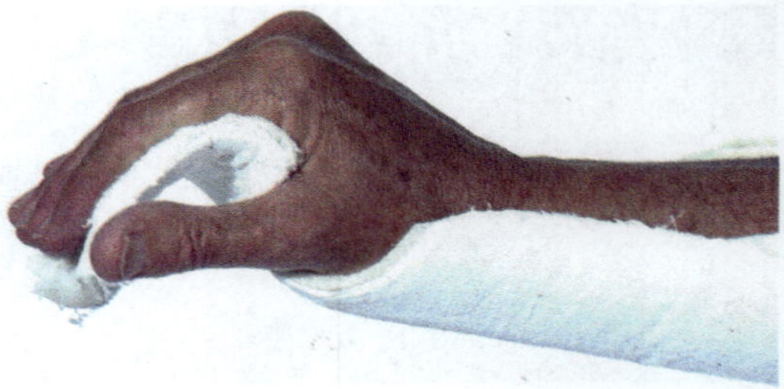

Fig. 17.6 The safe splinted position for the injured hand and digits

Appendix

Double Bandage Instructions for Leg and Foot Injuries (See Editors' Comments, Appendix p. 171)

Throughout Dr Chapple's book, there are frequent references to what she described as the 'Double Bandage Instructions', a technique she had devised for the follow-up management of leg and foot injuries, and lower extremity surgery.

The concept of the method is sound, in that it aims to reduce the potentially deleterious effects of hydrostatic venous pressure on healing wounds in the leg, when a patient is in the upright position, or walking during rehabilitation. It is clear that Dr Chapple placed almost obsessional importance on the use of the technique, but we have no idea how successfully it was actually implemented in her practice. The conditions of her hospital appointment within New Zealand's state-funded medical system were almost unique at that time, and certainly even then provided her with a greater ability to spend time with patients and follow them up meticulously than would have been possible for the vast majority of contemporary surgeons. However, suffice it to say that the straitened times health systems currently face would surely make the situation very significantly more constraining.

Well knowing the vagaries of patient behaviour, the Editors seriously question the practicality of the Double Bandage technique for the average person recovering at home, even perhaps with the support of (necessarily intermittent) domiciliary nursing care. It is possible that the system could be simplified by replacing the second outer bandage with an appropriate below-knee compression stocking, but even this option would pose major logistical difficulties for most people, especially without assistance.

Out of respect for Dr Chapple's original book and her firmly held philosophies of patient management, the Editors have elected not to remove reference to, and description of, the Double Bandage Instructions from this re-edition. However, we would ask readers to critically evaluate the primary reasoning behind Dr Chapple's recommended technique and, if possible, endeavour to implement this, in other ways that might be more practicable in the very different clinical world of today.

P. Charlesworth, M. F. Klaassen, *Chapple's Principles of Wound Care and Healing*,
https://doi.org/10.1007/978-3-031-53104-0

Two Bandage Instructions for Leg and Foot Injuries

1. Do not remove the inner bandage. It is holding the dressing on and its end is taped securely.
2. BEFORE you put your leg down always apply a firm second bandage, securing the end with a safety pin. This bandage is to prevent the wound bruising or bleeding when you are upright, but it also reduces the circulation considerably. Your wound will start to throb with it on, reminding you to put your leg up again as soon as you can.
3. Once your leg is elevated again, it is safe to remove the firm outer bandage, restoring full circulation immediately and dramatically relieving the throbbing pain.
4. You should rest up for the first 2–3 days, getting onto your feet only to use the bathroom or for a change of scenery. You can safely walk around more after the first few days, as long as the wound is comfortable in a modestly firm supportive bandage.
5. This regime will minimise swelling, pain and complications during your recovery and assist your wound to heal well.

GPSR Compliance

The European Union's (EU) General Product Safety Regulation (GPSR) is a set of rules that requires consumer products to be safe and our obligations to ensure this.

If you have any concerns about our products, you can contact us on ProductSafety@springernature.com

In case Publisher is established outside the EU, the EU authorized representative is:

Springer Nature Customer Service Center GmbH
Europaplatz 3
69115 Heidelberg, Germany

Batch number: 10731385

Printed by Printforce, the Netherlands